PEDIATRICS RECALL

PEDIATRICS RECALL

EUGENE D. McGAHREN III, M.D.
Assistant Professor
Division of Pediatric Surgery
Department of Surgery
University of Virginia Health Sciences Center
Charlottesville, Virginia

WILLIAM G. WILSON, M.D.
Associate Professor
Department of Pediatrics
University of Virginia Health Sciences Center
Charlottesville, Virginia

Williams & Wilkins
A WAVERLY COMPANY

BALTIMORE • PHILADELPHIA • LONDON • PARIS • BANGKOK
BUENOS AIRES • HONG KONG • MUNICH • SYDNEY • TOKYO • WROCLAW

Editor: Elizabeth Nieginski
Manager of Development Editing: Julie Scardiglia
Managing Editor: Amy G. Dinkel
Marketing Manager: Rebecca Himmelheber
Development Editor: Beth Goldner
Production Coordinator: Danielle Hagen
Text/Cover Designer: Karen Klinedinst
Typesetter: Port City Press, Inc.
Printer/Binder: Mack Printing Group

351 West Camden Street
Baltimore, Maryland 21201-2436 USA

Rose Tree Corporate Center
1400 North Providence Road
Building II, Suite 5025
Media, Pennsylvania 19063-2043 USA

Accurate indications, adverse reactions and dosage schedules for drugs are provided in this book, but it is possible that they may change. The reader is urged to review the package information data of the manufacturers of the medications mentioned.

Printed in the United States of America

First Edition,

Library of Congress Cataloging-in-Publication Data
McGahren, Eugene D.
   Pediatrics recall / Eugene D. McGahren, III, William G. Wilson.
      p.   cm. — (Recall Series)
   Includes index.
   ISBN 0-683-05855-X
   1. Pediatrics—Examinations, questions, etc. 2. Pediatrics—Outlines, syllabi, etc. I. Wilson, William G. (William Grady), 1949–   . II. Title. III. Series.
   [DNLM: 1. Pediatrics—examination questions. WS 18.2 M478p 1997]
RJ48.2.M37 1997
618.92′00076—dc21
DNLM/DLC
for Library of Congress   96-29736
                                                                          CIP

The publishers have made every effort to trace the copyright holders for borrowed material. If they have inadvertently overlooked any, they will be pleased to make the necessary arrangements at the first opportunity.

                                                              97 98 99 00
                                                          2 3 4 5 6 7 8 9 10

Contents

Contributors

Stephen Borowitz, M.D.
Associate Professor
Division of Gastroenterology
Department of Pediatrics
University of Virginia Health
   Sciences Center
Charlottesville, Virginia

Robert J. Boyle, M.D.
Associate Professor
Division of Neonatology
Department of Pediatrics
University of Virginia Health
   Sciences Center
Charlottesville, Virginia

Mark A. Brown, M.D.
Assistant Professor of Pediatrics
Pediatric Pulmonary Section
Department of Pediatrics
University of Arizona School of
   Medicine
Tucson, Arizona

Pamela Clark, M.D.
Assistant Professor
Division of Pediatric Endocrinology
Department of Pediatrics
University of Louisville School of
   Medicine
Louisville, Kentucky

William L. Clarke, M.D.
Professor
Division of Pediatric Endocrinology
Department of Pediatrics
University of Virginia Health
   Sciences Center
Charlottesville, Virginia

Michael D. Dickens, M.D.
Pediatric Associates
Charlottesville, Virginia

Kimberly Dunsmore, M.D.
Assistant Professor
Division of Hematology-Oncology
Department of Pediatrics
University of Virginia Health
   Sciences Center
Charlottesville, Virginia

Patricia Hagan, M.D.
Fellow in Neonatology
Department of Pediatrics
University of Virginia Health
   Sciences Center
Charlottesville, Virginia

Rajesh Malik, M.D.
Assistant Professor
Division of Hematology-Oncology
Department of Pediatrics
University of Virginia Health
   Sciences Center
Charlottesville, Virginia

Nancy L. McDaniel, M.D.
Associate Professor
Division of Cardiology
Department of Pediatrics
University of Virginia Health
   Sciences Center
Charlottesville, Virginia

Eugene D. McGahren III, M.D.
Assistant Professor
Division of Pediatric Surgery
Department of Surgery
University of Virginia Health
   Sciences Center
Charlottesville, Virginia

Robert S. Michel, M.D.
Assistant Professor
Department of Pediatrics
University of Virginia Health
  Sciences Center
Charlottesville, Virginia

Victoria Norwood, M.D.
Assistant Professor
Division of Nephrology
Department of Pediatrics
University of Virginia Health
  Sciences Center
Charlottesville, Virginia

W. Davis Parker, M.D.
Professor
Division of Pediatric Neurology
Department of Neurology
University of Virginia Health
  Sciences Center
Charlottesville, Virginia

Vito A. Perriello Jr., M.D.
Pediatric Associates
Charlottesville, Virginia

Alan R. Rogol, M.D., Ph.D.
Professor
Division of Pediatric Endocrinology
Department of Pediatrics
University of Virginia Health
  Sciences Center
Charlottesville, Virginia

Frank T. Saulsbury, M.D.
Professor
Department of Pediatrics
University of Virginia Health
  Sciences Center
Charlottesville, Virginia

Jocelyn Schauer, M.D.
Assistant Professor
Division of General Pediatrics
Department of Pediatrics
University of Virginia Health
  Sciences Center
Charlottesville, Virginia

Deborah E. Smith, M.D.
Associate Professor
Pediatric Adolescent Medicine
Department of Pediatrics
University of Virginia Health
  Sciences Center
Charlottesville, Virginia

Richard D. Stevenson, M.D.
Associate Professor
Department of Pediatrics
University of Virginia Health
  Sciences Center
Charlottesville, Virginia

Kathryn Weise, M.D.
Associate Professor
Department of Pediatrics
University of Virginia Health
  Sciences Center
Charlottesville, Virginia

William G. Wilson, M.D.
Associate Professor
Department of Pediatrics
University of Virginia Health
  Sciences Center
Charlottesville, Virginia

Paul Wisman, M.D.
Pediatric Associates
Charlottesville, Virginia

Claudia C. Zegans, M.D.
Unified Clinics of the Peninsula
San Bruno, California

Preface

Pediatrics Recall provides information in a concise question-and-answer format, which allows easy access to material that is essential for medical students during their third-year clinical clerkships in pediatrics. The book covers basic issues in neonatal and pediatric fluid management, blood products, nutrition, emergencies, growth, and intensive care. In addition, an entire chapter is devoted to issues relating to the adolescent patient. Disease entities are organized into chapters according to the systems involved. Descriptions of the individual diseases include signs, symptoms, essentials of pathophysiology, treatments, and possible outcomes. Students may use the question-and-answer format to work through each condition from presentation and diagnosis to therapy and outcome.

Pediatrics Recall is not intended to be used as a primary text. Rather, it allows students to review essential information in an efficient format that is designed to facilitate retention.

We have used input from students, residents, community physicians, and pediatric generalists and specialists in both the primary writing and review of the text. We feel that this input has greatly enhanced the ability of this book to address the needs of students and other learners in general pediatrics. We hope that this book is useful to you, and we welcome your questions and comments.

Acknowledgments

We would like to express our sincere gratitude to Peg Lascano, who tirelessly created order out of the massive amounts of drafts, dictations, and editing efforts that went into compiling this book. Her skills and humor helped get us all through.

Section 1

Overview and Background Information

1

Introduction

USING THE STUDY GUIDE

This study guide was written to accompany the pediatric clerkship, and we welcome any feedback (both positive and negative) or suggestions for improvement. The objective of the guide is to provide a rapid overview of common pediatric topics, but keep in mind that this **is NOT an all-encompassing source** (i.e., you will have to consult major textbooks to round out the information in this guide). The guide is organized in a self-study/quiz format. By covering the information/answers on the right side of the page with the bookmark, you can attempt to answer the questions on the left to assess your understanding of the information. Keep the guide with you at all times, and when you have even a few minutes (e.g., between cases), hammer out a page or at least a few questions.

PEDIATRIC NOTES AND PRESENTATIONS

DOCUMENTATION AND COMMUNICATION

For every patient, it is necessary to document the patient's status, plans for evaluation, previous medical and surgical treatments, test results, plans for treatment and discharge, and communication with other members of the health care team.

In addition to the documentation and communication functions, the content of admission and progress notes implies much about the medical student's and resident's ability to gather and analyze data and formulate a treatment plan. Therefore, pertinent negatives (i.e., the normal findings that the student chooses to include in the written notes) convey the student's problem-solving abilities. In addition, many pediatric, medical, or surgical services expect the medical students and residents to write a detailed discussion of the patient's condition at the end of an admission or progress note; make certain that you understand what is expected of you.

ADMISSION NOTES

The format of an admission note may vary in different institutions, but it generally contains the following information:
1. Name
2. Age
3. Gender
4. Reason for admission (presenting complaint or diagnosis)

5. Informant (historian)
6. Referring physician or health professional (if referred)
7. History of present illness
8. Past medical history (including, as indicated, prenatal and newborn history)
9. Immunizations
10. Allergies
11. Current medications
12. Hospitalizations
13. Surgeries
14. Developmental history
15. Review of systems
16. Physical measurements (height, weight, head circumference)
17. Vital signs (usually temperature, pulse, respiratory rate, blood pressure)
18. Physical examination
19. Assessment
20. Plan

The organization of the admission note may vary. Because pediatrics encompasses a broad age range with different issues, certain elements may be included or excluded, depending on the situation. For example, the elements of the history for a 3 year old with seizures and developmental delay may not be the same as that of a 16 year old with an ankle fracture.

PROGRESS NOTES

Progress notes should be concise and convey information about the patient's status, test results, and current treatments and plans. Editorial comments, criticisms of other services or the nursing staff, and humor should be avoided. Most hospitals use some modification of the **SOAP note**—subjective (what the patient says he/she feels), objective (what your physical exam reveals), assessment (interpretation of the information obtained), plan (treatment plan)—as the standard for progress notes.

ORAL PRESENTATIONS

The format of an oral presentation depends on the situation. Presentations are usually brief on work and check-out rounds and are more detailed during attending or teaching rounds. You must clearly communicate to your colleagues the important information needed for patient care. Presentations during teaching rounds usually allow more time for discussing differential diagnoses and basic science correlations.

Presentations, similar to written notes, convey information about the clinical and analytical skills of the student. A clear, well-organized presentation, with discussion of the patient's differential diagnosis and plans for evaluation and treatment, implies much about the student's ability.

COMMON ABBREVIATIONS

Although abbreviations are a part of the medical culture, they may be misinterpreted. A written note that does not use abbreviations is much less likely to be misinterpreted than one that is filled with abbreviations. For example, the abbreviation CP could mean cerebral palsy, cleft palate, chest pain, or carotid pulse. Most hospitals have a list of approved abbreviations; make certain that you use abbreviations that are approved in your hospital. Be careful in using abbreviations, because many have several different interpretations, depending on the context and the type of patient. When in doubt, write out the term. Remember that the purposes of written notes are documentation and communication.

Δ	Change
ā	Before
ABG	Arterial blood gas
As and Bs	Apnea and bradycardia
A and B spells	Apnea and bradycardia spells
ADH	Antidiuretic hormone
AF	Anterior fontanelle
AFO	Ankle flexion orthotic
AGA	Appropriate for gestational age
AI	Aortic insufficiency
ALL	Acute lymphocytic leukemia
AMA	Against medical advice
AML	Acute myelocytic leukemia
ANC	Absolute neutrophil count
ANLL	Acute nonlymphocytic leukemia
AP	Anterior-posterior
AS	Aortic stenosis
ASD	Atrial septal defect

BA	Bone age
BAER	Brain-stem audio-evoked response
BE	Barium enema
BID	Twice a day
BM	Bowel movement Bone marrow (aspirate)
BP	Blood pressure
BPD	Bronchopulmonary dysplasia
BUN	Blood urea nitrogen
c̄	With
CA	Cancer; chronologic age
C & S	Culture and sensitivity
CC	Cubic centimeter (milliliter) Clinical clerk
CDH	Congenital dislocation of the hip Congenital diaphragmatic hernia
CF	Cystic fibrosis
CHD	Congenital heart disease
CHF	Congestive heart failure
CMV	Cytomegalovirus
CN	Cranial nerve
CNS	Central nervous system
C/O	Complaint of
CP	Cerebral palsy Cleft palate
CPR	Cardiopulmonary resuscitation

C-spine	Cervical spine
CVA	Cerebrovascular accident (stroke)
CVP	Central venous pressure
C/W	Compatible with
CX	Culture
CXR	Chest radiograph
D/C (or DC)	Discontinue Discharge
DDST	Denver Developmental Screening Test
DI	Diabetes insipidus
DIC	Disseminated intravascular coagulation
DM	Diabetes mellitus
DNS	Dextrose in normal saline
DPT	Diphtheria/pertussis/tetanus immunization
DTRs	Deep tendon reflexes
D#W	Dextrose in water (#%)
DX	Diagnosis
ECG/EKG	Electrocardiogram
ECMO	Extracorporeal membrane oxygenation
EGA	Estimated gestational age
ESR	Erythrocyte sedimentation rate
ESRD	End-stage renal disease
ETT	Endotracheal tube
FiO$_2$	Fraction of inspired oxygen

FROM	Full range of motion
GBS	Group B streptococcus
G tube	Gastrostomy tube
GU	Genitourinary
HA	Headache
HAL	Hyperalimentation
HC	Head circumference Hydrocephalus
HFOV	High-frequency oscillatory ventilation
HMD	Hyaline membrane disease
HSP	Henoch-Schönlein purpura
HSV	Herpes simplex virus
IDDM	Insulin-dependent diabetes mellitus
IRDS	Infantile respiratory distress syndrome
ITP	Idiopathic thrombocytopenic purpura
IUGR	Intrauterine growth retardation
IVH	Intraventricular hemorrhage
IVP	Intravenous pyelogram
LA	Left arm Left atrium
LE	Lower extremity
LFTs	Liver function tests
LGA	Large for gestational age
LLL	Left lower lobe of lung
LP	Lumbar puncture

LR	Lactated Ringer's
LUL	Left upper lobe of lung
LV	Left ventricle
LVH	Left ventricular hypertrophy
ICH	Intracranial hemorrhage
I/O	Intake and output
IVIG	Intravenous immune globulin
MAP	Mean airway pressure
MD	Muscular dystrophy Medical doctor
MS	Mitral stenosis Multiple sclerosis Morphine sulfate
MSPN	Medical student progress note
MVA	Motor vehicle accident
NAD	No apparent distress No acute distress
ND	Nasoduodenal
NEC	Necrotizing enterocolitis
NG	Nasogastric
NGT	Nasogastric tube
NPO	Nothing by mouth
NSR	Normal sinus rhythm
OFC	Occipitofrontal circumference
OM	Otitis media
PA	Pulmonary artery; posterior-anterior

PAC	Premature atrial contraction
PDA	Patent ductus arteriosus
PE	Physical examination Pulmonary embolism
PEEP	Positive end-expiratory pressure
PEG	Percutaneous endoscopic gastrostomy
PID	Pelvic inflammatory disease
PIP	Positive inspiratory pressure
PO	By mouth
PPHN	Persistent pulmonary hypertension of the newborn
PR	Per rectum
PRN	As needed
QD	Daily
QID	Four times a day
QOD	Every other day
RA	Radial artery Right atrium
RAM	Rapid alternating movements
RDS	Respiratory distress syndrome
RLL	Right lower lobe of lung
RLQ	Right lower quadrant
RML	Right middle lobe
ROM	Range of motion Rupture of membranes
RSV	Respiratory syncytial virus

RUL	Right upper lobe of lung
RUQ	Right upper quadrant
RV	Right ventricle
RVH	Right ventricular hypertrophy
Rx	Treatment
s̄	Without
SCT	Sacral-coccygeal teratoma
SEM	Systolic ejection murmur
SGA	Small for gestational age
SIADH	Syndrome of inappropriate antidiuretic hormone secretion
SIDS	Sudden infant death syndrome
S/P	Status post
SVC	Superior vena cava
SVT	Supraventricular tachycardia
SX	Symptoms
TBW	Total body water
TEF	Tracheoesophageal fistula
TID	Three times a day
Tmax	Maximum temperature
TOF	Tetralogy of Fallot
TOGV	Transposition of the great vessels
TPN	Total parenteral nutrition
TRP	Tubular reabsorption of phosphate

UAC	Umbilical artery catheter
UPJ	Ureteropelvic junction
U/S	Ultrasound examination
UTD	Up to date
UTI	Urinary tract infection
UVC	Umbilical vein catheter
VCUG	Vesicocystourethrogram Voiding cystourethrogram
VER	Visual evoked response
VSD	Ventricular septal defect
VUR	Vesicoureteral reflux
WBC	White blood cell count
WNL	Within normal limits
$\bar{x}$	Except

2

Pediatric Procedures

VENIPUNCTURE/IVs

What are three indications for peripheral IVs in infants and children?

1. Administration of resuscitative fluids
2. Administration of maintenance fluids
3. Access for drugs

What are appropriate-size IVs for infants?

24 or 22 gauge

For toddlers?

22 gauge

For school-age children?

22 or 20 gauge

For older children and adolescents?

20, 18, or 16 gauge

What are the preferred sites for IVs?

Generally, you should start at a peripheral location to avoid using up potentially easier sites (e.g., the antecubital veins). In infants, multiple sites may be used, including the foot, the dorsum of the hand, and the scalp. If these sites are not useable, use the saphenous or antecubital vein. IV sites should be carefully secured so that an infant cannot pull the IV out. In toddlers and older children, hand and arm sites are generally best, because these patients can walk.

What is the best technique for placing an IV?

Most health care workers have a technique that works best for them. In general, it is important to hold the extremity still. (This will often require an assistant when placing IVs in neonates and toddlers.) The skin over the vein is pulled tautly, which allows the IV needle to puncture through the skin without creating redundancy. Once a flash of blood is obtained, the needle should be inserted approximately 1 mm further to ensure that the plastic catheter is in the vein. The catheter is then inserted over the needle. It is always important to have securing materials, including tape and an extremity board, ready when the IV is placed.

What are three complications of IVs?

1. Infiltration
2. Thrombophlebitis
3. Necrosis of surrounding soft tissue; usually occurs with infiltration of high-concentration calcium solutions or pressors administered through peripheral IVs

How are these three complications treated?

1. For infiltration, the IV is removed, the extremity is elevated, and a warm soak is applied.
2. For thrombophlebitis, removal of the IV with elevation of the extremity and warm soaks are usually adequate treatment. Occasionally, an associated cellulitis may need to be treated with antibiotics.
3. In cases of necrosis of surrounding soft tissue, the IV needs to be removed. These lesions are often treated like a burn by applying antibiotic ointments (e.g., Silvadine, bacitracin ointment). Any eschar should be removed. In rare cases, skin grafting may be necessary.

How can the pain of IV placement be minimized?

In infants and toddlers, Emla cream can usually be applied to the IV site before placement. In older, more cooperative children, Emla or subcutaneous 1% Xylocaine may make IV placement less painful.

LUMBAR PUNCTURE

What are indications for lumbar puncture (LP)?

Any suspicion of meningitis; other need to evaluate CSF; administration of intrathecal medications

What are three contraindications to LP?	1. Evidence of increased intracranial pressure 2. When position for an LP would risk cardiopulmonary compromise 3. Infection of the skin overlying the site of an LP
Should a contraindication to an LP delay any antibiotic treatment or other therapy that may be needed?	No
How is an LP performed?	Generally the patient is in a flexed lateral decubitus position. The needle is passed into the L3-L4 or L4-L5 interspace. Local anesthesia (1% Xylocaine) is provided. Usually a 22-gauge 1½-inch spinal needle is used. The needle is advanced very slowly until it feels as though it has entered the CSF space. When the CSF space is entered, it can usually be felt with a small "pop." This sensation may not be felt when performing an LP in a neonate.
What studies should be performed on a CSF specimen?	Culture and sensitivity, cell count, and glucose and protein levels
What is a traumatic LP?	It is a puncture contaminated by blood from a surrounding vessel. Usually this disrupts the neutrophil and protein count. It is best to rely on the bacterial culture of this kind of specimen, instead of adjusting the neutrophil or protein counts to account for the traumatic tap or obtaining another LP sample.

SUPRAPUBIC PUNCTURE

What is an indication for suprapubic puncture?	Requirement for a sterile urine collection; it is usually performed in infants and toddlers because it is difficult to obtain a midstream urine specimen

What is the technique for suprapubic puncture?

After adequate hydration is accomplished, a full bladder can be percussed. The skin is disinfected in the suprapubic region. A 22- or 25-gauge needle is then placed into the bladder approximately one finger-breadth above the pubis. One or two milliliters of fluid are then obtained for culture.

ARTERIAL PUNCTURE

What are indications for arterial puncture or catheter placement?

Arterial puncture is usually needed when an arterial blood gas is required. In rare instances in which a blood draw is needed and a vein cannot be accessed, an artery provides a good site, particularly in an infant.

Which arteries are preferred for blood draws in infants?

Usually the radial or the dorsalis pedis artery; access of the femoral artery is strongly discouraged because it may lead to thrombosis and arterial insufficiency to the leg

When should an arterial cannula be placed?

1. When constant monitoring of blood pressure is required
2. When frequent blood samples are required, especially in an infant or premature baby
3. When frequent arterial blood gases are required

What are the best sites for arterial catheters?

Again, the radial and dorsalis pedis arteries are the best sites. In the newborn, an umbilical artery catheter can be placed for a short period of time, about 3–5 days.

What is the technique for blood sampling via an artery?

Usually a thin needle (e.g., a 25- or 23-gauge needle) may be used. It is placed into the artery at a 45° angle facing toward the proximal end of the artery. It is usually best not to go "searching" for the artery with a needle; instead, make one clean pass and then pull the needle back until it is within the lumen of the artery. At that point, the sample can be taken.

What are the best techniques for placement of an arterial catheter?

Similar principles hold for placement of a catheter. Sometimes an angle of about 30° may be better. After blood is obtained, the catheter should pass easily over the needle. If it does not, it is helpful to have a small guidewire available. The needle can be removed, the guidewire can be passed through the plastic catheter, and the catheter can be advanced over the guidewire. Arterial catheters should be secured tightly with tape in neonates and usually with a suture in toddlers and older children. These materials should be ready at the time of cannulation.

What are complications of arterial catheters?

Thrombosis with ischemia to the affected extremity; this is quite rare when the radial or the dorsalis pedis artery is used, because there is usually excellent collateral flow to the palmar and plantar arches in the hand and the foot, respectively; umbilical catheters are discussed in Chapter 8

3   Fluids and Electrolytes

MAINTENANCE FLUID REQUIREMENTS

What are three primary methods for calculating maintenance fluid requirements?

By basing calculation on:
1. Body weight
2. Body surface area
3. Caloric requirements/expenditures

How do fluid requirements in children differ from those in adults?

Children are "dynamic"—i.e., fluid needs per kg and the ratio of body surface area to weight change with age. Therefore, adjustments are made as a child grows.

What are approximate maintenance fluid requirements for infants and toddlers?

Fluids
  100 ml/kg/24 hr for first 10 kg
  50 ml/kg/24 hr for second 10 kg
  25 ml/kg/24 hr for each subsequent
    10 kg
Electrolytes
  Na: 3 mEq/100 ml
  Cl: 2 mEq/100 ml
  K: 2 mEq/100 ml

What are approximate maintenance fluid requirements for older children (10–14 years of age)?

Water: 1500 ml/m^2/24 hr
Sodium: 30–50 mEq/m^2/24 hr
Potassium: 20–40 mEq/m^2/24 hr

DEHYDRATION

What is it?

Depletion of total body water

What are common pediatric causes of dehydration?

GI losses (e.g., gastroenteritis, diarrhea), inadequate fluid intake, excess renal losses, increased insensible losses (e.g., fever, sweating)

What are the findings in mild dehydration?

Loss of 3%–5% of body weight, normal hemodynamic parameters and skin turgor, dry mucous membranes, slight decrease in urine output, and decreased tearing

What are the findings in moderate dehydration?

Loss of 8%–10% body weight, decreased skin turgor, dry mucous membranes, relatively normal hemodynamic parameters, decreased urine output, and slight increase in heart rate

What are the findings in severe dehydration?

Loss of 10%–15% of body weight, abnormal skin turgor and color, dry mucous membranes, rapid heart rate, decreased blood pressure, and poor peripheral perfusion; no urine output or tears

ISOTONIC DEHYDRATION

What is it?

Dehydration with maintenance of normal Na^+ concentration; as dehydration worsens, K^+ and BUN tend to increase, and HCO_3^- tends to decrease

What will happen to urine specific gravity?

It will increase. However, infants have poor concentrating ability; thus specific gravity may reach only 1.020, even in cases of severe dehydration.

What is the most common cause of isotonic dehydration?

GI losses secondary to viral or bacterial enteritis

What is the treatment strategy?

Calculate fluid and electrolyte losses using body weight, electrolyte values, and estimated time of dehydration. Then, rehydrate with appropriate fluids over 24–48 hours. **Note:** Potassium losses should be replaced more slowly because K^+ needs time to move intracellularly, where it is the predominant electrolyte.

HYPERNATREMIC DEHYDRATION

What is it?

Loss of more body water than solute, or administration of excess sodium, resulting in elevated serum sodium (> 145 mEq/L)

What are four causes of hypernatremic dehydration?

1. **Increased Na,** which may be caused by excess Na^+ intake/administration or hyperaldosteronism
2. **Water loss,** which may occur through respiration and perspiration or because of diabetes insipidus
3. **Water loss that is greater than Na^+ loss,** which occurs with GI and renal losses
4. **Abnormal central control of osmotic balance,** which occurs in essential hypernatremia

What are the symptoms and signs?

Lethargy, irritability, muscle weakness, convulsions, coma

Why is hypernatremic dehydration dangerous?

Because losses are more from intracellular than intravascular spaces, the symptoms may be masked until dehydration becomes severe.

How is hypernatremic dehydration treated?

Rehydrate **slowly** with low sodium fluid to avoid rapid fluid shifts to the intracellular spaces. Usually replace deficit over 48 hours.

What may happen if correction is too rapid?

CEREBRAL EDEMA

HYPONATREMIC DEHYDRATION

What is it?

Relative depletion of sodium compared with total body water loss

What are four common etiologies?

1. GI losses
2. Renal losses, including those caused by diuretics
3. Adrenal insufficiency
4. Third-space losses (e.g., ascites, postsurgical, burns)

What are the symptoms and signs?

Anorexia, nausea, muscle cramps, lethargy, disorientation/agitation, diminished or pathologic reflexes, Cheyne-Stokes respiration, hypothermia, pseudobulbar palsy, seizures

What is the treatment?

Isotonic saline with rate determined by assessment of fluid and electrolyte losses and adequacy of rehydration; in some cases, judicious administration of hypertonic saline may be beneficial

4

Blood and Blood Products

What is whole blood used for?

It is sometimes used for **volume expansion** in emergencies in which there has been acute blood loss. However, since the advent of component therapy, whole blood has few uses.

What constitutes a unit of packed red blood cells?

One unit of packed cells = 300 ml ($\pm$50 ml) with a hematocrit of 65%–80%

What are the uses of packed red blood cells?

To **correct anemia;** to improve oxygen-carrying capacity of blood

What percent does a packed red cell transfusion of 3 ml/kg raise the hematocrit?

Approximately 3%

What constitutes a unit of platelets?

One unit of platelets = approximately 5×10^{10} platelets in 40–70 ml of plasma if stored at 20°C–24°C or 20–30 ml of plasma if stored at 1°C–6°C

What are the indications for platelet transfusions?

Treatment of **thrombocytopenia** or **severe platelet dysfunction**

How much of a platelet solution, stored at 20°C–24°C, is given to raise the platelet count by 50,000?

10 ml/kg should raise platelet count by about 5.0×10^4/ml.

What is fresh frozen plasma (FFP)?

Plasma from whole blood, containing about 80% of plasma proteins

How much FFP is needed to raise clotting factors by 10%–20%?

10–15 ml/kg

What are the therapeutic uses of immunoglobulin?

Replacement in immunodeficient patients; **treatment** of Kawasaki disease; convey **passive immunity** to susceptible patients exposed to a variety of specific infections, such as tetanus, hepatitis B, rabies, and varicella-zoster

What is cryoprecipitate?

A plasma preparation containing factor VIII, von Willebrand factor, and fibrinogen

What risks are associated with the use of blood products?

Risks vary with the type of product, clinical situation, and patient, but include **infection** (e.g., HIV, hepatitis B and C, CMV), **sensitization, immune response, graft-vs-host reaction.**

5   Pediatric Nutrition

Why do nutritional considerations in pediatric patients differ from those in adults?

Growth, maturation, and development are anabolic processes that increase the nutritional needs of children.

What is the caloric content of fat?

9 kcal/g

Of carbohydrates or protein?

4 kcal/g

What are the caloric requirements of a healthy term infant?

On average, **100 kcal/kg/day**

What are the fluid requirements if provided by an enteral route?

About **150 ml/kg/day**

Recommended protein intake of infants?

Approximately **2.0–2.2 g/kg/day**

What is the caloric content of breast milk?

It varies; averages about **20 kcal/30 ml**

Of commercial infant formula?

Most infant formulas contain **20 kcal/30 ml.**

What are some advantages of breast-feeding?

Easily available, inexpensive, promotes mother–child bonding, less immunogenic, contains antibodies (which may reduce incidence of infection)

Do breast-fed infants require supplementation?

Yes. Breast-fed infants require vitamin D, fluoride (after age 6 months), and iron (after age 4–6 months) supplementation.

Name four contraindications to breast feeding.

1. Medications the mother may be taking (e.g., antimetabolites, chloramphenicol)
2. Maternal infection—HIV, active TB in the mother

3. Maternal substance abuse
4. Abnormal gag reflex or swallowing in the infant

What is the best regimen for breast-feeding?

On-demand feeding early until the milk supply has been established and feeding is going well; intervals between feedings can be gradually increased as the length of each feeding increases

What is colostrum?

It is the first secretion produced by the breast during late pregnancy and soon after delivery.

How does it differ from breast milk?

Colostrum has a higher specific gravity, higher protein and vitamin content, and a lower fat content than breast milk. It contains secretory IgA and other immune substances.

At what age should breast-feeding stop?

It varies. Some parents wean the child around 9 months of age, as the child learns to drink from a cup. Others may continue breast-feeding longer. Usually, breast-feeding does not extend beyond 18 months of age.

What are essential amino acids?

Amino acids that cannot be synthesized and must be acquired through the diet

Which amino acids are essential?

Isoleucine, leucine, lysine, phenylalanine, threonine, tryptophan, and valine

What are essential fatty acids?

Fatty acids that cannot be synthesized and must be obtained from dietary sources

Name two essential fatty acids.

Linoleic and linolenic acid

What are symptoms of essential fatty acid deficiency?

Diarrhea, dermatitis, hair loss, and skin abnormalities (e.g., poor wound healing)

What is MCT oil?

A medium-chain triglyceride preparation

Uses of MCT oil?

Primarily as a caloric supplement

Name the fat-soluble vitamins.

Vitamins A, D, E, and K

Why is vitamin K given to newborns?

Newborns may be deficient in vitamin K, and administration helps prevent hemorrhagic complications caused by deficiency in vitamin K–dependent coagulation proteins.

What is the primary carbohydrate in breast milk and in cow milk–based formulas?

Lactose

Indications for using a lactose-free formula?

Galactosemia; lactose intolerance (either temporary or persistent); formula intolerance

When are solid foods introduced?

Usually around 4–6 months of age; this practice varies markedly, depending on the preferences of the parents and physician

What solid food is introduced first?

Usually an iron-fortified single-grain cereal

Why use single-grain cereals?

Allows easier identification of specific foods or ingredients that may not be tolerated by the infant

What foods should be avoided in young children?

Foods that are easily aspirated (e.g., nuts, popcorn, chunky foods that need to be chewed by molar teeth)

Do older infants need vitamin supplementation?

Children on a well-balanced diet probably do not need vitamin supplements.

Do vitamin supplements have a role in treating children with mental retardation?

Although some have advocated the use of vitamin and other nutritional supplements, there are few scientific studies to support their general use in treating children with mental retardation. Children whose diets are inadequate or who have specific nutritional needs (or deficiencies) may benefit from specific supplements.

What is marasmus? Wasting of muscle and subcutaneous fat from malnutrition

What is kwashiorkor? Malnutrition in which there is relative protein deficiency; affected children are usually edematous

Are vegetarian diets safe for children? A well-planned vegetarian diet that contains all essential amino acids is probably safe for children.

Will a vegetarian diet provide an adequate amount of vitamin B_{12}? Because vitamin B_{12} comes from animal sources, strict vegetarians may be at risk for vitamin B_{12} deficiency.

INTRAVENOUS AND PARENTERAL ALIMENTATION

Note: Most hospitals have established intravenous alimentation protocols, many using computer templates for calculation of components. Students and house officers should familiarize themselves with these protocols.

What are indications for intravenous alimentation? Broadly speaking, an inability to maintain adequate fluid or nutritional balance by oral fluid or nutrient intake

What is TPN? Total Parenteral Nutrition—implies a goal of sufficient calories and nutrients for growth and weight gain

Components of TPN? Nitrogen source (amino acids)
Calories (primarily from glucose)
Electrolytes
Vitamins
Minerals
Water
(Lipids are administered in a separate preparation.)

What are some indications for TPN? Severe GI disease, extensive bowel resection, inflammatory bowel disease, conditions that necessitate bowel rest or prohibit oral intake for an extended period of time

When should total (central) parenteral nutrition be used? When a period of greater than 2 weeks of intravenous alimentation is anticipated

When should peripheral hyperalimentation be used?

Usually when a short-term need is anticipated, or when the peripheral alimentation is used as a supplement to enteral nutrition

What is the main limiting factor of peripheral hyperalimentation?

The high osmotic content of hyperalimentation solutions may be irritating to peripheral veins and necessitate a higher flow vein for fluid administration. Generally, 10%–12.5% dextrose is the upper limit for peripheral infusion.

What is D10?

10% dextrose (in water or another solution). This means 10 g of dextrose per 100 ml of fluid.

What is the caloric density of dextrose monohydrate?

3.4 kcal/g; for D10, this means 34 kcal/100 ml fluid

What is Intralipid?

A fat emulsion that serves as a source of fatty acids and calories

Caloric density?

A 10% solution of Intralipid contains 1.1 kcal/ml.

How is Intralipid administered?

Intralipid cannot be mixed in the hyperalimentation solution and is usually given via a Y-connector.

Source of protein in TPN?

Usually a commercially prepared amino acid or protein solution, of which there are several

How is TPN initiated?

Usually begin with a 10% dextrose solution (with electrolytes) as maintenance fluid, with incremental increases (by 2.5%/day) as tolerated, up to a 20% dextrose solution. The amino acid mixture is then added, and the infusion rate is increased until the desired intake is achieved. Intralipid is usually administered in an amount to provide appropriate balance of sugar, protein, and fat calories.

How are vitamins administered?

Usually in a mixture prepared for this purpose and added to the TPN

How are TPN patients monitored?

1. Daily weights
2. Strict intake and output measurements
3. Test urine for glucose and ketones each shift until regimen is established; then test daily
4. Daily electrolytes and glucose until regimen is established, then every 3 days (or weekly, depending on the protocol of the institution)
5. CBC, total protein, calcium, magnesium, phosphorus, hepatocellular enzymes, bilirubin, and creatinine weekly
6. Zinc, copper, iron levels monthly
7. Visual checks for lipemia daily
8. Serum triglycerides weekly (if using lipids); obtain sample immediately before infusion

What are some complications of TPN?

1. Infection (particularly line infections)
2. Hyperglycemia
3. Hypoglycemia (if TPN is stopped too quickly)
4. Acidosis
5. Abnormal liver function
6. Hypocalcemia, hypomagnesemia
7. Trace metal deficiency
8. Hyperlipemia
9. Hyperammonemia
10. Thrombosis
11. Hyperbilirubinemia

6

Pediatric Emergencies

What basic premise should be applied in approaching all pediatric emergencies?

Remember the **ABCs**—**A**irway, **B**reathing, and **C**irculation must be confirmed or established before further interventions. This may require placement of an oral airway or endotracheal tube and will almost always require placement of an IV or intraosseous catheter.

RESPIRATORY DISTRESS

What is respiratory distress?

A set of clinical signs observed when increased breathing work is required to compensate for hypoxia, hypercarbia, or airway obstruction

What are five common clinical signs of early respiratory distress?

1. Anxiety or irritability
2. Use of accessory muscles of respiration (e.g., sternocleidomastoid, intercostals, abdominal musculature)
3. Tachypnea
4. Tachycardia
5. Hypertension

What are three clinical signs of respiratory failure?

1. Severe anxiety or lethargy
2. Labored or sometimes slowed respirations
3. Pallor or cyanosis

Are there any absolute laboratory or radiographic findings that define respiratory distress or failure?

NO. Laboratory studies may help determine the cause or show trends, but they must be placed in the context of the physical findings and history.

What are common postoperative causes of respiratory distress?

Atelectasis, pulmonary edema, pleural effusion, pneumothorax, malpositioned endotracheal tube, aspiration

Posttraumatic causes?	Pulmonary contusion, pneumothorax/hemothorax, disruption of an airway
Infectious causes?	Pneumonia, pleural effusion, empyema, croup, epiglottitis
Primary lung disease causes?	Asthma, cystic fibrosis
Other causes?	Foreign body, anatomic airway anomaly
What happens if respiratory distress is not treated?	Patient may progress to **respiratory failure.**

TREATMENT

What is the initial management and evaluation?	Do not be afraid to use oxygen liberally outside of the immediate newborn period; children do not develop retinopathy of prematurity! Identify probable cause and tailor treatment to etiology. Evaluate: 1. Airway patency 2. Adequacy of air movement 3. Oxygenation
When should intubation be undertaken?	Support airway and/or breathing (i.e., intubate) if child is showing progression toward respiratory failure after simple interventions. **Intubation is necessary whenever a child shows clinical signs of respiratory failure, even if laboratory values (ABG) are acceptable.**
What happens if respiratory failure is not treated?	Untreated respiratory failure is the most common cause of **cardiac arrest** in the pediatric population.

HYPOTHERMIA

What is hypothermia?	Core body temperature below 36°C
What are common early signs and symptoms?	Shivering, vasoconstriction, elevated blood pressure

Late signs and symptoms?	Lethargy, dysarthria, decreased deep tendon reflexes, sluggish pupillary reactions, anisocoria, decreased heart rate and cardiac output (but elevated blood pressure), ECG abnormalities, dysrhythmias, respiratory depression
What are the physiologic results of moderate hypothermia?	Increased metabolic rate Increased cardiac output and oxygen consumption Increased respiratory effort
What are the physiologic results of severe hypothermia?	Decreased cerebral metabolic rate Decreased cardiac output Respiratory acidosis Loss of protective airway reflexes Hypoglycemia (in infants)
What are three common causes of hypothermia?	1. Induced hypothermia (e.g., intraoperative or infusion of large volumes of cold fluid) 2. Exposure (especially after trauma) 3. Near drowning
How is it diagnosed?	Obtain rectal or other core temperature.
How is it treated?	1. Eliminate ongoing heat loss. 2. Gradually rewarm patient at approximately 1°C/hr.
What are three methods for rewarming?	**Surface rewarming:** blankets, heat lamp **Core rewarming:** warm inhaled gases, warm IV fluids, peritoneal lavage **Extracorporeal techniques:** cardiopulmonary bypass
What is carefully monitored during rewarming?	**Electrolytes** and **acid–base status** are monitored carefully; acidosis and associated hyperkalemia may worsen during rewarming. Avoid burning tissue with heat lamps. Perfusion is already compromised!
How long should a patient with accidental hypothermia be resuscitated?	This issue is controversial. Neurologic signs are absent at < 25°C–27°C; defibrillation is difficult at temperatures < 30°C. Exercise clinical judgment. Usually a rule of thumb is that **a patient is not dead until they are warm and dead!**

MAJOR TRAUMA: PEDIATRIC ASPECTS

UPPER AIRWAY OBSTRUCTION

What are the major points to remember in any pediatric trauma situation?

The **ABCs**—Airway, Breathing, Circulation

How is an airway established in an infant or child?

1. Inline cervical spine immobilization should be accomplished.
2. The jaw may be thrust forward to eliminate occlusion from the tongue.
3. An oropharyngeal airway may be placed.
4. An endotracheal tube may be placed if needed.

How is an airway established if a child has severe facial fractures or if an endotracheal tube cannot be placed?

A 14-gauge needle is used to pierce the trachea at the cricothyroid membrane. Jet ventilation is then accomplished up to 60 breaths/minute. This procedure is best performed in the infant or small child. In an adolescent, a surgical cricothyroidotomy may be made.

Once an airway is established, how are oxygenation and ventilation maintained?

1. In some cases, the child may breathe spontaneously and supplemental oxygen may be the only additional measure needed.
2. Hand ventilation may be accomplished with an ambo bag.
3. A mechanical ventilator may be used if available.
4. In the absence of these conditions, mouth-to-tube ventilation can be accomplished. The health care worker should be aware of secretions in this situation.

Circulatory Support

What is the best way to establish access for circulatory resuscitation in the event of trauma?

Establishment of two large-bore peripheral IV lines. The size of the IV line should be appropriate for the size of the infant or child.

What access route is used if IVs are unsuccessful?

An intraosseous line; this can be accomplished by placing a 16-gauge IV needle or a bone marrow aspiration needle directly into the bone marrow

What are the preferred sites for this?

The most preferred site is the proximal tibia, approximately 1finger-breadth below the tibial tuberosity. The second preferred site is the distal femur, approximately 1finger-breath above the knee.

How long may intraosseous lines stay in place?

No longer then 6 hours

What is the circulating blood volume of an infant or toddler?

80 ml/kg

What resuscitative strategy should be used in the infant or child who has experienced trauma?

The first IV bolus should consist of 20 ml/kg of lactated Ringer's. A second bolus should be given if hemodynamic stability is not obtained. If there is still doubt about adequacy of resuscitation, 20 ml/kg of blood should be administered and sources of ongoing blood loss should be sought. Surgical exploration should be consideration for ongoing blood loss.

What are the most likely sites of ongoing blood loss after trauma?

1. Abdomen
2. Chest
3. Retroperitoneum
4. Femur fracture
5. Intracranial loss in the infant whose fontanels are not yet closed. (**Note: In all patients except for infants,** intracranial bleeding alone does not account for hemodynamic instability.)

What is characteristic about the child's ability to compensate for intravascular volume loss?

Generally, blood pressure is maintained until 25%–40% of intravascular volume is lost. Therefore, major signs to watch for are tachycardia and decreased urine volume. When blood pressure begins falling, the child may be exhibiting circulatory collapse.

What are the best signs of adequate circulatory resuscitation?	Adequate urine output Adequate pulse and blood pressure

HEAD TRAUMA

What injury is most responsible for childhood deaths beyond 1 year of age?	Head trauma
What percent of children with head trauma have a skull fracture?	Approximately 35%
How should a child with a severe head injury be approached?	As with any trauma victim, the ABCs—Airway, Breathing, and Circulation are the top three priorities. However, cervical spine immobilization must be maintained.
What percent of children who die of brain injury have NO evidence of a skull fracture?	50%
What percent of children with epidural hematoma do NOT have a skull fracture?	50%
What is the most common cause of head trauma?	Automobile accident
What are four other causes?	1. Bicycle accidents 2. Motorcycle accidents 3. Falls 4. Child abuse
What is a concussion?	A brief, variable, reversible alteration in consciousness with amnesia of the events immediately surrounding the injury
What are indications for hospitalization after a concussion?	In many centers, any child who suffers a concussion is observed in the hospital overnight. However specific indications are: 1. Deterioration in the level of consciousness

2. Persistent confusion and lethargy
3. Excessive vomiting
4. Lack of an accurate history of the trauma
5. Focal neurologic signs
6. Seizures
7. Presence of a skull fracture

What is a subdural hematoma?

A collection of blood between the dura and cerebral mantle

What are typical physical signs?

Poor feeding, failure to thrive, irritability, lethargy, vomiting, and fever; the child's eyes may also show a "setting sun" position because of increased intracranial pressure (ICP)

What does the eye exam show?

Fifty percent of children have retinal or subhyaloid hemorrhages.

How is the diagnosis made?

With CT or MRI scan

What is an epidural hematoma?

A collection of blood in the extradural space, usually caused by a rupture of the middle meningeal artery or tears in the dural vein; therefore, blood usually collects rapidly

What is a typical symptom course?

A child will suffer a brief concussion. Often there is a lucid interval before the onset of vomiting, headache, and focal neurologic signs.

What is the treatment for a subdural or an epidural hematoma?

Decompression of the hematoma

What is the prognosis?

Usually good, unless there is underlying brain injury or the hematoma was not recognized in a timely fashion

What types of insults lead to potential severe brain dysfunction?

Penetrating injury, contusion, intracranial bleeds, shear injuries, and the subsequent cerebral edema that can result from all of these injuries

Can intracranial blood loss cause hypotension?

In the infant it can. In an older child with hypotension, another source of blood loss must be sought.

What are specific interventions to treat cerebral edema?

The following interventions must be individualized according to the needs of the patient:
1. Oxygenation
2. Elevation of the head of the bed
3. Judicious use of IV fluids
4. Hyperventilation
5. ICP monitoring
6. Administration of mannitol

What is the prognosis for seizures that develop within a few minutes or hours of head trauma?

These are usually brief and do not have long-term sequelae.

What is the prognosis if seizures develop within 24–48 hours of injury?

These are called **early posttraumatic seizures,** and the affected child should be treated for the seizures. Most children are treated with phenytoin to prevent further brain injury from secondary seizure.

What is the most important determinant of neurologic outcome following head injury?

Duration of coma

How does the outcome for children compare with that of adults if the brain injuries are similar?

Children do better.

How does the outcome for children younger than 2 years of age compare with that of children who are older than 2 years of age if the brain injuries are similar?

Children less than 2 years of age do worse.

SEIZURES

What is a seizure?

Clinical manifestation of synchronized electrical discharges of CNS neurons

What are signs and symptoms of motor seizures in children?

They are characterized by patterns of movement that relate to the patterns of electrical discharges and are usually, but not always, accompanied by impaired consciousness.

Of nonmotor seizures?

They may be manifested only by loss of responsiveness to the environment and may be mistaken for coma without seizures.

How are seizures classified?

Table 6–1. International Classification of Epileptic Seizures

Classification	Subclassification
Partial (focal, local)	
Simple partial seizure	With motor signs
	With somatosensory or special sensory symptoms
	With autonomic signs or symptoms
	With psychic symptoms
Complex partial seizure	Simple partial onset followed by impairment of consciousness
	With impairment of consciousness at onset
Partial seizures evolving to secondarily generalized seizures	Simple partial seizures evolving to generalized seizures
	Complex partial seizures evolving to generalized seizures
	Simle partial seizures evolving to complex partial seizures evolving to generalized seizures
Generalized (Convulsive and Nonconvulsive)	
Absence seizure	Typical absence
	Atypical absence
Myoclonic seizure	
Clonic seizure	
Tonic seizure	
Tonic–clonic seizure	
Atonic (astatic) seizure	
Unclassified epileptic seizure	

What are the physiologic results of brief seizures (seconds to a few minutes)?

It is believed that brief seizures do not harm brain tissue, but the child may sustain secondary injury (e.g., may aspirate, strike head, drown, become hypothermic) through loss of protective reflexes.

What are the physiologic results of prolonged seizures (> 30 minutes)?

They may cause direct injury to brain tissue through electrolyte shifts, including excessive calcium entry into neurons. They may also enhance brain damage by increasing cerebral blood flow and elevating ICP.

What are common physiologic causes of seizures?

A unifying physiologic cause is unknown, but most seizures are probably associated with an imbalance between effects of excitatory neurotransmitters (e.g., glutamate) and inhibitory neurotransmitters (e.g., GABA).

What are common pathologic causes?

Table 6–2.
Common Pathologic Causes of Seizure

Fever

Infection
  Encephalitis
  Meningitis
  Abscess

Traumatic brain injury

Hypoxic–ischemic injury

Metabolic disorders
  Acute electrolyte abnormalities
  Genetic metabolic disease

Drugs or toxins

Infantile spasms

Brain malformations or tumors

Primary or idiopathic syndromes
  Benign neonatal seizure
  Absence epilepsy
  Generalized tonic–clonic seizure
  Myoclonic seizure

What characterizes a simple febrile seizure?

It tends to be generalized tonic–clonic and occur in children 3 months to 5 years of age; lasts < 15 minutes; occurs on day 1 of illness with high fever; family history common

What characterizes a complex febrile seizure?

Lasts > 15 minutes; multiple seizures in 1 day; partial or focal seizures; family history of nonfebrile seizures; neurologic deficits or developmental delay

What diagnostic studies are used?

Physical examination during episode may be diagnostic of type of seizure, but not of cause. Electroencephalography, with or without video monitoring, may be useful but should not delay treatment.

Treatment

What is the main goal of treatment?

Stopping seizure activity rapidly without compromising patient

What are immediate treatment procedures?

1. Evaluate and support airway and breathing.
2. Draw blood to evaluate electrolytes (e.g., calcium, sodium, glucose), drug levels, and suspected toxins. Send bedside glucose screen.
3. Gain venous access; begin infusion of dextrose in normal saline or lactated Ringer's solution. Avoid hypotonic solutions until electrolytes available.

What are the next treatment procedures (10–30 minutes) postpresentation?

Administer anticonvulsants:
1. **Rapid-onset, short-acting agents** include:
   Lorazepam—0.03 to 0.05 mg/kg, **slow** IV push
   Diazepam—0.2 to 0.5 mg/kg, **slow** IV push
   (Repeat dose three times as needed at 5–10-minute intervals. Give over several minutes to minimize respiratory depression.)
2. **Delayed-onset, long-acting agents** include:
   Phenytoin—20 mg/kg IV; delivered at < 1 mg/kg/min, with cardiovascular monitoring
   Phenobarbital—15 to 20 mg/kg IV, monitoring cardiorespiratory status

What are later (30–60 minutes) treatment procedures postpresentation?

1. Consider increasing long-acting anticonvulsant levels or using additional medications if seizures persist.
2. Pursue diagnostic workup:
   Evaluate initial laboratory studies
   Obtain further history
   Consider CT or other imaging studies, especially if seizures were focal
   Consider obtaining CSF if no evidence of increased ICP

Complications of treatment?	Respiratory depression from anticonvulsant drugs; other drug toxicity, such as cardiac depression; failure to secure compromised airway
What is the outcome?	**Brief seizure**—good if no iatrogenic complications occur; damage may still occur because of underlying cause **Prolonged seizure**—variable, but should be anticipated to be worse than that from a brief seizure

CARDIAC ARREST

What is cardiac arrest?	Pulseless cardiac arrest is a clinical diagnosis based on the absence of a palpable central (femoral, brachial) pulse. It is accompanied by apnea. It may exist in the presence of electrocardiographic complexes.
What are common causes in children?	The vast majority of pulseless arrest in children is a result of **severe hypoxemia** and **acidosis,** secondary to **respiratory failure or shock.**
What are causes of electromechanical dissociation?	1. Hypoxia 2. Volume loss 3. Tension pneumothorax 4. Cardiac tamponade 5. Electrolyte imbalance 6. Profound hypothermia 7. Drug overdose
What are common causes of primary cardiac failure?	Common causes are associated with poor ventricular function or severe dysrhythmias: 1. Chronic: cardiomyopathy, structural heart disease 2. Acute: myocarditis, endocarditis
What are the physiologic consequences?	Absent cardiac output causes underperfusion of all organs within minutes. Because cardiopulmonary failure in children is usually the result of prolonged, worsening tissue perfusion, organ damage may exist before the arrest, making full recovery unlikely even if spontaneous circulation is rapidly

recovered. Neurologic recovery is usually poor after cardiopulmonary arrest.

What is the initial approach to and treatment of cardiopulmonary arrest?

The presence of cardiopulmonary arrest is a clinical diagnosis based on absence of pulses which signifies undetectable cardiac output.

1. Confirm cardiopulmonary arrest and begin CPR. (**Remember, airway is always secured first!!** Airway, Breathing, Circulation—the ABCs!)
2. Apply monitoring leads and confirm rhythm.
3. Obtain venous or intraosseous access.
4. Identify and treat causes.
5. Perform repeated cardiopulmonary assessments and respond to changes accordingly. [**See Decision Tree from Pediatric Advanced Life Support (PALS) manual**]

What should be done after initial treatment for cardiac arrest?

1. Perform serial rapid physical assessments of respiratory, cardiovascular, and neurologic systems.
2. Evaluate available history.
3. Assimilate ongoing assessments of response to treatment to identify probable etiology of arrest.
4. Obtain ancillary studies: measure bedside glucose (from fingerstick); obtain arterial blood if possible to measure ABG, electrolytes and glucose, CBC, liver and renal function studies, toxins, and blood cultures
5. Consider radiographic studies.
6. Alert any pertinent consultants.

What should be done after stabilization?

1. Continue resuscitative efforts until cardiorespiratory status is satisfactory.
2. If cause is still undetermined, continue laboratory, radiologic, and subspecialty evaluation.
3. Ensure secure venous access for transport to receiving unit or facility.
4. Administer antibiotics if infection is a possible cause. In most cases, delay

lumbar puncture until patient is stable in receiving unit.

How should transport be arranged?

Contact receiving unit, copy pertinent records, obtain permission to transport, and remain with patient while awaiting transport to perform and respond to continuing assessments.

Complications of treatment?

Iatrogenic complications include injury to respiratory, cardiac, and neurologic systems through inappropriate actions or failure to identify further deterioration.

What is the outcome?

Survival with an intact neurologic status after out-of-hospital cardiopulmonary arrest is rare. Organ systems other than the CNS are more resilient and may recover if the brain survives. Witnessed in-hospital arrest has a better, but still poor, prognosis for intact survival. **Poor prognosis after arrest makes identification of impending arrest crucial for early intervention.**

SHOCK

What is shock?

A clinical state in which delivery of oxygen and metabolic substrates to tissues is inadequate to meet tissue metabolic demands

What are the two stages of stock?

Compensated shock—blood pressure is maintained within a normal range for age
Uncompensated shock—hypotension, with or without low cardiac output, is present

What are the causes of hypovolemic shock?

Inadequate intravascular volume to support cardiac output, which may result from diarrhea/dehydration, poor intake or output > intake, or blood loss

Causes of distributive shock?

Total body fluid may be adequate, but has left the intravascular space; it may be septic or anaphylactic.

What is "cardiogenic shock"?

Cardiac pump failure; volume status may be low, adequate, or excessive.

What are common causes of pump failure?

1. **Intrinsic cardiac disease**, including cardiomyopathy, myocarditis, structural heart disease, and dysrhythmia resulting in poor output
2. **Toxin-mediated,** including drug-induced state and sepsis-related mediators
3. **Hypoxia**
4. **Acute volume loss in trauma**

What are clinical signs of compensated shock in children?
  Cardiovascular signs?

Blood pressure normal or high
  (Children maintain blood pressure well until late in shock!)
Heart rate usually above normal range for age
Decreased peripheral perfusion (peripheral pulses thready or absent; capillary refill time > 2–3 seconds; skin temperature cool)

  Respiratory signs?

Respiratory rate often increased as compensation for metabolic acidosis
Work of breathing may be increased

  Renal signs?

Decreased urine output

  CNS signs?

Child may be agitated, combative, or lethargic; seldom playful

What are the clinical signs of uncompensated shock?
  Cardiovascular signs?

Blood pressure below normal range for age
Heart rate may remain elevated, or bradycardia may occur in late shock.
Decreased peripheral and central perfusion (peripheral signs of hypoperfusion combined with thready central pulses)

Respiratory signs?	Respiratory rate may remain elevated, or may have fallen despite metabolic acidosis.
	Work of breathing may be elevated or inappropriately low.
Renal signs?	Decreased urine output
CNS signs?	Child is usually combative or lethargic; may fail to recognize parent or appear apathetic with painful stimuli; and may be unresponsive or comatose.
What are laboratory signs of shock in children?	**Metabolic acidosis,** with or without respiratory compensation; elevated lactate implies poor tissue perfusion
	Hypoglycemia may occur in infants and children in shock, or may be a primary cause of shock.
What are physiologic consequences of shock?	Inadequate tissue perfusion causes end-organ dysfunction and eventually irreversible organ damage if untreated.
What is the diagnostic approach?	Identification of shock should be clinical, based on interpretation of the physical findings outlined above. Determination of the cause is useful in later treatment, but should not delay initial stabilization efforts.
Why must cardiogenic shock be differentiated from other forms of shock?	Because **although cardiogenic shock is relatively rare in children,** it requires a different treatment approach after initial interventions. Cardiogenic shock should be suspected when signs of congestive heart failure (e.g., enlarged liver, pulmonary congestion, signs of poor cardiac output) are present on initial evaluation or after initial fluid resuscitation.

Treatment

What is needed for definitive treatment of shock?	Identification of the cause, but basic interventions should be used in all cases of shock.

What are the basic interventions?

Remember the ABCs!

1. Immediately provide oxygen through an adequate airway (native or artificial) to optimize oxygen delivery to underperfused tissues.
2. If patient is both bradycardic and poorly perfused, proceed as if patient is in cardiac arrest.
3. Achieve vascular access when shock is recognized.
4. Provide an initial fluid bolus of 20 ml/kg, using an isotonic crystalloid without dextrose (normal saline or lactated Ringer's solution). Preferred method of administration in infants and children is pushing fluid using a large syringe and stopcock, **not** a "wide open" infusion, in order to allow rapid administration while avoiding inadvertent overhydration.
5. Obtain a bedside glucose measurement, and treat with 0.5–1.0 g/kg of IV dextrose if patient is hypoglycemic. Consider obtaining other diagnostic studies (e.g., blood studies, radiographs), but do not delay treatment of Airway, Breathing, and correction of Circulatory deficit during this process.
6. Reassess peripheral perfusion (pulse strength and capillary refill time), fluid balance (liver size, urine output); breath sounds (work of breathing); and vital signs. Repeat fluid boluses with frequent reassessment until patient is no longer in shock or until signs of fluid overload are noted. Colloid may be required as a fluid replacement if colloid (e.g., blood) has been lost.
7. Remain aware that shock may recur until the predisposing condition has been corrected.

What do you do if patient displays signs of cardiogenic shock during resuscitation?

Initiate inotropic support via intraosseous or central venous access.
Doses:
   Dopamine: 5–20 mcg/kg/min
   Epinephrine: 0.05–1.0 mcg/kg/min

Consult pediatric cardiologist or intensivist to assist in further management of cardiogenic shock.

Complications?

The primary shortcoming in the treatment of shock is failure to correct tissue oxygenation and perfusion deficit before end-organ damage occurs. Conversely, overzealous treatment can cause fluid overload with resulting pulmonary compromise or, rarely, congestive heart failure. Either poor outcome is usually avoided by constant observation and reassessment of the results of interventions.

What are the outcomes?

They depend on the underlying cause and on the phase of shock at which intervention begins. Outcomes are improved by rapid recognition of shock and correction of tissue underperfusion before tissue damage becomes irreversible.

UNEXPLAINED COMA

What is coma?

A state of unconsciousness from which one cannot be aroused by stimulation of any magnitude

What is the differential diagnosis of coma in an infant or child?

Structural lesions resulting in increased ICP or seizures, including:
1. Trauma, resulting in shear injury, generalized edema, or an expanding mass lesion
2. Tumor
3. Abscess
4. Hemorrhage
5. Infarction

Functional disorders resulting in bilateral hemispheric dysfunction, including:
1. Hypoxic/ischemic injury
2. Ingestion or poisoning
3. Remote or CNS infection
4. Metabolic derangements, such as hypoglycemia, hyponatremia (usually < 120 mEq/L), severe

hypernatremia (cerebral edema), uremia, hyperammonemia, extreme hypercalcemia, severe hyperglycemia
5. Seizures: postictal state; ongoing electrographic (nonconvulsive) status epilepticus

What are important elements of the physical examination of the comatose infant or child?

1. **Rapid evaluation of the ABCs!**
2. **Rapid neurologic examination,** looking for signs of trauma, increased ICP, or specific toxidromes
3. If elements of ABCs appear acceptable and maintainable, proceed with examination for localized lesions, signs of infection, and associated conditions (e.g., cervical spine injury) that may cause morbidity.
4. Assigning a **Glasgow Coma Score** may aid in serial evaluations and determining prognostication.

What are appropriate initial interventions?

Remember the ABCs!
1. Stabilize the patient's airway and breathing. The deeply comatose patient usually requires intubation because of diminished or absent airway protective reflexes, or because of poor pharyngeal muscle tone that results in upper airway obstruction. Consider mild hyperventilation ($PaCO_2$ 30–35 mm Hg) and/or mannitol administration (0.25–0.5 g/kg IV) if increased ICP is suspected clinically.
2. Obtain intravenous access, obtain a rapid bedside glucose determination, and consider administering dextrose (0.5–1 g/kg) and naloxone (0.10 mg/kg, up to 2 mg) as a therapeutic and diagnostic trial, as indicated by findings.
3. Continue with more detailed physical examination, and delegate someone to obtain a rapid and pertinent history from the best available source.
4. Initiate appropriate consultations (e.g., neurosurgery, neurology, pediatrics, trauma surgery), laboratory evaluations, and imaging studies.

5. Avoid unnecessary procedures (e.g., an immediate lumbar puncture) until the patient is stable.
6. Evaluate for signs of associated shock and treat if present; brain perfusion must be maintained while avoiding fluid overload if increased ICP exists.
7. Long-term care approach is dictated by the patient's underlying cause of coma.

What initial laboratory and imaging studies are appropriate?

The choice of laboratory studies and imaging studies will be guided by your physical examination findings and by the patient's history. First-priority studies should be expedited while maintaining appropriate vigilance over the patient's evolving status.

First priority in metabolic/toxin evaluation?

Immediate bedside glucose determination and electrolyte panel, including calcium

Second priority in metabolic/toxin evaluation?

Consider ammonia level; urine toxicology screen, or specific toxin levels if history or physical examination findings are suggestive; consider studies for inborn errors of metabolism if suggested by history, in consultation with a medical geneticist.

First priority of imaging studies (CT, MRI)?

Rule out rapidly progressive CNS lesion.

Second priority of imaging studies?

Define subtle lesions(s) or repeat initial studies to define progression of an identified lesion.

After initial stabilization and evaluation, what are the monitoring and intervention procedures?

Ongoing monitoring and interventions are determined by initial findings and the patient's evolving status.
1. Consider ICP monitoring in consultation with a neurosurgery team if clinical or imaging evidence of increased ICP exists or if there is a high likelihood of development of elevated ICP based on history.
2. If hyperventilation is pursued, an arterial line or calibrated end-tidal

carbon dioxide monitoring is advisable to avoid extreme hypocarbia.

3. The nature and frequency of laboratory studies are determined by your findings. **Hypoglycemia** should be **corrected immediately,** whereas severe **hyperglycemia** and **hypernatremia** should be **corrected slowly.** Correct severe hyponatremia rapidly to a level of approximately 120 mEq/L; then proceed slowly. Electrolyte corrections must be monitored frequently to avoid complications of therapy.

4. Consider obtaining EEG if nonconvulsive status epilepticus is a possible cause of coma based on history.

5. If toxic exposure or ingestion is determined, specific therapy (if available) should be initiated in consultation with a toxicologist.

What are the outcomes?

Outcomes depend on the underlying cause of the coma, any associated comorbidity (e.g., secondary hypoxic–ischemic injury, progression of increased ICP), and the ability to reverse the progression of disease.

NEAR DROWNING

What is near drowning?

A submersion incident followed by survival for at least 24 hours, regardless of the ultimate outcome

What is drowning?

A submersion incident that results in death **within** the first 24 hours

What is the epidemiology of near drowning in children and infants?

Near drowning is more common in males than in females. High-risk pediatric groups include toddlers, adolescent males, and children with seizure disorders. Most drowning or near drowning in small children occurs during brief periods (< 5 minutes) without supervision, not as a result of neglect. Most near-drowning incidents occur in residential swimming pools, but can occur in any available body of water, **including standing water** on pool covers, lakes and rivers, 5-gallon industrial buckets (often used for storing liquids), bathtubs, toilet bowls, and hot tubs.

What determines outcome after a near-drowning incident?

Duration of the hypoxic insult during submersion, associated morbidities (e.g., aspiration injury, electrolyte abnormalities), and complications of therapy. Although greater than 90% of pediatric submersion injuries have a good outcome, in some states drowning and near drowning are leading causes of fatal injuries in young children.

What is the pathophysiology of submersion injury?

1. The initial response to unexpected submersion is thought to involve **aspiration** of small amounts of water, which triggers **laryngospasm.** As hypoxia and panic ensue, reflex swallowing of water into the stomach occurs. When hypoxia becomes severe, most victims have resolution of laryngospasm, followed by active or passive aspiration of water.
2. During resuscitative efforts, **emesis and aspiration** of swallowed water and gastric contents may occur.
3. **Hypoxic injury to the brain** and other organ systems occurs, the extent depending on the length of submersion and the water temperature.
4. **Lung injury** may be related to contents of the aspirated water. Surfactant washout is a theoretic concern in massive aspiration episodes.
5. **Electrolyte disturbances** may occur but are rarely observed in patients who survive until arrival at a hospital, unless the victim has aspirated extremely hypertonic solutions.
6. **Infection** may ensue, although not commonly from direct aspiration.

More likely, hypoxic injury to the gut may be followed by translocation of bowel flora into the bloodstream, resulting in sepsis and associated hematogenous spread of infection.

What are appropriate initial interventions (before child is at ER)?

1. **On-site basic life support,** including ABCs with stabilization of the cervical spine, is initially appropriate for all cold water (temperature < 5°C) submersion victims and arguably for all warm-water submersion victims, unless the submersion is known to be exceptionally prolonged.
2. Avoid increasing the risk of emesis and aspiration of gastric contents by avoiding excessive airway manipulation or pressure on the abdomen.
3. Escalate to advanced life support measures if needed, continuing until the patient is evaluated in the ER. Many clinicians recommend continuing resuscitative efforts until the patient's core temperature exceeds 32°C, because existence or maintenance of a spontaneous cardiac rhythm may not occur below this temperature.

What are appropriate interventions at the ER?

Decisions about level of further care are based on level of neurologic function and presence or absence of lung abnormalities. Patients with neither history of diminished mental status nor abnormal lung exam may develop pulmonary edema up to 12 hours after submersion, and therefore careful observation for at least 4–8 hours is recommended before discharge. All patients with altered mental or pulmonary status should be admitted, because the natural history of either is to worsen before resolution can be anticipated.

How long should cardiopulmonary resuscitation be continued in a submersion victim who arrives in the ER without spontaneous circulation?

This issue is controversial. Many clinicians recommend discontinuing efforts if advanced life support measures fail to restore spontaneous circulation once the patient has reached a core temperature of 28°C; others suggest using 32°C as a temperature goal.

What management approaches should be taken for the submersion patient who is admitted to the hospital?

Patients will have different treatment and monitoring needs, depending on the degree of hypoxic–ischemic insult and on comorbidities.

Respiratory care?

1. Oxygen is given to maintain saturations > 90%
2. If intubation is required, PEEP may be required to minimize intrapulmonary shunt.
3. ABG monitoring is indicated for the intubated patient.
4. Antibiotic coverage is indicated if the patient has clear signs of pulmonary infection.

Neurologic care?

1. If the patient is obtunded or has a declining mental status, intubate the trachea to protect the airway.
2. Although increased ICP may occur secondary to the hypoxic–ischemic insult, ICP monitoring has **not** been shown to alter ultimate neurologic outcome in this patient group, presumably because the global hypoxic–ischemic insult occurred long before the patient arrived at the hospital. However, efforts to avoid further CNS damage from fluid overload, hypoperfusion, hypoxemia, and seizure activity should be maximized.
3. Other rescue therapies that have not proven helpful include prolonged hypothermia, barbiturate coma, and steroids.

Cardiovascular care?

1. After stabilization of initial cardiac dysfunction associated with hypoxia

and acidosis, further impairment of cardiac dysfunction is associated with hypoxic cardiomyopathy or sepsis. Management of the depressed myocardium requires arterial and central venous pressure monitoring, and may require thermodilution cardiac output monitoring in severe cases. Catecholamine support may be needed.

Infection management?

It is managed symptomatically. Infection is secondary to translocation of gut flora through ischemic bowel, or it is caused by aspiration of grossly contaminated water. Multiple organ system failure may result from prolonged hypoxia or shock.

What are common complications of therapy?

Respiratory complications are usually due to barotrauma and may include acute pneumothoraces or fibrosis if prolonged mechanical ventilation is needed, and/or if high levels of PEEP are required.
Neurologic complications are largely due to progressive cerebral edema secondary to the initial hypoxic insult, but may be exacerbated by shock, fluid overload, and prolonged seizures.
Nosocomial infection may occur during prolonged invasive monitoring, which may be required in an unstable patient.

What are indicators of poor outcome after near drowning?

1. Documented submersion > 5 minutes
2. The need for CPR in the emergency setting
3. A serum pH < 7 or fixed and dilated pupils in the emergency setting
4. Need for cardiotonic drugs during resuscitation

However, the only factor consistently predicting poor outcome is the need for continued CPR in the ER for nonhypothermic patients.

What is the role of prevention?

Because near-drowning outcomes are largely determined by the degree of the **initial** hypoxic insult (assuming you are able to minimize complications of therapy), prevention is of paramount importance. Current areas of focus include improved legislation for barrier requirements around pools, education about drowning risks in the home and around natural bodies of water, and encouragement of CPR training for pool owners.

7

Growth and Development

GROWTH

Why is growth an important pediatrics issue?

Physical growth, maturation, and neurologic development (with its social and behavioral correlates) distinguish children from adults and are important areas of clinical study in pediatrics.

Most important feature of growth?

Growth is a **dynamic, not a static, process.**

Best way to evaluate growth?

Longitudinally along a time line, either by direct observation or by evaluation of accurate historical data

Why are growth charts important?

They facilitate growth data analysis and they are a record of data points, allowing easy comparisons with previous points and standard growth patterns.

What is growth rate?

Change in a growth parameter over time; when evaluating growth abnormalities, the growth rate is frequently more important than an isolated data point

When is growth most rapid?

Relative growth is most rapid during fetal development. Adolescence is the time of greatest postnatal growth.

What is the normal rate of weight gain for infants?

After the initial postnatal water loss (about 5%–10% of birth weight) during the first few days of life, an infant should gain about 1 oz (30 g) per day.

At what age does an infant double the birth weight?

Usually at 6 months of age

What height and weight should a normal child be at 4 years of age?

About 40 inches tall and 40 pounds

What is the upper:lower segment ratio?

The ratio between the upper segment (i.e., distance from top of the pubis to the top of the head) and the lower segment (i.e., distance from the top of the pubis to the bottom of the feet)

How do upper:lower segment ratios vary with age?

Infants are relatively short limbed compared with older children and adults.

What is the normal upper:lower segment ratio at birth?

1.7:1

What is the normal upper:lower segment ratio at 10 years of age?

1

What other variables are important in interpreting upper:lower segment ratios?

Normal values for upper:lower segment ratios can vary with **gender** and with **race/ethnicity.**

At what age do teeth usually erupt?

About 5–8 months

Which primary teeth usually appear first?

Central mandibular incisors

Which permanent teeth usually appear first?
  At what age?

First molars (6-year molars)

5–7 years

DEVELOPMENT

Why is development an important pediatrics issue?

Because it reflects neurologic maturation and social and sensory development in the child; abnormal development may reflect a neurologic, medical, or social problem

How does sensory impairment affect development?

Children with undetected hearing or visual deficits may not develop certain skills at the appropriate age because of these deficits.

At what age does an infant smile responsively?	6–8 weeks
At what age does an infant follow past midline?	2 months
At what age does an infant grasp an object (e.g., a rattle)?	3 months
At what age does an infant sit alone without support?	6 months
At what age does an infant transfer an object from hand to hand?	6 months
At what age does an infant begin to put objects in the mouth?	6–7 months
At what age does an infant demonstrate a pincer grasp?	9–10 months
At what age does an infant begin to babble?	5–6 months
At what age does an infant say "mama" or "dada" (nonspecifically)?	9 months
At what age does an infant crawl?	9–10 months
At what age does an infant pull to stand?	8–10 months
At what age does an infant walk without support?	13 months
At what age does an infant drink from a cup?	12 months
At what age does an infant use one or two words specifically?	12 months

At what age does an infant combine words into two- or three-word phrases?

24 months

At what age does a child run?

24 months

What is the Denver Developmental Screening Test?

A screening test developed for the quick assessment of developmental milestones

Does developmental delay imply later mental retardation?

No. Mental retardation usually refers to cognitive and problem-solving deficits, whereas developmental delay includes a wide range of skills that may be adversely affected by medical or neurologic problems that may not affect cognition.

PUBERTY

What is puberty?

The development of secondary sexual characteristics and the maturation of gonadal function

What is usually the first sign of puberty in boys?

Enlargement of the testes

When does puberty usually begin in boys?

Around 11.5 years of age

What is the normal age range of onset of puberty in boys?

Approximately 9.5–13.5 years

What is the normal progression of puberty in boys?

Usually enlargement of the testes, then appearance of pubic hair, then linear growth spurt

What is the first sign of puberty in girls?

Breast enlargement

When does puberty usually begin in girls?

Around 10.5 years of age

What is the normal age range of onset in girls?

8–13 years

What is the normal progression of puberty in girls?

Usually appearance of breast buds (thelarche), followed by appearance of pubic hair, growth spurt, and then menarche

When does the maximum growth velocity occur?

Usually 1.5 years after the beginning of puberty

When does menarche occur?

Usually 2 years after appearance of breast buds

Is precocious puberty more common in boys or girls?

Girls

What is the most common cause of precocious puberty in girls?

Idiopathic precocious puberty

Section II   Newborn Care

8

Perinatal Care and Evaluation of the Newborn

APGAR SCORES

What is the Apgar score?

It is a method of evaluating a newborn and was introduced in 1953 by Dr. Virginia Apgar. Five physical signs are identified and a score of 0, 1, or 2 is given to each sign at 1 and 5 minutes after birth.

What are the five signs evaluated, and what constitutes a score of 0, 1, and 2 for each sign?

Heart rate: absent (0); less than 100 beats/min (1); greater than 100 beats/min (2)

Respiratory effort: absent (0); irregular or weak cry (1); regular or strong cry (2)

Muscle tone: none (0); with some flexion (1); well flexed or spontaneous movement (2)

Reflex irritability: no response (0); grimace (1); cough or sneeze (2)

Color: central cyanosis (0); peripheral cyanosis (1); completely pink (2)

APGAR mnemonic?

Appearance, **P**ulse, **G**rimace, **A**ctivity, and **R**espirations

What do the 1- and 5-minute scores imply?

The 1-minute score indicates the infant's well-being; a score of less than 3 implies asphyxia.

The 5-minute score indicates the infant's continued well-being or subsequent decline. Alternatively, it may be an indication of improvement with resuscitation efforts if the 1-minute score was poor.

63

<table>
<tr><td>**Should additional Apgar assessments be made after 5 minutes?**</td><td>If the Apgar score is still less than 7 at 5 minutes, additional compilation of Apgar scores every 5 minutes for the subsequent 20 minutes is helpful to assess resuscitation efforts.</td></tr>
</table>

NEWBORN RESUSCITATION

INITIAL ASSESSMENT

What are the five components of initial assessment and management of a newborn?

1. Gentle suction of the mouth, nose, and pharynx with a bulb syringe or suction catheter
2. Clamping and division of the umbilical cord
3. Drying of the infant to minimize evaporative heat loss with subsequent warming via radiant heat
4. Auscultation and mild stimulation, such as flicking the soles of the feet, rubbing the back, or directing an oxygen stream toward the face
5. Assessment of Apgar criteria

What are the potential risks of suctioning?

Deep suctioning should be avoided in the initial resuscitation because this may induce laryngeal spasm, increase vagal tone resulting in apnea and bradycardia, or result in trauma to the pharynx or esophagus.

How should the infant be positioned as it is transferred from the mother to the resuscitation table and while on the resuscitation table?

The head should be placed in the dependent position (approximately 20°–30° below horizontal) to facilitate drainage of secretions from the pharynx.

INTUBATION

What is the primary indication for intubation?

Inability to oxygenate and ventilate an infant adequately via bag-and-mask ventilation

What are four signs of inadequate oxygenation and ventilation?

1. Poor color and poor or lack of responsiveness
2. Lack of movement of chest with bag-and-mask ventilation

3. Falling oxygen saturation
4. Falling heart rate

What is appropriate positioning for bag-and-mask ventilation?

Placement of a 0 or 00 oral airway; placement of the mask over the mouth and nose with the head and neck slightly extended

What are appropriate-size endotracheal tubes for infants?

Uncuffed tubes with internal diameters of 2.5, 3.0, or 3.5 mm, depending on the infant's size

What are important anatomic and position considerations during intubation?

1. The head and the neck should be slightly extended.
2. The larynx is more anterior in the neonate than in the older child or adult.
3. The epiglottis tends to hang over the vocal cords and, therefore, a straight blade laryngoscope is usually more useful for holding the epiglottis away from the cords during intubation.
4. The endotracheal tube should be placed only 1–1.5 cm beyond the cords to avoid main-stem intubation.
5. Once intubation has been accomplished, holding the tube against the roof of the mouth keeps the tube stable until it can be adequately secured with tape.

UMBILICAL VESSEL CATHETERIZATION

When are umbilical vessel catheters used?

These are generally used in acutely ill newborn and premature infants.

What are the purposes of an umbilical vein catheter?

This catheter may provide:
1. Central venous pressure monitoring
2. A conduit for administration of intravenous fluids, hyperalimentation, and medications
3. A means for sampling blood when needed

Where should the tip of the umbilical vein catheter lie?

Generally at the junction of the right atrium and inferior vena cava at the level of T10–T11

What are complications of an umbilical vein catheter?	Vascular embolization, vascular spasm, vascular perforation, infection, hemorrhage, venous congestion of the lower extremities, thrombosis (e.g., thrombosis of the portal vein, resulting in portal hypertension)
What are uses for an umbilical artery catheter?	1. Pulse and blood pressure monitoring 2. Access for blood samples and arterial blood gases 3. Administration of medications and hyperalimentation as well as intravenous fluids
Where should the tip of an umbilical artery catheter be placed?	Either just above the bifurcation of aorta at the level of L3–L5 or above the celiac axis at the level of T6–T10
What are complications of an umbilical artery catheter?	Vascular embolization, thrombosis, vascular spasm, vascular perforation, ischemic or chemical necrosis of abdominal viscera, infection, hemorrhage, impaired circulation to the leg, renovascular hypertension
How long may umbilical vein or artery catheters remain in place?	Generally, umbilical vein catheters should be removed within 7 days and arterial catheters within 10–14 days.

EVALUATION OF THE NEWBORN

How are newborns classified?	By **gestational age** and **size**
What gestational ages are considered preterm, term, and postterm?	Preterm is less than 37 weeks gestation; term is 37 weeks to less than 42 weeks; and postterm is 42 weeks and beyond.
What is SGA?	Small for Gestational Age
Is SGA a concern?	Yes. Infants who are SGA have increased caloric needs (relative to their weight), a higher mortality, and are at increased risk for malformations, hypoglycemia, and congenital infections.

What is symmetric growth retardation?	Growth retardation of all growth parameters (i.e., length, weight, and head circumference)
Implications of symmetric growth retardation?	It may imply an insult early in the pregnancy (e.g., teratogen), a malformation syndrome (including chromosome abnormalities), or early infection.
Implications of asymmetric growth retardation?	If weight is disproportionately low (relative to length and head circumference), it implies an insult later in pregnancy (e.g., maternal hypertension, placental insufficiency).
What is LGA?	Large for Gestational Age
What are some causes of LGA?	Maternal diabetes (including gestational diabetes), Beckwith-Wiedemann syndrome, twin–twin transfusion (recipient twin)
Do all LGA infants have an obvious cause?	No
Complications of LGA?	Hypoglycemia, increased incidence of injury at birth, complications related to underlying cause
What is an IDM?	Infant of a Diabetic Mother
What are risks of IDM?	Hypoglycemia, hypocalcemia, malformations (particularly congenital heart disease and variants of caudal regression syndrome), polycythemia, renal vein thrombosis
What are three tests that assess gestational age?	New Ballard Score, Lubchenco charts, Dubowitz exam
What is the significance of meconium staining?	It may reflect in utero stress and places the infant at risk for meconium aspiration.
What is the normal newborn heart rate?	Greater than 100 beats/min; usually 120–160 beats/min

When should a newborn be examined?

Newborns should be assessed in the delivery room and have a complete physical examination within 12 hours of birth.

What is the purpose of the delivery room assessment?

To determine if the infant will need resuscitation, to assess for obvious malformations or abnormalities, to estimate gestational age, and to ease the transition from the intrauterine environment to the "outside world"

What is the purpose of the later, more complete exam?

To evaluate infant for malformations, establish normalcy of growth and function, and document physical findings

What three physical measurements are routinely taken?

Head circumference (using greatest occipital-to-frontal diameter), weight, and crown-to-heel length

How should the newborn's temperature be measured?

Usually axillary or rectal

Which is more accurate?

Rectal

What is the normal newborn respiratory rate?

40–60 breaths/min

How should the complete physical exam of the newborn proceed?

After noting the vital signs and general appearance, the examiner should take advantage of the infant's current state. If the infant is sleeping or is quiet, begin with auscultation of the chest, and palpation and auscultation of the abdomen. Then proceed in a head-to-toe direction with inspection and palpation. Ophthalmologic and otoscopic evaluations are usually performed later in the exam, with the formal part of the neurologic exam at the end.

What is vernix caseosa?

A white greasy coating on the skin of newborns; more common in preterm infants

What is lanugo?

Fine hair that covers the body of infants; more common in premature infants

What are mongolian spots?	Bluish discolorations of the skin, usually over the buttocks and lower back; more common in racial groups with darker skin pigment
Is palpable breast tissue normal in newborns?	One centimeter of palpable breast tissue may be present in normal newborns (male and female) as the result of stimulation by maternal estrogens.
Are heart murmurs common in newborns?	No
Name five heart defects associated with cyanosis.	Tetralogy of Fallot, total anomalous pulmonary venous return, truncus arteriosus, transposition of the great vessels, tricuspid atresia
What lesion is associated with absence of or diminished femoral pulses?	Coarctation of the aorta
How is the fontanel measured?	From broad side to broad side
What disorders are associated with an enlarged anterior fontanel?	Hypothyroidism, hypophosphatasia, hydrocephalus, osteogenesis imperfecta, other skeletal dysplasias
What disorders are associated with a small fontanel?	Craniostenosis, including craniosynostosis syndromes, and microcephaly
What is molding?	Temporary misshaping of the cranium, usually related to position during the latter part of pregnancy and labor
What is a cephalohematoma?	A hematoma beneath the periosteum of the cranium
What is caput succedaneum?	Edema of the soft tissues of the scalp
How can cephalohematoma and caput succedaneum be differentiated?	Cephalohematomas do not cross suture lines.

What is hypertelorism? True hypertelorism is an increased distance between the orbits.

What is telecanthus? Increased distance between the medial canthi, frequently associated with the presence of epicanthal folds

What is the red reflex? The red reflection of the retina through the lens of the eye; a normal red reflex implies that there are neither large lens opacities nor large retinal tumor

Why is a catheter passed through both sides of the nose? To rule out choanal atresia or stenosis

Why not do this immediately after birth? There is concern that this procedure might cause a vagal response, with bradycardia.

Why is it important to have patent choanae? Infants are obligate nose breathers, so choanal atresia can cause respiratory distress.

What is the most common fracture during delivery? Fracture of the clavicle

How large is the newborn liver? The liver may be palpable 1–2 cm below the right costal margin.

What is the significance of a scaphoid abdomen? It may indicate a diaphragmatic hernia.

What is the normal number of vessels in the umbilical cord? Three vessels (i.e., two arteries and one vein)

When does the umbilical cord usually dry and fall off? Usually before 3 weeks of age

What is acrocyanosis? Bluish discoloration of the hands and feet; not rare in newborns but may be abnormal in older infants

What is harlequin color change?	Reddening of one side of the infant, with a sharp line of demarcation at the midline; may be related to autonomic factors; usually benign and self-limited
What is cutis marmorata?	Reticulated mottling of the skin; may be seen transiently in infants who are cold; also seen as a more persistent finding in infants with Down syndrome and several other disorders
What is the normal penis length in a term male infant?	About 3–4 cm shaft length
What is hypospadias?	Abnormal location of penile urethral meatus along the ventral aspect of the shaft
What is chordee?	Bowing or bending of the penile shaft
How do the labia minora vary with gestational age?	The labia minora are prominent in preterm females, usually protruding beyond the labia majora. They regress as the infant enlarges.
What is the significance of hair at the base of the spine?	This is sometimes associated with spina bifida.
What is syndactyly?	Cutaneous fusion of the digits
What is polydactyly?	Extra digits
What are the postaxial and preaxial sides of the hand?	Postaxial is the ulnar side of the hand, whereas preaxial is the radial side.
What is developmental dysplasia of the hip?	This term is sometimes used synonymously with congenital dislocation of the hip; however, it is a broader term that accounts for hip dislocation that may not be evident immediately at birth.
How do you screen for it?	Observation—asymmetry of fat folds, leg length discrepancy Passively abducting the hips (i.e., Ortolani maneuver) or adducting and rotating each hip (i.e., Barlow test)

Which gender is affected more often?	Females
Why give a newborn vitamin K?	Newborns may be deficient in vitamin K; it prevents hemorrhagic disease due to deficiency of vitamin K–dependent coagulation factors
Why put prophylactic antibiotics in the infant's eyes?	To prevent gonococcal and chlamydial eye infection (ophthalmia neonatorum)
What antibiotic is used?	0.5% erythromycin ophthalmic ointment or 1% silver nitrate solution
Is circumcision of males routine?	No. The indications for circumcision are primarily cultural and religious. There are few clinical indications for circumcision.
What about nonretractile foreskins?	Most foreskins will not retract completely in the newborn, but this improves with age.
Are there benefits of circumcision?	Some authors suggest a reduction in penile inflammation, cancer, STDs, and urinary tract infections in boys and men who are circumcised.
Contraindications to circumcision?	Hypospadias, chordee, micropenis, ambiguous genitalia; bleeding disorder (or family history of a bleeding disorder) is a contraindication until the child has been tested, and any deficiencies are accounted for
Why is imperforate anus important?	It may be an isolated finding or it may be associated with urinary tract abnormalities (including fistulae), cardiac anomalies, or any other malformations seen in the VACTERL association.

NEWBORN NURSERY ORDERS

[**Note:** These are examples for a normal term newborn. Preterm infants or critically ill infants will have different orders, depending on their gestational age and underlying illness.]

Admit to:	Newborn Nursery
Attending physician:	Dr. _____
Vital signs:	On admission, q 1 hour × 2, then q shift

Medications:	Vitamin K: 1 mg/0.5 ml IM
	Erythromycin ointment to each eye
	Males undergoing circumcision:
	    Vaseline, 3 tubes, 30 gm each; apply
	    to circumcision site
	Males undergoing circumcision:
	    Lidocaine 1%, 2 ml (used during
	    circumcision)

Feedings:	**Bottle:** nursery formula q4 hours ad lib (beginning when respiratory status is stable) **Breast:** breast feed immediately after delivery and prn
Labs:	1. Capillary hematocrit and bilirubin at 4 hours when Rh sensitization is known, or newborn is pale color, twin gestation, infant of a diabetic mother, or SGA. Call house officer for hematocrit < 40 or > 70 and bilirubin > 4. 2. Dextrostix within 1 hour and prn if weight < 2500 g or > 90th percentile for gestational age (LGA); or if newborn is jittery, has unstable temperature, or has apnea. Call house officer for dextrostix < 60. Hematocrit and state newborn screen at discharge.
Notify house officer for any of the following:	Weight < 2500 g or > 4000 g, feeding intolerance, temperature instability, apnea, cyanosis, resting respiratory rate consistently > 70, signs of respiratory distress, abnormal tone, jaundice, malformations, heart murmur
Car seat:	Required for discharge; seat insert for infant weighing < 3000 g

9   Common Clinical Problems

JAUNDICE

What is it?	Accumulation of bilirubin in the epidermal tissues of the body resulting in a yellowish tinge to the skin, sclera, and mucosa
At what level is jaundice usually evident?	Serum levels > 5.0 mg/dl
What type of bilirubin is most commonly elevated in the neonate?	Unconjugated bilirubin
What is the physiology of elevated bilirubin?	Unconjugated hyperbilirubinemia is secondary to increased production of bilirubin (e.g., excess RBC destruction), decreased hepatic conjugation of bilirubin, and/or decreased hepatic uptake of bilirubin. Conjugated hyperbilirubinemia is caused by hepatobiliary dysfunction.
Complications of hyperbilirubinemia?	Persistent and pathologic elevation of bilirubin in the newborn may cause an excess of free bilirubin (unconjugated bilirubin not bound to albumin or other serum proteins). This potential neurotoxin may cause kernicterus, an often irreversible phenomenon characterized by jaundice, alteration of neurobehavioral status, and injury to selected neuronal pathways in the brain (e.g., basal ganglia, hippocampal cortex, cranial nerve VIII). Long-term sequelae of kernicterus may include deafness, cerebral palsy, or death.

What level of bilirubin is excessive in neonatal jaundice?

It remains controversial. In healthy term infants, an unconjugated bilirubin concentration > 20 mg/dl is potentially concerning. Prematurity, acidosis, and other conditions may lower the threshold at which hyperbilirubinemia will cause damage.

Differential Dx?

Unconjugated hyperbilirubinemia may be physiologic (i.e., caused by immature hepatic enzyme pathways in the newborn) or may be associated with breast feeding. More pathologic causes include:

1. Rh, ABO, or other RBC isoimmunization complications
2. RBC membrane defects (e.g., congenital spherocytosis)
3. RBC biochemical defects (e.g., G-6-PD deficiency)
4. Deficiency in glucuronyl transferase (e.g., Crigler-Najjar syndrome)
5. Hypothyroidism
6. Infants of diabetic mothers
7. Bacterial or viral sepsis

Conjugated hyperbilirubinemia may be caused by direct hepatic insult from asphyxia, sepsis, or congenital metabolic toxins, or by intrahepatic or extrahepatic biliary obstruction.

What are important components of the clinical evaluation?

1. Pertinent history should identify maternal complications with pregnancy or delivery; maternal and neonatal blood types, and direct Coombs' results; feeding history; time of onset and duration of jaundice.
2. Clinical examination should be thorough and should include a neurobehavioral exam and evaluation for signs of sepsis.
3. Pertinent studies include fractionated bilirubin level, hematocrit, and evaluation of a blood smear for evidence of hemolysis; evaluation of liver function and hepatocellular integrity are necessary with conjugated hyperbilirubinemia.

4. Liver and biliary tree ultrasound exam or nuclear medicine excretion studies may be needed to rule out anatomic abnormalities (e.g., biliary atresia).
5. Liver biopsy may be needed in certain cases.

What is the treatment?

Unconjugated hyperbilirubinemia: prophylactic or therapeutic phototherapy applied to the entire body of the infant; infants at high risk of kernicterus may need exchange transfusions of whole blood

Conjugated hyperbilirubinemia: treat the underlying liver disease or other disease process

NEONATAL SEIZURES

What is the incidence in neonates?

0.8%–1.0% of all live births; more common in preterm infants

What do seizures reflect?

Seizures may indicate underlying illness or metabolic derangement. All seizures require prompt evaluation!

What are common manifestations of seizures in a neonate?

Sudden onset of apnea; intermittent vasomotor phenomena; oromotor, ocular, or facial tics; repetitive motion of facial muscle groups

Seizure activity in the extremities of the newborn is commonly a focal clonic movement often followed by multifocal clonic, tonic, and myoclonic seizures.

Complications of seizures?

May cause permanent brain injury if undiagnosed or untreated; subtle seizures may place infant at risk for acute life-threatening events (ALTEs)

What is the most common cause of seizures?

Hypoxic–ischemic encephalopathy (HIE), which is caused by intrauterine or birth-related insult

What are other common causes of seizures?	Infection Imbalances in the blood concentrations of glucose, Na^+, Ca^{2+}, and Mg^{2+} Intracranial hemorrhage CNS malformation Drug withdrawal Inborn errors of metabolism Benign neonatal epilepsy
What are the important factors in the history when evaluating a seizure?	Must evaluate for complications during pregnancy or delivery, maternal drug use, family history of seizures, and the risk factors for sepsis
What diagnostic studies should be performed?	1. Blood chemistries (e.g., electrolytes, calcium, magnesium, glucose, arterial blood gas) 2. Evaluation for sepsis, including lumbar puncture 3. Cranial ultrasound or CT to evaluate for hemorrhage or CNS malformation 4. EEG for detecting subtle seizures
What do skin vesicles or mucosal lesions suggest?	Herpes is the most commonly diagnosed cause of any seizure in an infant with vesicular skin or mucosal lesions, or occurring after 7 days of age (until proven otherwise).
What is the treatment for neonatal seizures?	1. Electrolyte replacement as needed 2. Antibiotics and acyclovir therapy as clinically indicated 3. Surgical procedures for certain malformations or hemorrhages 4. Anticonvulsant therapy (e.g., phenobarbital and phenytoin) titrated for effect
What is the prognosis?	Depends on etiology of seizure
What are poor prognostic signs?	Seizures caused by HIE or CNS malformation Seizures initially occurring before 12 hours of life Refractory seizures persisting past 24 hours of life

What percent of infants with seizures will have cerebral palsy?	30%
What percent of infants with CP will have neonatal seizures?	30%

NEONATAL ANURIA AND OLIGURIA

What is neonatal oliguria?	Urine output of < 15–20 cc/kg/day in the first 24–48 hours of life
What is neonatal anuria?	Failure to void by 48 hours of life
What percent of neonates void within 24 hours?	92%
Within 48 hours?	99%
What are causes of oliguria?	Prerenal in origin until proven otherwise! It is usually secondary to hemodynamic compromise caused by sepsis, congenital heart disease, dehydration, hypoxia, or (rarely) renovascular accident.
What are causes of oliguria due to urinary retention?	Maternal or neonatal drug exposure; CNS disease (e.g., meningitis) or spinal cord malformation (e.g., myelomeningocele); renal malformation; or urinary outflow tract obstruction (e.g., posterior urethral valves)
What are causes of intrauterine anuria?	Bilateral renal agenesis, severe congenital polycystic kidney disease, posterior urethral valves
What can be associated with intrauterine anuria?	Oligohydramnios and pulmonary hypoplasia
What is the incidence of renal malformations, and what is the most common one?	5–6 per 1000 live births; horseshoe kidney is most common

What are some primary renal causes of anuria?

Horseshoe kidney, renal agenesis, multicystic renal disease, infantile polycystic kidney disease, nephritis, exposure to nephrotoxins

What are important obstructive lesions?

Duplication of the calyces, renal pelvis, or ureters
Ureteropelvic junction obstruction
Posterior urethral valves
Urethral atresia
Urethral diverticula

Why is family history important?

Many congenital renal disorders are inherited.

What are important aspects of prenatal history?

Maternal history of oligohydramnios or history of drug use

How can suspected prerenal compromise be evaluated?

1. Fluid bolus challenge of 10–20 cc/kg
2. Single-dose furosemide therapy (1.0 mg/kg) following a bolus dose of isotonic fluids may help rule out more severe pathology.

What are important laboratory values in evaluating a neonate with oliguria or anuria?

1. Blood chemistries
2. BUN and creatinine concentrations (**IMPORTANT:** neonatal electrolytes and chemistries typically reflect the mother's values in the first 24 hours of newborn's life)
3. Urinalysis

What are the most helpful imaging studies?

1. Renal ultrasound
2. Nuclear medicine excretion studies may help assess the relative function of each kidney. Any infant with multiple congenital anomalies should have the kidneys evaluated.

What may management of neonatal oliguria or anuria include?

1. Judicious use of IV fluids and diuretics to maintain adequate urine output
2. Maintenance of normal blood pressure; renovascular accidents, renal dysplasia, and postobstructive disorders are associated with severe hypertension
3. Peritoneal or arteriovenous dialysis if renal failure ensues

4. Transplantation of kidneys in the neonate has been successfully performed.

What is the outcome?

Outcome varies depending on the etiology. Prerenal injury is often reversible but depends on the type and duration of initial insult. Prompt diagnosis and treatment of oliguria and anuria prevent continued renal deterioration.

What is the infant mortality for renal malformations?

1 in 1000 live births

FAILURE TO PASS MECONIUM

When is meconium normally passed?

First 24–48 hours of life; sick term infants and healthy preterm infants may not pass meconium for 3–5 days

What are the signs and symptoms of failure to pass meconium?

Abdominal distention, feeding intolerance, emesis, aspiration; any bilious emesis requires prompt evaluation and should be considered volvulus until proven otherwise

Differential Dx?

1. Hirschsprung disease
2. Meconium ileus
3. Meconium plug
4. Anorectal outlet obstruction or atresia
5. Malrotation
6. Duodenal webs, annular pancreas
7. Atresia of the duodenum, jejunum, ileum or colon
8. Intestinal duplication
   In any of these conditions except meconium ileus or imperforate anus, meconium may still pass appropriately!

What are important aspects of the clinical evaluation?

1. Confirming patency of rectum with digital exam or passage of soft catheter
2. Water-soluble contrast study of lower and upper GI tract to determine if obstruction is present
3. Rectal biopsy if Hirschsprung disease is suspected
4. Assessing for cystic fibrosis

| What is the treatment? | 1. Water contrast enema may alleviate meconium plug or ileus. (Must consider cystic fibrosis or Hirschsprung disease in these infants!) |
| | 2. Surgical exploration and repair may be necessary for obstructing pathology. Maintenance of fluid and electrolyte homeostasis and hemodynamic status is imperative in these cases. |

NEONATAL CYANOSIS

What is it?	Bluish tint of the skin—reflects the presence of 3–5 g/dl of reduced hemoglobin in the blood
What must the O_2 saturation be for an infant with polycythemia to demonstrate cyanosis?	< 88%
An anemic infant?	< 70%
What are common causes of cyanosis?	Primary lung disease Poor cardiac output Congenital cyanotic heart disease Pulmonary hypertension of the newborn Methemoglobinemia
Why are prenatal and perinatal histories important?	Intrauterine or birth-related complications may indicate sepsis, asphyxia, or pulmonary insult as causes of cyanosis.
What are significant findings on clinical examination?	Heart murmurs, absent distal pulses, respiratory distress
Why is a chest radiograph important?	It allows evaluation of the lung fields for evidence of primary lung disease, and of cardiac size and shape for evidence of congenital heart disease.

What are significant findings on ABG?	PaO_2 level > 60 torr on room air virtually excludes cyanotic heart disease.
What is the significance of chocolate-colored blood?	It may indicate methemoglobinemia.
What condition may cause a 5%–10% O_2 saturation difference between the right and left arms?	Pulmonary hypertension
Why?	It may cause shunting through a patent ductus arteriosus. Blood supply to the right arm is preductal and to the left arm is postductal.
What is the treatment for cyanosis?	Treat the underlying disease. Antibiotics are useful in fighting infection. Oxygen and ventilatory support may be required for noncyanotic heart disease and primary lung disease. Extracorporeal membrane oxygenation (ECMO) therapy may be needed for refractory pulmonary disease, sepsis, and persistent pulmonary hypertension.

NEONATAL RESPIRATORY DISTRESS

What is the most common reason for admitting a newborn to a level II or III neonatal intensive care unit?	Respiratory distress
Features of respiratory distress?	1. Tachypnea (i.e., > 60 breaths/min in any infant) 2. Use of accessory muscles of respiration (e.g., nasal flaring, intercostal retractions, grunting) 3. Hypoxia or hypercapnia
What is the most common cause of neonatal respiratory distress?	Primary lung disease

What are three types of restrictive (poor lung compliance) conditions?	1. Pneumonia 2. Surfactant deficiency 3. Malformation of the lung or chest wall
What are types of obstructive (normal compliance) conditions?	Aspiration syndromes—e.g., aspiration of blood, amniotic fluid, meconium, or gastric contents
What are other common causes of respiratory distress?	CNS injury Obstruction of upper airway by nasopharyngeal tissues (as in choanal stenosis or atresia) or the tongue (as in severe micrognathia) Primary malformations of lung tissue Pulmonary edema Retained fetal lung fluid following precipitous vaginal delivery or cesarean section Pleural effusion Excessive incursion of abdominal contents Diaphragmatic hernia Hypoplastic lungs (caused by renal dysfunction or other causes of oligohydramnios) Infection
What are important factors in evaluation?	1. Clinical history and examination 2. Chest radiograph 3. ABGs 4. Blood chemistries 5. Hematocrit 6. Assessment for cardiac disease 7. Evaluation for sepsis Chapter 10 discusses specific management.

NEONATAL HYPOTONIA

What is the normal resting position for a newborn?	Elbows and knees flexed; hands most often in the fisted position
For a premature newborn?	Flexed and fisted less frequently

How does hypotonia present?	1. Extension of extremities 2. Open hands 3. Occasionally exaggerated "frog-leg" position when supine 4. Child not withdrawing into flexion with noxious stimuli 5. Diminished primitive reflexes because of poor truncal tone
What causes hypotonia?	Insults that are genetic or acquired in the intrauterine environment or during the birth process
What are causes of hypotonia without weakness?	Maternal disease and/or medication Placental insufficiency Sepsis Direct CNS injury Severe respiratory disease
What are causes of hypotonia with weakness?	Nervous system impairment—specific disorders in the neonate include: 1. Direct CNS or spinal cord injury 2. Anterior horn cell degeneration (e.g., Werdnig-Hoffmann syndrome) 3. Variants of congenital myasthenia gravis 4. Myotonic dystrophy and other muscular dystrophies 5. Myotubular myopathy 6. Arthrogryposis multiplex congenital— a diagnosis of exclusion characterized by fixed joint contractures at birth Congenital metabolic disorder should be suspected in any infant with sudden onset of lethargy, hypotonia, or seizures.
Why is family history important?	Because of possible genetic etiology
What laboratory studies are important?	1. Blood chemistries 2. Sepsis evaluation 3. Acid–base status 4. Plasma ammonia concentration 5. Creatinine phosphokinase (CPK) levels
What imaging studies are helpful?	Cranial and spinal MRI or CT

Why are EEG and EMG important?

They can help rule out seizures and skeletal muscle innervation abnormalities.

What is another important test?

Muscle biopsy

What can rule out myasthenia gravis?

Neostigmine and atropine challenges

What consultants are commonly needed?

Neurologists and genetic consultants provide workups of specific congenital metabolic disorders.

What is the treatment?

Must be tailored to underlying etiology

What is the prognosis?

The outcome depends on specific disease present; genetic counseling may be helpful in certain cases.

10

Diseases of the Newborn

PERIVENTRICULAR–INTRAVENTRICULAR HEMORRHAGE

What is it?

Intracranial bleeding that most commonly arises from the capillary network of the subependymal germinal matrix layer; arises less frequently from the choroid plexus or the roof of the fourth ventricle

How are these hemorrhages classified?

Small hemorrhage
  Grade I: isolated germinal matrix hemorrhage
  Grade II: intraventricular hemorrhage with normal ventricular size
Moderate hemorrhage
  Grade III: intraventricular hemorrhage with acute ventricular dilatation
Severe hemorrhage
  Grade IV: intraventricular hemorrhage with parenchymal hemorrhage

What is the incidence?

Approximately 40%–50% of infants who weigh < 1500 g and are < 35 weeks gestation have some degree of hemorrhage. Most hemorrhages occur within the first week of life, usually within the first 2 days. Although essentially a condition of premature neonates, it is seen occasionally in full-term infants.

What is the physiology of this condition?

The germinal matrix is a periventricular structure, containing a rich vascular network of primitive vessels prominent from 26 to 34 weeks from conception. Bleeding from the matrix ruptures into the lateral ventricles and spreads, creating an arachnoiditis. Severe bleeding may penetrate into the periventricular white matter.

What are predisposing conditions and events?

1. Most commonly, prematurity and acute respiratory failure requiring mechanical ventilation
2. Others include pneumothorax, hypotension, acidosis, coagulopathy, volume expansion, bicarbonate infusion, and the stress of transport between institutions

What are signs and symptoms?

The spectrum includes hypotension, apnea, metabolic acidosis, and bulging of the anterior fontanel in severe cases; however, at least **50% of infants have no clinical symptoms.**

What methods are used for Dx?

Ultrasound is usually preferred. The first ultrasound should be performed at the end of the first week of life, with follow-up at the end of the second week of life. CT may also be used.

What is the treatment?

Supportive care. Anticonvulsants may be required for seizures or seizure prophylaxis. If posthemorrhagic hydrocephalus ensues, treatment options include:
Lumbar punctures
Drugs (e.g., acetazolamide, furosemide) that induce hyperosmolarity to decrease CSF production
Ventriculostomy
Ventriculoperitoneal shunt placement

RESPIRATORY DISTRESS SYNDROME (RDS)

What is it?

Pulmonary disease associated with prematurity and surfactant deficiency; previously called hyaline membrane disease

What is the incidence?

Age dependent: 60% at 29 weeks gestation; decreases to less than 1% by 39 weeks gestation

What infants are most commonly affected?

1. Infants who have diabetic mothers
2. Infants who have siblings who had RDS
3. Males
4. Infants born by cesarean section without labor
5. Infants who experience perinatal asphyxia
6. Infants who had prolonged rupture of membranes or intrauterine growth retardation, or mothers who experienced physiologic "stress" are relatively spared

What are the classic features?

1. Onset of grunting respirations, retractions, and increased oxygen requirements; characteristic radiographic changes within 6 hours of symptoms
2. Other features include systemic hypertension, fine inspiratory rales, hypothermia, peripheral edema, and pulmonary edema.

What are the acute and long-term complications?

Acute: alveolar rupture leading to pneumothorax, pneumomediastinum, pneumopericardium, or interstitial emphysema; infections, especially those associated with instrumentation; intracranial hemorrhage; PDA

Long-term: bronchopulmonary dysplasia (BPD); retrolental fibroplasia (also called retinopathy of prematurity); possible neurologic impairment

How is pulmonary immaturity detected prenatally?

Because fetal lung fluid enters the amniotic cavity, amniocentesis provides a means for assessing pulmonary maturity via analysis of phospholipids in the amniotic fluid. Lecithin–sphingomyelin (L/S) ratio of < 2:1 and a saturated phosphatidylcholine (SPC) concentration of < 500 are associated with insufficient surfactant, and therefore potential RDS.

What is the treatment?

Stabilization of the premature infant, including:

Skilled resuscitation to prevent hypoxia
Early surfactant administration
Lung expansion, using intubation,
  mechanical ventilation, and PEEP
Thermal neutrality, usually a skin
  temperature of 36.5°C
Administration of oxygen as required to
  keep PaO_2 at 50–80 torr
Cardiovascular support
Acid–base and electrolyte therapy as
  indicated

How can RDS be prevented?

1. Administer surfactant to the infant by
   1–2 hours of life via the airway.
2. Treat mother with glucocorticoids >
   24 hours before delivery if premature
   delivery is anticipated or inevitable.

TRANSIENT TACHYPNEA OF THE NEWBORN (TTN)

What is it?

Early onset of mild respiratory distress

What causes TTN?

Any circumstance delaying the clearance
of lung liquid by the lymphatics,
including elevation of central venous
pressure by late clamping of the cord,
prematurity and administration of
surfactant, or cesarean section without
labor

What is the clinical presentation?

Classically, an extremely tachypneic
infant with 60–120 shallow respirations/
min, mild grunting, flaring and
retractions, mild cyanosis; infant may
have a mild respiratory acidosis and
mild-to-moderate hypoxemia without
evidence of persistent fetal circulation

What are radiographic signs?

Changes include hyperaeration of the
lungs, prominent pulmonary vascular
markings, and mild cardiomegaly, all of
which resolve within 24–48 hours.

What is the treatment?

As a self-limited condition, it requires
supportive care with supplemental
oxygen. Diuretics are not helpful.

MECONIUM ASPIRATION SYNDROME

What is meconium?

A thick, blackish-green material that accumulates in the fetal intestines beginning at the end of the first trimester; it is the accumulation of debris from the developing GI tract

What is caused by meconium aspiration?

Significant pneumonia or pneumonitis can be caused by an infant inhaling meconium peripartum.

Who is at risk?

Meconium-stained fluid is seen in 8%–20% of all deliveries, especially in small-for-gestational-age and post-date infants. Passage of meconium accompanied by fetal heart rate changes may indicate fetal distress and result in a higher rate of complications. Meconium staining rarely occurs before 34 weeks gestation.

How can this syndrome be prevented?

Maternal management: amnioinfusion of 1000 ml normal saline to relieve cord compression if fetal distress is evident
Infant management: obstetrician suctions the mouth and nose of the infant before delivery of the thorax or the pediatrician immediately intubates and suctions the trachea before the initiation of spontaneous respirations if the meconium is thick or particulate

What is the treatment?

1. When all meconium cannot be removed from the airway and respiratory distress develops, supportive care, especially directed at oxygenation, is established. Asphyxiated infants or those who do not respond to oxygen therapy with or without CPAP may require intubation, mechanical ventilation, sedation, and neuromuscular blockade. Special attention is then required because of the substantial risk of pneumothorax and pneumomediastinum.
2. Antibiotics often are given after bacterial cultures are obtained,

because meconium may promote bacterial growth, and sepsis may have contributed to the initial passage of meconium.

3. Difficulty with oxygenation may persist as a result of either worsening pneumonia or the development of persistent pulmonary hypertension; these infants may be referred for ECMO. Corticosteroids have not proven useful.

What are the outcomes?

Historically, meconium aspiration syndrome is associated with a high mortality—up to 30% in infants who require mechanical ventilation. ECMO saves 85%–95% of infants who would have probably otherwise died. Morbidity is less associated with pulmonary complications than with the hypoxic insult the infant sustained.

PERSISTENT PULMONARY HYPERTENSION OF THE NEWBORN (PPHN)

What is it?

PPHN, or persistent fetal circulation (PFC), implies pulmonary hypertension, right-to-left shunting at the level of the PDA and PFO, and a structurally normal heart. The constellation causes severe hypoxemia.

What is the etiology?

Primary or idiopathic; it may also be secondary to:
Meconium aspiration or other aspiration syndromes
Hyperviscosity of blood
Neonatal sepsis
Intrauterine or perinatal asphyxia
Myocardial dysfunction
Congenital diaphragmatic hernia
Neonatal pulmonary disease

What are the signs and symptoms?

Affected infants usually have respiratory distress and cyanosis. Other signs include a gallop rhythm with a blowing murmur of tricuspid regurgitation, shock, and heart failure.

What are the EKG findings?

Usually consistent with RVH but can vary from normal-for-age to showing signs of ischemia or infarction

What are radiographic findings?

May illustrate underlying lung disease; may be normal or show diminished pulmonary markings

Differential Dx?

1. Cyanotic congenital heart disease, including transposition of the great arteries, total anomalous pulmonary venous return, pulmonic stenosis or atresia, and Ebstein anomaly
2. Severe left ventricular dysfunction caused by ischemia or obstruction, such as hypoplastic left heart syndrome, coarctation of the aorta, and critical aortic stenosis

What is the treatment?

Goal is to decrease pulmonary vascular resistance and right-to-left shunting:
1. Supportive management is directed at correcting acidosis and hypoxemia (100% oxygen by hood should be initiated ASAP).
2. If conservative therapy fails, intubation, mechanical ventilation, sedation, and neuromuscular blockade with 100% oxygen are initiated; the goal is to hyperventilate to P_{CO_2} 20–30 mm Hg and pH 7.45–7.55.
3. Tolazoline, a pulmonary vasodilator, has been used with mixed results; nitric oxide is currently being evaluated for its efficacy.
4. ECMO may be indicated if conventional therapy fails.

What are the outcomes?

Mortality ranges from 20%–40%.The incidence of neurologic sequelae ranges from 12%–25% for survivors; neurosensory hearing loss has been reported in up to 20% of affected survivors.

NEONATAL PNEUMONIA

What is the incidence?

The lung is the most commonly recognized site of infection within 24 hours postdelivery, affecting up to 0.5% of all live births.

What is the etiology?

Infection may be bacterial or viral and may be acquired transplacentally, through the birth canal, or postdelivery.

What is the most common bacterial agent?

Group B Strep, affecting 1–4 in 1000 live births

Other common bacterial agents?

E.coli
Klebsiella species
Group D streptococci
Listeria species
Pneumococci
Staphylococcus and *Pseudomonas* species can cause slightly later onset disease, and *Chlamydia trachomatis* can cause pneumonia as late as 3–4 weeks after birth.

What are common viral agents?

Viral pneumonia may be associated with the **TORCH** infections, but most are acquired postnatally.
Respiratory syncytial virus (RSV) and **adenovirus** have been associated with significant morbidity and mortality in this population.

What are four predisposing factors?

1. Premature labor
2. Rupture of membranes before onset of labor or prolonged rupture of membranes
3. Prolonged active labor with cervical dilatation
4. Frequent obstetric digital exams

What are the signs and symptoms?

Nonpulmonary symptoms include lethargy, thermal instability, apnea, abdominal distention, and jaundice.
Pulmonary symptoms include tachypnea, cyanosis, and respiratory distress.

What are radiographic findings?

Chest radiograph can vary from bilateral streaky density, to diffuse opacification, to a granular appearance.

What are some important studies to be obtained during the evaluation?	Blood and CSF cultures as well as culture of gastric aspirates, latex agglutination of CSF or blood, nasopharyngeal culture for chlamydia or viruses, and measurement of cord blood immunoglobulins as indicated by clinical scenario
What is the treatment?	Initial treatment includes a penicillin (usually ampicillin) and an aminoglycoside because broad-spectrum coverage is indicated for early-onset condition. Treatment for later onset pneumonia should also include coverage for *Staphylococcus* organisms. When the causative organism is identified, treatment may be narrowed and continued for a minimum of 10 days.

NEONATAL SEPSIS

What is it?	A generalized bacterial infection in a clinically ill infant with a positive blood culture during the first month of life
What is the incidence?	It occurs in 1 in 500 to 1 in 600 live births and is influenced by maternal factors, including active infection at delivery, and neonatal (especially prematurity) and environmental factors.
When can infection occur?	1. Before labor—it can occur transplacentally or through the amniotic fluid with or without intact membranes 2. During delivery—as the infant passes through the birth canal 3. Postdelivery
What are the most common bacterial agents?	Group B streptococcus *E. coli* *Listeria monocytogenes* Group A streptococcus Group D streptococcus *Streptococcus viridans* *Staphylococcus* species

Other bacterial agents?	Less common agents include: *Pseudomonas* species *Haemophilus influenzae* *Klebsiella pneumoniae* *Citrobacter* species
What are the signs and symptoms?	Onset of symptoms may occur at any time (early signs usually are subtle) and include lethargy, irritability, poor feeding, temperature instability, possible fever if fulminant, tachypnea, hypotension, cyanosis, apnea, tachycardia, seizures, vomiting, diarrhea, hepatomegaly, jaundice, petechiae, and bleeding.
Differential Dx?	Because of the nonspecificity of symptoms, differential may include hemolytic anemia, hypovolemic shock, intracranial hemorrhage, respiratory distress syndrome, pneumonia, GI anomalies, ITP, neonatal leukemia, hypoglycemia, or other metabolic disease.
What is the treatment?	1. After blood and CSF cultures have been obtained, broad-spectrum coverage is initiated with ampicillin and an aminoglycoside, usually gentamicin; when an organism has been identified, coverage is narrowed based on sensitivities and a 7- to 10-day course can be completed. 2. Granulocyte transfusions may be required for desperately ill newborns with neutropenia. 3. Immunoglobulin transfusions are still being studied (without promising results) for this population. 4. ECMO may be employed for infants suffering pulmonary failure secondary to neonatal sepsis.
What is the outcome?	Mortality can be as high as 13%–50%.

NEONATAL BACTERIAL MENINGITIS

What is the incidence?	It develops in approximately 2–10 of 10,000 live births and is responsible for 1%–4% of neonatal deaths.

What are the most common infecting agents?

Same as those discussed in neonatal sepsis; most common are group B streptococcus, *E. coli*, and *Listeria monocytogenes*; *F. meningosepticum* is associated with epidemic disease and *Citrobacter* species are associated with CNS abscess formation

What are the risk factors?

They are the same as those associated with neonatal sepsis. Meningitis is associated with up to 33% of the cases of newborn septicemia. Local infections of the skin, respiratory tract, and urinary tract are also associated with bacteremia and thus the possibility of developing meningitis. Infants with meningomyelocele and premature infants are at increased risk. Certain strains of bacteria are associated with increased risk—specifically, *E. coli* containing capsular polysaccharide K1, group B strep serotype III, and *L. monocytogenes* type IV.

What are the signs and symptoms?

Same as those for sepsis
Seizures, paralysis of cranial nerves, abnormal cry, focal neurologic signs may be seen.
Bulging fontanel may be a late sign.
Stiff neck and positive Kernig or Brudzinski signs are rarely seen in this age-group.

What are the important factors in the evaluation?

Every infant with subtle signs of sepsis requires a **lumbar puncture** with Gram stain, cell count, protein and glucose analysis, and culture of the CSF. Blood and urine cultures should also be obtained. Interpretation of the CSF cell count may be difficult because normal newborns may have up to 32 WBC in their CSF; however, the complete profile of the CSF must be evaluated with the patient and the culture.

What is the treatment?

Broad-spectrum antibiotic therapy is initiated with ampicillin and an aminoglycoside. When an organism and its sensitivities are identified, treatment should be tailored to that organism—gram-positive meningitis is treated for a minimum of 14 days whereas gram-negative meningitis is treated for 2 weeks after the infection is cleared or 3 weeks minimum, whichever is longer.

What are the outcomes?

Mortality ranges from 20%–50%. Morbidity is also substantial and includes hydrocephalus, subdural effusions, ventriculitis, deafness, and blindness. Neurologic impairment is evident in 40%–50% of survivors. All survivors require audiologic and neurologic follow-up.

APNEA OF INFANCY/SIDS

What is apnea of infancy?

Pause in breathing, usually ranging from 5 to > 20 seconds in duration, which arises from a central event, an obstructive event, or a combination of both

What is the normal physiology of infantile breathing?

Infants < 6 months of age may experience periodic breathing or isolated, asymptomatic apneas of 5–15 seconds in duration while the respiratory system matures.

When are apneic periods of clinical importance?

When unexplained apneas are > 20 seconds or are symptomatic

What is an acute life-threatening event (ALTE)?

Prolonged apnea resulting in bradycardia and color change that requires vigorous stimulation or positive pressure ventilation; it is also know as a near-SIDS event

What are the causes of ALTE?

Apnea, GE reflux, inborn errors of metabolism, seizures, sepsis, heart disease, Munchausen syndrome by proxy or child abuse, apnea of prematurity, breath holding, poisoning

What are the treatment options?	Up to 30% of cases may be treatable as they are secondary to sepsis, GE reflux, metabolic disorders, apnea of prematurity; for remaining cases, apnea monitoring and CPR training of the parents may be recommended.
What is SIDS?	Sudden infant death syndrome
What is the incidence?	**2 in 1000 live births;** results in 6000–10,000 deaths yearly, with a peak incidence between 2–4 months
What is the etiology?	Unknown
What are the risk factors?	Infants who have had an ALTE are at increased risk for dying from SIDS; however, **93% of infants who die of SIDS have never had such an event.** Infants of substance-abusing mothers Infants put to sleep on their abdomens Infants who are stressed (e.g., with a URI)
How can SIDS be prevented?	Placing infants **"back to sleep,"** or in a **supine** sleeping position, is recommended nationally. Also, parents are advised to have infants on **firm** rather than soft bedding and to avoid stuffy, overly warm sleeping quarters. Parents are also advised to refrain from smoking around their infants.

NEONATAL DIARRHEA

What is it?	Abnormally frequent, loose stools in an infant; may be associated with dehydration, failure to thrive, or systemic illness
What are the complications?	Profound dehydration and nutritional deprivation, which is particularly dangerous for the developing nervous system

What are common causes?   Infectious causes are most common, especially **rotavirus** (after 4 months), but also *Salmonella, Campylobacter,* and *E. coli* (during the first 2 months).

Primary or secondary carbohydrate malabsorption

Fat malabsorption, as with **cystic fibrosis** or other cause of pancreatic insufficiency

Congenital malformations of the intestines (e.g., malrotation)

Acquired defects of the bowel (e.g., short-gut syndrome)

Hormonal abnormalities (e.g., thyrotoxicosis, congenital adrenal hyperplasia)

Allergic conditions (e.g., intolerance to cow's milk protein)

How should neonatal diarrhea be evaluated?

1. History and physical examination are most important and should include family history, birth history, and a chronology of the illness.
2. Physical examination should be detailed after an initial assessment of hemodynamic stability and hydration status.
3. Pertinent laboratory tests include serum electrolytes, BUN, and creatinine levels; CBC to assess for a coinciding anemia; and stool studies for culture, rotavirus antigen, electrolytes, WBC and occult blood, and reducing substances.

What is the treatment?   Following fluid and electrolyte stabilization, therapy is determined by underlying condition. Antimotility agents are **NOT** used in infants and have a significant morbidity in this age-group.

UMBILICAL ABNORMALITIES

OMPHALITIS

What is it?   Infection of and around the umbilicus and the retained umbilical remnant in the infant

What are the signs and symptoms?	Fever, possibly signs of sepsis
What does the umbilicus look like?	Erythema around umbilicus; may spread within hours to become a frank **fasciitis** with crepitus and tissue necrosis!
What is the treatment?	Broad-spectrum antibiotics as soon as condition is recognized; umbilical remnant may need to be removed and, if omphalitis has progressed to fasciitis, more extensive surgical debridement may be needed
How can it be prevented?	Hand washing, asepsis in handling of fresh cord, washing infant with antiseptic soaps
What may be a significant associated condition?	There appears to be a link between delayed separation of the cord, omphalitis, and defective neutrophil motility.

UMBILICAL HERNIA

What is it?	Congenital fascial defect that persists in the umbilical region; cause unknown
What is the incidence?	1 in 6 children
Who are they most common in?	They are nine times more common in **African-American children** and also common in **premature** infants.
What is the natural history of an umbilical hernia?	Umbilical hernias usually close spontaneously by 3–5 years of age; however, fascial defects > 1.5 cm are not likely to close.
What is the treatment?	Surgical fascial closure via infraumbilical curvilinear incision, usually with excision of the sac
What are indications for surgery?	1. Lack of closure by 5 years of age 2. Fascial defect 1.5 cm or greater 3. Large umbilical proboscis resulting in skin excoriation or other difficulty 4. Incarceration (rare)

UMBILICAL GRANULOMA

What is it?

Persistent granulation tissue on umbilicus after separation of umbilical cord

What are signs and symptoms?

Persistent discharge or oozing at site of granuloma; may develop surrounding cellulitis, leading to omphalitis

What is the treatment?

Mild cases respond to 1–2 applications of silver nitrate. Some granulomas require surgical excision. If cellulitis begins, infant should be treated with intravenous antibiotics and observed for any progression of infection.

OMPHALOMESENTERIC REMNANT

What is it?

It may take various forms:
Omphalomesenteric duct
Omphalomesenteric cyst
Omphalomesenteric sinus
Mucosal polyp on umbilicus (can look like a granuloma)

What are they remnants of?

Embryologic connection between gut and umbilicus (**vitelline duct**)

What are the signs and symptoms?

1. Persistent pink excrescence on umbilicus
2. Persistent discharge of mucus, pus, succus entericus at umbilicus
3. Palpable mass (sometimes tender) at umbilicus
4. Possible cellulitis around umbilicus
5. Nausea and vomiting if bowel has volvulized around persistent remnant

How is it diagnosed?

1. Usually by physical examination
2. Abdominal film may suggest obstruction if volvulus is present.
3. Sinogram or upper GI may reveal connection between intestine and skin.

What is the treatment?	Surgical excision; polyp may be removed as a granuloma would be; other remnants may be removed via infraumbilical incision; excision may require removal of a wedge of bowel with closure

PERSISTENT URACHAL REMNANT

What is it?	It may take various forms: Urachal cyst Urachal sinus Urachal fistula
What are they remnants of?	The embryologic connection of the umbilicus to the bladder (**allantois**)
What are the signs and symptoms?	1. Persistent discharge of mucus, pus, frank urine from umbilicus 2. Cellulitis or sepsis if remnant becomes infected 3. Possible mass (may be tender) in infraumbilical midline position
How is it diagnosed?	Usually by physical examination; sinogram or cystogram may reveal sinus or fistula
What is the treatment?	Surgical excision, usually through infraumbilical midline or curvilinear incision; remnant must be removed down to level of bladder

11

Newborn Intensive Care: General Considerations

RESPIRATORS

What are the basic modalities of oxygen therapy?

1. Nasal cannula with oxygen flow
2. Head box with humidified, heated oxygen to prevent excessive heat loss in the infant, with continuous and frequent monitoring of FiO_2
3. **CPAP:** Continuous positive airway pressure administered through nasal cannulae or endotracheal tube
4. Endotracheal intubation with mechanical ventilatory support

What are two types of respirators?

Conventional: oxygen is delivered 20–40 cycles/min and may be pressure limited, time cycled, or volume limited
High-frequency: facilitated diffusion of gases in lung at 600–900 cycles/min; may be a jet ventilator or oscillator

MONITORS

How are infants monitored in the intensive care setting?

1. Cardiorespiratory (CR monitor): apnea and bradycardia are common in severely ill infants
2. Arterial blood gases: indwelling catheters may be placed in an umbilical or peripheral artery for frequent blood gas or chemistry sampling and for continuous blood pressure monitoring
3. Pulse oximetry: continuous transcutaneous monitoring of arterial oxygen saturation; less useful in the hyperoxic infant

4. Transcutaneous oxygen (TcO$_2$): heated electrode applied to skin measures oxygen crossing skin membrane; continuous measurement; correlation with arterial Po$_2$ varies with infant; good for monitoring trends; unreliable with poor perfusion
5. Transcutaneous carbon dioxide: same issues as TcO$_2$

NUTRITION

What IV fluids are appropriate for the newborn infant?

D$_{10}$W in first 24 hours, except for the very low birth-weight infant who may require only D$_5$W; add ¼ normal saline after 24 hours

At what rate?

80–100 cc/kg/day

When is hyperalimentation used?

For the low birth-weight infant or ill term infant

What are hyperalimentation goals?

Goal: ~ 80–120 kcal/kg/day, including 3 g/kg amino acids, 3–4 g/kg fat; calcium, phosphorus, and other electrolytes and vitamins are added

What are administration routes for hyperalimentation?

It may be administered by peripheral IV (limited to 12.5% dextrose) or central line (up to 25% dextrose).

What are routes of enteral feeding?

Gavage: feedings administered through nasogastric tube every 2–4 hours or by continuous infusion

Nasoduodenal: continuous feeding through transpyloric duodenal tube

Gastrostomy: gastrostomy tube may be placed when infants undergo abdominal surgery and a quick return to oral feeding is not anticipated, or when infant feeding skills are poor

What are standard categories of formula?

Standard formula: 20 kcal/oz iron-fortified for term infants (same caloric concentration as breast milk)

Premature formula: 24 kcal/oz with increased concentration of Na, Ca, PO$_4$ vitamins for improved growth and bone mineralization

Elemental formula: hydrolyzed protein and modified fat blend for improved absorption in infants with malabsorption or feeding intolerance

Formulas may be milk or soy based.

COMMON QUESTIONS PARENTS ASK

What are survival rates for premature babies?	Less than 750 g:< 40% 750–1250 g: 90% More than 1250 g: 95%–98% Congenital malformations and chromosomal anomalies impact these data.
What are some common complications of prematurity?	Cerebral palsy, developmental delay, visual impairment, hearing loss, learning disability, chronic lung disease, mental retardation
What is the incidence of a premature infant having complications?	Less than 1000 g: 25%–30% More than 1000 g: 15%–20% Incidence depends on birth weight, perinatal asphyxia, and intraventricular hemorrhage.
When can an otherwise healthy premature baby be discharged?	Without major complications, a premature infant is expected to be discharged shortly before its term due date.
Can a mother still provide breast milk for a premature baby?	Yes. Although the infant may not be able to breast feed initially, the mother should begin pumping her breasts shortly after delivery at least every 3 hours.
Can the mother's milk be supplemented with calories and minerals?	Yes

Section III

Ambulatory Pediatrics

12

The Pediatric Physical Examination

THE WELL-CHILD VISIT

What is the purpose of the well-child visit?

To identify physical, psychosocial, and developmental problems; to prevent unnecessary morbidity; and to provide guidance and advice to parents, helping assure that the child grows and develops to full potential

What are seven components of the well-child visit?

1. Identifying and responding to parental concerns
2. Historical assessment of physical and psychosocial growth and development
3. History of family–child interactions and/or problems
4. Age-specific physical examination to look for previously undiagnosed problems, assess previously identified problem areas, and assess normal neurologic development
5. Screening laboratory tests
6. Immunizations
7. Anticipatory guidance

At what ages should visits be scheduled?

1 month, 2 mos, 4 mos, 6 mos, 9 mos, 1 yr, 15 mos, 18 mos, 24 mos, 2 yrs, 3 yrs, 4 yrs, 5 yrs, and every other year thereafter

Who recommends these intervals?

The American Academy of Pediatrics (AAP)

What other visits may be needed for a newborn?

1. A baby who is discharged before 36 hours of age should be seen within 48 hours of discharge.
2. If the mother is breast-feeding for the first time or had a problem feeding a previous child, the infant should be seen at 2 weeks of age.

How long should the well-child visit last?   20–30 minutes

What are common parental concerns for an infant:

Newborn to 2 months of age?   Sleep schedules, feeding, crying

2–3 months of age?   Sleep, interpreting cries, initiation of solid foods, effect of mother going to work

4–6 months of age?   Sleep, scheduling naps, initiation of solid foods, effects of day care

6–9 months of age?   Motor development, child's tolerance of solid foods, patterns of discipline

9–12 months of age?   Motor development, temper tantrums, fear of strangers

12–18 months of age?   Temper, limit setting, night walking

18–24 months of age?   Temper and violence toward other children, limit setting, language abilities

24 months of age?   Toilet training, playing with others

36 months of age?   Social skills

What physical measurements should be recorded?

1. **Weight:** at every visit, with the child unclothed
2. **Length:** until the child is old enough to stand cooperatively; then **height** is recorded
3. **Head circumference**
4. **Blood pressure:** in all four extremities at 1 month of age to assess for coarctation of the aorta; routine single extremity blood pressure at every visit beginning at 3 years of age

How are these parameters tracked?   Using standardized growth curves expressed in percentiles

When is physical growth considered abnormal?

If the child's growth pattern deviates by **more than one standard deviation from its previous percentile** or is **more than two standard deviations from the mean**

What areas of development are monitored?

Gross motor, fine motor, social, and language development

What are representative gross motor milestones at:

    1 month?

Lifts head from prone position

    2 months?

Holds head upright without wobble

    3 months?

Regards hand

    4 months?

Purposeful grasp; rolls front to back

    6 months?

Sits up with support; rolls back to front

    9 months?

Sits without support; up on all fours; crawls

    12 months?

Pulls to standing; walks with support

    15 months?

Walks independently

    18 months?

Walks up and down stairs

    24 months?

Jumps in air

    36 months?

Peddles wheel toy

What are representative fine motor milestones at age:

    2 months?

Follows visually past midline

    3–4 months?

Grasps objects and brings to mouth

    6 months?

Places objects carefully rather than dropping them, transfers hand to hand

    9 months?

Clasps hands

10 months?	Pincer grasp
15 months?	Scribbles; stacks two cubes
18 months?	Stacks four cubes
24 months?	Stacks eight cubes

What are representative social milestones at age:

2 months?	Smiles when seeing mother
4 months?	Smiles spontaneously
6 months?	Copies facial expressions
9 months?	Fears strangers; separation anxiety; plays interactively (peekaboo, patty-cake)
12 months?	Drinks from cup and finger-feeds self
15 months?	Uses spoon; imitates adult actions
18 months?	Removes clothing; uses cup
24 months?	Begins toilet training; puts on clothing

What are representative language milestones at age:

2 months?	Coos responsively
4 months?	Social laughter
6 months?	Makes nonspecific vowel sounds
9 months?	"Dada" and "Mama" (nonspecific)
12 months?	"Dada" and "Mama" plus two other words
15 months?	Several more words
18 months?	Combines two words into phrases
24 months?	Combines three or more words

36 months?	Most speech clear to strangers
48 months?	Toddler stuttering subsiding
What is the most commonly used developmental screening test?	The **Denver Developmental Screening Test**

What other specific areas should be addressed?

At what age should malformation of fetal development or stigmata of syndromes be looked for?	Birth
At what age should intra-abdominal masses be looked for?	Birth to school age
At what age should retinoblastoma be looked for?	Throughout the first year
At what age should cardiac murmurs be looked for?	During the first 3 months
At what age should visual function be assessed?	By 3–4 months
At what age should congenital hip dysplasia be looked for?	Until child is walking
When does normal tooth eruption occur?	First tooth averages 6 months; normal up to 15 months
What are normal hearing milestones?	Responds to sound by 2 months; orients to sound by 4 months; play audiometry at 3 years; pure tone audiometry at 4 years; brain stem–evoked audiometry if in high-risk group by age 6 months

When does normal development of secondary sexual characteristics begin?

Between 8 and 12 years in girls and 10 and 14 years in boys

When does scoliosis commonly become apparent?

Beginning with the onset of puberty through Tanner stage IV

What are common screening laboratory tests, and when are they performed?

1. Screening for a variety of **metabolic diseases** (e.g., PKU, hypothyroidism, sickle cell disease, biotinidase deficiency, galactosemia) is performed at birth on a state-by-state basis; these tests may need to be repeated
2. Screening for **sickle cell disease** (based on ethnicity) at 9 months of age, if not done at birth
3. Screening for **anemia** between 9 and 12 months of age, at entry to school, once in midchildhood, and once in adolescence
4. Screening for elevated **lead** levels as per current AAP/CDC protocols
5. **Urinalysis** is controversial, but infants are often screened once in infancy and again at school entry

When is screening for TB performed?

Frequency of screening depends on the area of the country and the child's background. Most children are screened at 12 or 15 months of age and again at school entry.

IMMUNIZATIONS

What diseases are children routinely immunized against?

Diphtheria, pertussis, tetanus, polio, measles, mumps, rubella, influenza type B, and hepatitis B

What source is the authority on immunization schedules?

The AAP's Redbook is the ultimate authority on childhood vaccination principles and is updated every other year.

What other vaccines may be administered?

Influenza types A and B, meningococcus, pneumococcus, and varicella

ANTICIPATORY GUIDANCE

What anticipatory guidance may be given to parents?

Injury and poison prevention, development stimulation, nutritional advice, behavioral development advice, advice on adjusting to family disruptions (e.g., new siblings, moves, illness)

Guidance about accident prevention?

1. Use a proper **infant car seat** from birth to 4 years of age (or 40 pounds), followed by **seat belt** use thereafter
2. **Poison prevention** advice beginning at 6 months (including distribution of ipecac) with reinforcement thereafter; formal safety check of home before 6 months; discuss drugs, household chemicals, and plants
3. **Firearm safety** advice in the home beginning at birth
4. **Swimming lessons** beginning by 3 years of age
5. **Bike helmet use** beginning with first tricycle
6. **Burn prevention** advice throughout childhood; adjust water heater temperature at birth
7. **To avoid use of walkers**

Guidance about child's development?

Discuss milestones achieved and those to be achieved in the interval before next checkup. Discuss ways to help the child achieve the next milestone in a fun way.

Guidance/advice about nutrition?

1. Breast feed until 1 year; use formula if breast milk is unavailable.
2. Start solid foods about 4 to 6 months of age (preferably 6 months).
3. Review the principles of a balanced diet regularly.
4. Review the elements of a heart-healthy diet.

5. Review proper elements of food preparation and storage to avoid food poisoning
6. Avoid constant overfeeding
7. Discuss fluoride supplementation when necessary
8. Monitor for nutritional practices that lead to iron deficiency

Advice about smoking/ tobacco products?

Begin discouraging parental smoking at the prenatal visit and every visit thereafter. Offer to prescribe nicotine patch withdrawal systems for the parents.

What are some time milestones for how the child sees the world around him/her and for the beginning of common areas of conflict?

6 months—exploring as a way of learning and how to set limits
9 months—separation anxiety and stranger fear
12 months—temper tantrums
18 months—developing language and independence
24 months—playing together with other children and conflict resolution
36 months—language and abstract concepts

What major family stresses should be evaluated?

Divorce; separation; absence of a parent (e.g., at work) for prolonged periods; parental or sibling illness or disability; move from one house to another; death of family member, close friend, or pet; natural disasters affecting the family, such as fire, flood, or hurricane

How should these stresses be addressed?

Be sensitive and take the time to counsel the parents about how much children are affected by these events; discuss impact of stresses during more than one visit

THE SCHOOL PHYSICAL

What is a "school physical"?

The formal assessment of a child just before entering kindergarten

When is it performed?

Usually within 6 months of school entry; individual state laws vary; usually at 4 ½ to 6 years of age

In what three ways is the school physical different from a well-child visit?

The school physical:
1. Focuses on health and development as it relates to school readiness
2. Seeks to identify problems that may impair educational functioning of the child
3. May be considered (by some parents) as the last of the mandatory well-child examinations; special care should be taken to identify problem areas

What are eight general components of the school physical?

1. Immunization record review and completion
2. Developmental history and assessment
3. Screening hearing test
4. Screening vision test
5. Screening laboratory tests
6. Complete physical examination
7. Discuss school placement and the child's potential strengths and weaknesses with parents
8. Completion of school form giving direction and advice to the school system about the child's unique needs, if any

What immunizations are given at the school physical?

1. Final dose of polio vaccine
2. Final dose of DTP vaccine, either regular DTP or DTaP vaccine
3. Second dose of MMR
4. Completed vaccination against influenza type B
(**Note:** State laws vary and dictate which immunizations are required for school entry. It is likely that hepatitis B and varicella vaccinations will be required for school entry.)

What certification must the physician sign?

Usually the physician must certify that the child has received all appropriate immunizations, has a medical or religious contraindication, or, if not fully immunized, has a plan to complete the required vaccines and by a given date.

What screening labs are performed?

Usually **hemoglobin, urinalysis,** and a **TB skin test;** in addition, **lead level** should be tested if there is any history of lead exposure, developmental delay, or anemia

What hearing test is used?

A pure tone audiometry test is performed in a quiet place.

  How does this test work?

Each ear is tested individually over a frequency range of 500–4000 Hz, with a minimal threshold of 15–20 decibels for the child to pass.

How is vision tested?

Visual acuity is tested in each eye separately and in both eyes together using a Titmus vision testing machine or a method of equal accuracy. Color vision should be tested. An assessment of strabismus, including a cover test, is also important.

What are the components of speech evaluation?

The child should speak clearly with little hesitation, using complete sentences. Clarity is evident if the physician readily understands what the child is saying. Occasional stutter may be normal particularly if the child is excited, but facial grimacing, explosive speech, or frustration associated with the stammering is not normal. The vocabulary should be in excess of several hundred words, and the child should know colors and body parts and readily identify most objects to which the tester points.

What are the standards for math readiness?

The child entering kindergarten should already understand the concept of more versus less and above versus below. The child should also be able to count and correctly identify the number of raised fingers (up to five). The child should be able to recite back to you three number sequences presented orally.

What questions should the physician ask the parents about the child's social, behavioral, and developmental history?

Does the child play regularly with other children and does he/she look forward to these activities?
Does the child get frustrated and cry easily?

Is the child prone to violent outbursts of temper?

How does the child handle conflict resolution in the family?

Does the child have trouble separating from the parents?

Is the child incontinent when napping during the day?

Is the child clumsy or physically awkward?

Is the child overly quiet and shy around strangers?

Does the child have older siblings in the school?

Does the child already like to read and does he/she have the ability to sustain concentration over a given task long enough to complete it?

Were the parents worried about this child's development either in the past or presently?

Has the child ever had a preschool experience and, if so, were the teachers there at all concerned about the child?

Does the child speak English fluently?

What should the physician do if concerned about the child based on the school physical?

Medical problems should be addressed. The physician should alert the school to the potential problem so the school can perform an evaluation at the earliest possible date.

Is the child's size important?

Yes. A child who is unusually small or large may be subject to extra emotional stress from classmates. This issue should be foreseen and discussed with the parent. Also, a child who is unusually small may be underestimated and treated like a younger child. If there has been a recent change in growth pattern greater than one standard deviation, then the child should be assessed for comorbid illnesses associated with growth delay or with overgrowth.

How are medications at school addressed?

A note is given to the school indicating the medication the child is taking, its therapeutic usefulness, possible side effects, and dosage schedule. The note should also indicate the primary illness that requires medication, whether it is contagious, and what effect it may have on the child's school performance.

What are causes of fatigue in a school-age child?

Fatigue affects school performance and increases irritability. Major sources of fatigue in a school-age child include late bedtime, getting up too early, an overly long bus ride, skipping meals, lack of time to rest or nap at school when the body is tired, frequent intercurrent mild respiratory viral illness contracted in the school setting, and overinvolvement in after-school organized activities.

How are physical handicaps addressed?

A child with a physical handicap needs special communication with the school to ensure appropriate treatment. An honest but upbeat appraisal of the child's abilities is critical. Point out any activity that may put the child at risk and consult with the teacher for alternative strategies. The teacher's fears about the child with special physical needs in the classroom should be addressed. Any special help the child may need, such as adaptive physical education and time for trips to a physical therapist, should be described in detail.

Advice to parents with a physically handicapped child?

Stay involved in your child's daily classroom activities. Don't be shy and assume that everything will turn out well. If the child is not doing well academically, is fearful of school, doesn't want to discuss school, or seems to have undergone negative personality changes, then the parent should contact both the teacher and physician immediately.

What are common specific reasons for physical exams?

The most common are the preparticipation sports physical (see Chapter 13) and the every-3-years' physical required for children receiving special educational assistance.

What is the purpose of the sports physical?

To discover any problems that may increase the child's risk of injury in certain sports and to allow the physician to discuss with the child and parents proper preparation for a sports activity (e.g., conditioning exercises, fluid and nutritional guidance, special equipment, and injury prevention techniques unique to the sport).

What is the purpose of the every-3-years' physical?

It focuses on an assessment of any new or changed physical or developmental limitations, including changes in physical functioning (e.g., vision and hearing) and new information about a child's chronic illness (e.g., new medications or complications), that affect the child's school performance.

COMMON CLINICAL PROBLEMS

WHEEZING

What are common causes of wheezing in the infant?

Tracheal malformations, vascular rings, T-E fistula, mediastinal masses, aspiration, reflux, cystic fibrosis (CF), infections

In toddlers?

Infection (especially RSV and adenovirus), asthma, CF, foreign body aspiration, tumor

In older children?

Infection (especially viral), asthma, CF, tumor (especially lymphoma)

FEVER

What temperature is a fever?

Generally, a rectal temperature of > 37.8°C is considered a fever, but some authors use a higher figure (38.0°C–38.2°C). Interpretation of fever may vary with the patient's age.

Does fever equal infection?

No, but the concern about infection depends on the patient's age and clinical status. **Infants with fever should be carefully evaluated for meningitis or septicemia.**

RESPIRATORY DISTRESS

What are causes of respiratory distress in the child?

1. **Upper airway obstruction,** including epiglottitis, peritonsillar or retropharyngeal abscess, foreign body, edema, malformations, intrinsic or extrinsic masses
2. **Lower airway obstruction,** including foreign body and bronchiolitis/reactive airways disease
3. Pneumonia
4. Congestive heart failure/pulmonary edema
5. Trauma
6. Metabolic diseases
7. Muscle diseases

ABDOMINAL PAIN

What are some causes of abdominal pain in the child?

Viral gastroenteritis, appendicitis, mesenteric lymphadenitis, bacterial enterocolitis, Meckel diverticulitis, inflammatory bowel disease, hernia with incarcerated bowel, food poisoning, intussusception, abdominal adhesions, pneumonia, acute intermittent porphyria, trauma, volvulus, functional; in girls who have begun menstruating, pregnancy must also be considered as a cause for abdominal pain.

DIARRHEA

What are some causes of acute diarrhea?

1. Bacterial infections, such as *Salmonella, Shigella, E. coli, Campylobacter,* and *Yersinia*
2. Viral gastroenteritis
3. Food poisoning

What are some causes of chronic diarrhea?

Fat malabsorption, CF, dietary allergy, lactose intolerance, bacterial infection, celiac disease, malnutrition, antibiotic use, inflammatory bowel disease

VOMITING

What are some causes of vomiting?

Viral gastroenteritis, food poisoning, upper GI obstruction, inborn error of metabolism, CNS tumor, motion sickness, sepsis, paralytic ileus, adhesive obstruction (if previous operation), malrotation, appendicitis, intussusception, incarcerated hernia

ACNE

What is it?

It is a skin condition commonly affecting adolescents, consisting of four basic types of lesions: Open and closed comedones, papules, pustules, and nodular-cystic lesions.

What causes it?

During adolescence, androgens stimulate the growth of sebaceous glands as well as the production of sebum. Some of these materials are hydrolyzed to free fatty acids, which can cause inflammation. Characteristic abnormal keratinization of skin cells at this time also contributes to the lesions.

What are open comedones?

Commonly called **blackheads,** the orifice of the follicular duct is open and the involved sebum has been oxidized to the black color. There is usually not any surrounding inflammatory reaction.

What are closed comedones?

Commonly called **whiteheads,** these do cause surrounding inflammatory reaction because the follicular duct is occluded.

How may the development of acne by minimized?

General cleansing of the face two to three times daily with a mild soap; avoidance of oil-based skin preparations and makeup

How is acne treated?

The most common topical agents are benzoyl peroxide and retinoic acid. Systemic antibiotics, such as tetracycline or erythromycin, may be needed in more severe cases. 13-cis-Retinoic acid is used for the most severe cases of acne (**cystic acne** or **acne conglobata**).

What are potential side effects of retinoic acid preparations?

There may be carcinogenic effects from the combination of light and retinoids. Therefore, avoidance of sun or, alternatively, the use of sunscreen is recommended for patients using retinoic acid. Retinoic acid also may cause hyperpigmentation in patients with darkly pigmented skin. Retinoic acid and related compounds may be teratogens.

INGESTION OF POISONOUS AGENTS

How important are ingestions of poisonous agents in pediatrics?

They are the fourth most common cause of death in children.

What is the peak age of ingestions?

2 years of age; however, teens also are prone to ingesting caustic substances as suicide attempts or gestures

What are commonly ingested items?

Cleansers (e.g., sodium hydroxide), batteries (potassium hydroxide), and miscellaneous acidic agents (e.g., sulfuric acid)

How should a child who has ingested something be evaluated?

Esophagoscopy within 24 hours and barium swallow within 48 hours to assess degree of injury, stricture, and esophageal motility

What is the treatment?

Begin ampicillin and gentamicin with hydration when ingestion is suspected. Strictures may require dilation, feeding tube (NG or gastrostomy), or anatomic replacement.

What are the best methods of prevention?

"Childproofing" the home and educating children and parents

DEVELOPMENTAL DELAY

What is it?

Delay in attaining developmental milestones at the appropriate age

Does developmental delay equal mental retardation?

No. There may be reasons for developmental delay that are unrelated to cognitive skills.

How does a physician screen for developmental delays?

Careful history and physical; use of screening test (e.g., Denver Developmental Screening Test)

What laboratory, radiographic, or other tests are indicated for developmental delay?

This part of the evaluation should be individualized, using the history and physical examination and the developmental evaluation as starting points.

SHORT STATURE

What is it?

Height less than the second percentile for age (**Note:** definitions may vary)

What are the most common causes?

Normal variation and constitutional delay

Other causes?

Endocrine abnormalities, metabolic diseases, genetic syndromes, skeletal dysplasias, chromosome abnormalities, chronic diseases, pyschosocial short stature

How is it evaluated?

History (including family history), review of growth data, physical exam, appropriate radiographic and lab studies as indicated

Why are previous measurements so important?

Growth is a **dynamic** process; evaluation of change over time gives more information than isolated growth points

OBESITY

What causes obesity?

Caloric intake exceeds caloric expenditures.

What is the most common cause of childhood obesity?

Exogenous obesity (excessive intake)

What is the relationship of obesity to height?

Children with exogenous obesity tend to be taller than average. Most endocrine disorders and syndromes in which obesity is seen are associated with stature that is shorter than average.

Name some syndromes associated with obesity.

Prader-Willi syndrome, Cushing syndrome, pseudohypoparathyroidism type I, growth hormone deficiency

FAILURE TO THRIVE

What is it?

Usually failure to gain or maintain weight adequately

What are some causes?

GI disorders, immune disorders, chronic diseases, inborn errors of metabolism, inadequate intake, CNS abnormalities, psychosocial problems

How is it evaluated?

Careful history, physical exam, weight measurements, review of growth data, lab and radiographic studies as indicated

ENCOPRESIS

What is it?

Fecal incontinence due to overretention of stool

What are the causes?

Psychological problems, Hirschsprung disease, chronic stool retention, neurologic abnormalities, hypothyroidism

How is it evaluated?

Careful history, physical exam, review of growth data, lab and radiographic studies as indicated

What is the treatment?

Depends on the etiology; educating and supporting the parents and child are key, regardless of the etiology; a clean-out regimen, followed by a program to maintain regularity, is usually helpful; attention must be given to emotional and behavioral issues

ENURESIS

What is it?

Urinary incontinence in child 5 years of age or older

Differential diagnosis?

Urologic abnormalities, neurologic abnormalities (including seizures), diabetes mellitus, diabetes insipidus, psychosocial stress

How is it evaluated?	Careful history, physical exam, review of growth data; lab evaluation (including urinalysis, regardless of suspected cause) and radiographic studies as indicated
What is the treatment?	Depends on the etiology; therapies of nonorganic enuresis may include medications, alarms, and behavioral modification

SCHOOL PHOBIA

What is it?	Fear of or refusal to attend school
What are the causes?	Many potential causes, including real fear of the school environment (e.g., bullies, violence), fear of a teacher, and fear of separation from the parent or family
How is it evaluated?	If somatic complaints are present, a good history and physical exam are indicated, along with a detailed interview with the parents and child.
What is the treatment?	The goal is to normalize the child's school experience, which usually involves returning the child to the classroom as soon as possible. Parental education is important, as well as additional counseling if the school phobia is a manifestation of more serious emotional problems.

ATTENTION DEFICIT HYPERACTIVITY DISORDER (ADHD)

What is it?	A disorder characterized by limited capacity for attention, overactivity, and impulsivity; it is distinct from abnormal conduct behavior and specific learning disabilities
What is the etiology?	This is still not fully known.
What is the prevalence?	1.5%–4%
Is it more common in boys than girls?	Boys, by a 5:1 ratio

What is the age of onset?	Usually before 4 years of age
Is family history important?	Yes. ADHD is more common in children who have had family members with ADHD.
What are typical clinical manifestations?	A history of **behavior in specific situations** is very important. Also, birth and neonatal histories are important. There is often a history of difficult birth, colicky behavior as an infant, sleep and feeding difficulties as an infant, and excessive temper tantrums as a toddler. The diagnosis is usually first entertained when the child is in school and is uncontrollable, refuses to sit still, intrudes upon other children, and refuses to follow instructions. During formal examination, symptoms may be difficult to detect because these children can behave well in significantly structured situations.
How is the diagnosis made?	Usually it is on a clinical basis. Children with symptoms of ADHD should be tested for other causes, such as specific learning disabilities, hearing impairment, petit mal epilepsy, side effects of medication, anxiety or depressive disorders, or poor living situations.
What is the treatment?	Behavioral and psychosocial therapy with a confirmed structure to the child's environment. Stimulants, including methylphenidate (Ritalin), dextroamphetamine, pemoline, and clonidine, are sometimes used in conjunction with these therapies. Tricyclic antidepressants may also be efficacious.
What is the prognosis?	Prognosis appears to be better if a child with this condition does not exhibit aggression. There are concerns that children with ADHD may be more prone to alcoholism, sociopathy, and hysteria in adulthood; steady gainful employment seems to be helpful.

LIMP

What are some causes of limp?	Foot problems (e.g., calluses, foreign bodies, warts, shoe problems)
	Sprains, strains
	Fractures
	Dislocated hip
	Toxic synovitis
	Osteomyelitis
	Soft tissue trauma
	Arthritis (septic, inflammatory)
	Cancer (e.g., osteosarcoma, leukemia, neuroblastoma)
How is it evaluated?	Begin with a careful history and physical exam; lab and radiographic studies as indicated

HEADACHE

Are headaches a sign of dangerous disease?	Very rarely
What are signs that a headache may be serious?	Excruciating pain, stiff neck, accompanying neurologic findings, impairment of consciousness
What are the characteristics of migraine?	Rapid onset
	Pain often hemicranial and behind the eye
	Visual changes (e.g., seeing flashing lights, black spots)
	Pain is intense and pounding.
	Photophobia
	Child sleeps and awakens without headache.
Is a family history of migraine common?	Yes
What is the treatment?	Sleep is the best treatment. Other therapies include ergot derivative, isometheptene, and analgesics. Some patients may require chronic treatment with β-blockers, tricyclic antidepressants, or calcium channel blockers. Biofeedback or relaxation therapy may be helpful.

What are characteristics of tension headaches?

Slow onset of pain
Bifrontal distribution
Pain is not really debilitating
Pain is squeezing in quality and may have a throbbing component
No visual changes or photophobia
Gradual remission of pain
May be associated with definable psychological stress

What is the treatment of tension headaches?

Analgesics, biofeedback, or relaxation therapy

13

Pediatric Sports Medicine

PREPARTICIPATION SPORTS ASSESSMENT

What are the three primary goals of a sports physical exam (PE)?

1. Identify youngsters at high risk for injury because of disqualifying factors or because of predisposing conditions.
2. Recommend rehabilitative measures to correct or minimize the risk factor or condition.
3. If rehabilitation is not possible, redirect the athlete to another sport in which his/her risk is lessened.

Maximize the opportunity for a happy successful student athlete while minimizing the likelihood of injury.

What two secondary goals or benefits are derived from a sports PE?

1. Educates youngsters about nutrition, fitness, and their connection to sports
2. Introduces many youngsters to health care; the sports PE is frequently the only contact adolescents have with a physician

Is there a standard form or set of requirements for sports PE?

No. Although the American Academy of Pediatrics and American Academy of Family Practice have made recommendations on this issue, state requirements vary.

Why should the sports PE be comprehensive?

It is usually the only physical a youngster receives.
In order to identify relevant important historical information
In order to determine appropriate participation

What particular factors are important during a comprehensive sports PE?

In addition to the components of a standard PE, a sports PE should focus on:
1. **History**—provides highest yield of

factors that might affect an athlete's participation

2. **Physical maturity**—one of the most common factors for disqualifying a youngster from participating in a collision sport

3. **Musculoskeletal examination**— most common area of physical findings predisposing a youngster to recurrent injury

4. **Measure of fitness and state of nutrition**—especially important in sports in which weight loss is common (gymnastics and wrestling) and where obesity might predispose to heat injury (football practice in August)

5. **Analysis of history and physical and knowledge of nature of sports**— needed to make an appropriate recommendation for specific sports participation

How is physical maturity measured?

By determining the youngster's Tanner stage of pubertal development; another popular method is to measure hand grip strength with a hand ergometer

Boys and girls should reach what Tanner stages to participate in vigorous competition?

Boys at less than Tanner stage 4 should not participate in collision sports (e.g., football, lacrosse, ice hockey) with fully mature boys because of increased risk for injury, especially to epiphyseal plates. Physical maturity is much more relevant to injury risk than weight or size.

Girls who reach 15 years of age and are still at Tanner stage 2 or less should receive close scrutiny and evaluation before participation in "weight conscious" sports, such as gymnastics, dancing, or cross-country running.

As a nonorthopedist, how does a physician conduct a musculoskeletal examination?

Evaluate all joints and muscle groups for symmetry of range of motion, strength, muscle mass, and bony structures. The same evaluation should be performed on the neck. Special attention should be paid to any area with a history of previous injury.

How is an athlete's fitness determined at the time of the sports PE?

How is cardiovascular fitness measured?

1. Blood pressure
2. Cardiac examination for murmur and rhythm
3. Exercise: Listen for abnormal sounds to evaluate cardiovascular fitness. One practical method is a 2-minute jumping jack task at 1 jump/sec. Measure resting pulse, pulse immediately after exercise, and pulse after a 1-minute recovery period. A rise in pulse to > 95 beats/min during exercise, or a drop to < $\frac{2}{3}$ of the resting level on recovery is grounds for slow and cautious advancement to full practice and activity.

How is general health, fitness, and nutrition measured?

1. **Height/weight proportions** on standard growth chart
2. **Body fat:** In females, body fat is between 10%–25%; in males, it is between 7%–20%. Body fat below these ranges is considered unhealthy in most individuals and should raise concerns about malnutrition or eating disorders. Body fat above the upper limits indicates obesity and could be a problem in acclimatization to heat, requiring close scrutiny and slower adaptation to full-speed participation.

How is body fat determined?

1. Determining body density by water immersion (most accurate); however, this is impractical in routine sports PEs
2. Measuring skinfold with calipers; the most common sites utilized are the triceps, abdominals, pectorals, and iliac crest area

How is pulmonary fitness measured?

Some sports medicine specialists recommend including a pre- and post-exercise FEV_1 to identify a treatable condition of exercise-induced bronchospasm. Early studies have shown as much as 10% of the athlete population experiences this to a degree enough to affect performance.

To provide the best quality of evaluation for a youngster, when should a sports PE be performed?

Ideally, 2–4 weeks before practice begins so that if a mild abnormality is noted (whether it be loss of full range of motion of a joint, poor cardiac fitness, or obesity), there is time for appropriate conditioning and/or rehabilitation

Where should a sports PE be performed?

In a private, quiet, and convenient location that will accommodate the needs of a comprehensive physical examination; a doctor's office is usually best; a school can be set up for quality mass screening

What format should be used for a sports PE?

The one-on-one, physician–athlete examination is a desirable method. However, most youngsters in the United States receive sports PEs in a mass screening format, usually at their school. If stations are set up, different health care providers perform different aspects of the examination, with a final station for recommendation for participation, as well as to give the youngster an opportunity to ask health-related questions. The station format can provide a high-quality, efficient method of preparticipation sports PEs.

How frequently should a sports PE be given?

Significant data exist suggesting that a yearly physical is unnecessary; however, there is no standard recommendation for frequency. The current mode is for a yearly physical.

By whom should a sports PE be performed?

The athlete's individual physician has the advantage of knowing the youngster well, including history and family, and should be more likely to uncover undue family pressure to participate or know of history that the youngster might choose not to report. Still, the physical should be performed by the physician most interested and tuned into the demands of various sports.

What laboratory tests should be included in a sports PE?

There is no need for doing routine laboratory tests on all youngsters. If the history or PE raises questions, then these may be indicated.

Urinalysis test?

It is reasonable to perform test as a baseline in case of future injury to the kidney or if the youngster has not had a urinalysis in the last 2 years and is receiving no other health care.

Hemoglobin/hematocrit?

Anemia has been shown to affect athletic performance. An Hct/Hgb count is reasonable to perform if the youngster is not receiving any other health maintenance.

Free erythrocyte protoporphyrin/ferritin?

These probably are the most valuable tests that can be performed, although not practical in many mass screening situations. Studies have shown that low iron stores, even with normal hemoglobin or hematocrit, occur in certain sports fairly commonly and are especially problematic in female athletes.

What are the four possible recommendations to an athlete following preparticipation evaluation?

1. Full participation—history and PE are normal
2. Limited participation—everything is in normal range, but some factor recommends against participation in a certain sport (e.g., a boy in Tanner stage 3 is recommended for all sports except a collision sport)
3. Conditional participation—youngster is allowed to participate, but some restrictions or precautions are recommended (e.g., an obese, out-of-shape athlete is required to lose a certain amount of weight before putting on football pads, or a cross country runner with tight hamstrings may require some additional stretching before competing at full speed)
4. No participation—youngster may be required to get clearance from an orthopedist before playing because of

knee surgery or from a cardiologist because of previous syncope

What recommendation should be made if a youngster only has one kidney or has had five or six concussions?

The physician should probably make a **strong recommendation not to participate in collision sports.** If the family insists, precedents have been set so that courts will allow a youngster to participate over a physician's recommendation.

What are the key ingredients to an excellent sports preparticipation evaluation?

1. Thorough sports-specific and traditional medical and family history
2. Thorough traditional physical and neurologic exam
3. Additional examination includes:
   - Tanner staging
   - Body fat measurements
   - Resting, exercise, and recovery pulse
   - FEV_1 pre- and postexercise
4. Some measure of iron stores and/or anemia
5. Performed 2–4 weeks before practice begins
6. Performed in a quiet and private environment convenient for the athlete, conducive to a good examination and an opportunity for conversation with the athlete
7. Performed by individual(s) knowledgeable and interested in all aspects of sports and athletes
8. Followed by summation and appropriate recommendation and follow-up for the athlete, family, coach, and school

SPRAINS AND STRAINS

What is a sprain?

Injury to a ligament or joint capsule

What is a strain?

Injury to a muscle

Acute treatment of sprains and strains?

RICE—Rest, **I**ce, **C**ompression, and **E**levation

What is the most common lower extremity injury?

Ankle sprain

What is an indication for radiographs?

Suspicion of a fracture, which may be difficult to diagnose clinically

Does taping the ankle help prevent sprains?

It may help patients who have recurrent sprains, if the coach or trainer is skilled in the proper use of tape.

What is the most common finger injury?

Finger sprain (sometimes called a "jammed" finger)

How are these injuries evaluated?

Carefully, to exclude disruption of the tendons

Are radiographs indicated?

Usually with significant finger injuries

What is the most common shoulder injury?

Acromioclavicular sprain

What is the most common shoulder dislocation?

Anterior (90%)

What is the most common knee injury?

Medial collateral ligament sprain

EYE INJURIES

Should eye injuries be evaluated by an ophthalmologist?

Injuries with significant trauma to the globe or the periorbital tissues should be evaluated by an ophthalmologist.

Concerns?

Hemorrhage, retinal detachment, hyphema, lens dislocation, orbital floor fracture

How can eye injuries be prevented?

Protective eyewear, especially in children with visual impairment

14   Adolescent Medicine

PUBERTY AND GROWTH

What is adolescence?	The period between childhood and adulthood (*adolescere* means "to grow up")
When does adolescence occur?	From 10–21 years of age; exact limits vary
What are the five tasks of adolescence?	Identity formation, autonomy, separation from family, vocation, and internal moral standards
What is puberty?	Biologic maturation (*pubescere* means "to grow hair")
When does puberty occur?	Onset in early adolescence; 8–13 years of age in girls; 9–14 years of age in boys
When is menarche?	10–15 years of age (average age is 12); ovulation usually occurs within 2 years after menarche
When does sperm production begin?	13–14 years of age
What are Tanner stages?	Stages of external physical (sexual) maturation
What is Tanner stage 1?	Prepubertal
Stage 2?	Onset of any sign of sexual change; in girls—breast buds, sparse pigmented pubic hair; in boys–enlargement of testes, scrotum, and penis, with sparse pigmented pubic hair
Stages 3 and 4?	Increased pubic hair; other findings in girls include increased breast tissue, raised areola (stage 4); other findings in boys include enlargement of genitalia

Stage 5?	Adult secondary sexual characteristics; areola now continuous with the breast, pubic hair on the inner thighs
What is precocious puberty?	Onset before 8 years of age in girls and before 9–10 years of age in boys
What is delayed puberty?	No development before 14–15 years of age In girls, no menarche after 3 years of onset of secondary sexual characteristics or no menarche before 15–16 years of age
What are the causes of precocious puberty?	Idiopathic (most common), endocrine abnormalities, CNS abnormalities
What are the causes of delayed puberty?	Idiopathic (most common); Turner syndrome (in girls); Klinefelter syndrome (in boys); chronic illness; weight problems; CNS abnormalities, including secondary abnormalities; psychological or psychosocial problems
What are five important factors in the evaluation of abnormal timing of puberty?	1. Careful history 2. Careful physical exam 3. Plot longitudinal growth data 4. Bone age 5. Lab tests as clinically indicated
How do you assess growth at puberty?	Using longitudinal data
What is a normal growth rate?	Prepubertal: about 5 cm/year During puberty: 9 cm/year for girls; 10 cm/year for boys (boys also have a "strength spurt" near the end of puberty)
What are causes of a delayed growth spurt or strength spurt?	Idiopathic, stress, chronic illness, nutritional deficiencies, genetic disorders, endocrine disorders

LEGAL ISSUES

What is emancipation?	Fiscal and physical independence

What is the legal age of emancipation?	Usually 18 years of age; may vary with states (check local statutes)
For what types of procedures can minors consent?	In most states, minors can consent to: 1. Emergency care 2. Diagnosis, treatment, and prevention of STDs 3. Contraception, but not sterilization 4. Diagnosis and management of pregnancy 5. Management of rape or sexual abuse 6. Diagnosis and treatment of mental health problems, including substance abuse **NOTE:** State laws vary and may change regarding these issues.
Who is an emancipated minor?	A minor who is currently or was married; a teenage parent; a self-supporting minor living away from home; a minor in the armed forces

BASIC ISSUES OF TEEN HYGIENE

When does a woman have her first pelvic exam?	1. By 18 years of age 2. Before initiation of sexual intercourse 3. If there is a gynecologic problem
What three immunizations are given to adolescents?	1. Second MMR (if not received earlier) 2. Tetanus booster (10 years after previous booster) 3. Hepatitis B series (if not already received)
When is adult dentition present?	By midpuberty
How often is routine dental care needed?	Routine dental hygiene every 6 months; routine check-up yearly
How often are eye exams needed?	Every 1–2 years during adolescence, more often if indicated
What are the causes of acne?	Androgens, abnormal keratinization of sebaceous ducts and hair follicles, and bacterial colonization; acne may be affected by stress and hormones

Does diet affect acne?   Usually not

What are the five types of   1. Closed comedones (whiteheads)
acne?   2. Open comedones (blackheads)
                                       3. Pustules
                                       4. Nodules
                                       5. Cystic acne

How is acne managed?   Maximize skin hygiene with:
                                       Nonperfumed, antibacterial soaps
                                       Skin-drying agents
                                       Benzoyl peroxide (5% or 10%)
                                       Topical retinoic acid or oral antibiotics
                                           may be recommended for severe
                                           cases. Refer to dermatologist as
                                           needed.

MENSTRUATION

What are the   Flow < 8 days
characteristics of a normal   Duration of 21–35 days
menstrual period?   Blood loss of 50 ml

OLIGOMENORRHEA

What is oligomenorrhea?   Too little bleeding; skipping months

What are the causes?   Anovulatory cycles, stress, pregnancy,
                                       weight change (i.e., loss or gain),
                                       polycystic ovary syndrome, thyroid
                                       disease, increased prolactin production,
                                       androgen excess

What is the treatment?   Regulate periods with Provera or oral
                                       contraceptives, and treat underlying
                                       cause.

What causes secondary   Pregnancy and stress are most common
amenorrhea?   causes; other causes, as per
                                       oligomenorrhea

POLYMENORRHEA

What is polymenorrhea?   Excessive bleeding

What are the causes?	Anovulatory cycles, pregnancy problems (e.g., ectopic, miscarriage), STDs, endocrine causes (similar to oligomenorrhea), diabetes, blood dyscrasias, iron deficiency
What are the important factors in evaluation?	History, physical and pelvic exams, hematocrit, platelet count
What is the treatment?	Same as for oligomenorrhea

DYSMENORRHEA

What is dysmenorrhea?	Cramping, colicky pain immediately before or during menses
How common is it?	It is the most common cause of school absence in adolescent females.
What are some associated symptoms?	Headache, irritability, emotional lability, nausea, vomiting, diarrhea, backache
What are important factors in the evaluation?	History, physical and pelvic exams
What is the treatment?	Nonprescription analgesics, NSAIDs, oral contraceptives

SEXUALLY TRANSMITTED DISEASES (STDs)

How common is sexual activity among teenagers?	Varies widely with the population—some studies show 50% by 16 years of age and 90% by 19 years of age
How common are sexually transmitted diseases (STDs)?	Present in 25% of sexually active teenagers
What is the most common STD?	Human papillomavirus (HPV)
What does HPV cause?	Genital warts, abnormal pap smears, cervical cancer
What are other viral STDs?	Herpes (herpes simplex virus) HIV Hepatitis B virus (HBV)

Are there other nonviral STDs?	Gonorrhea, chlamydia, syphilis, trichomonas
How does gonorrhea present?	Males present with urethritis. Females present with mucopurulent cervicitis or PID. Both may be asymptomatic.
How does chlamydia present?	Similar to gonorrhea
What are some infestations that may be transmitted by close contact?	Pubic lice ("crabs"), body lice, scabies
What are some genital infections that are *not* sexually acquired?	Monilia, bacterial vaginosis, folliculitis
What are six methods of diagnosing of STDs?	1. History and physical exam 2. Bacterial cultures 3. Fluorescent antibody studies for syphilis, chlamydia, and herpes 4. ELISA for HIV, chlamydia, and herpes 5. DNA probe tests (as indicated) for HIV, papillomavirus, chlamydia, and herpes 6. Wet preps of discharges: KOH for *Gardnerella*; saline for *Trichomonas* 7. VDRL for syphilis
What are treatment standards for STDs?	1. As per Center for Disease Control (CDC) recommendations 2. Partner(s) need treatment. 3. Report "reportable" diseases to Public Health Department.
How can STDs be prevented?	Education Abstinence Use of latex condoms with nonoxynol 9 Use of female condoms Avoidance of multiple sexual partners

PREGNANCY AND CONTRACEPTION

How common is teenage pregnancy?	About 1 million/year in the United States; 50% result in spontaneous or elective abortion and 50% result in live birth

What are the hazards of teenage pregnancy?

For parents (i.e., the adolescent), it may lead to:
Dropping out of school
Poor development of job skills
Short- or long-term welfare dependency
Parenting difficulties

What are the hazards for children of teenagers?

Increased incidence of low birth weight
Prematurity
Health and/or psychosocial problems related to poverty or poor parenting skills
ADHD

How is teenage pregnancy managed?

Teen-oriented obstetric care; promote family and community involvement; long-term follow-up and support after birth of child

How can teenage pregnancy be prevented?

1. Education
2. Building skills to enhance self-esteem, self-efficacy, and decision making
3. Understanding of abstinence and/or delayed sexual intercourse as appropriate courses
4. Knowledge and availability of birth control

Name nine methods of birth control.

1. Abstinence
2. Condom (with spermicide)
3. Oral contraceptives (birth control pills)
4. Diaphragm (with spermicide)
5. Rhythm method
6. Norplant
7. Female condom
8. Depo-Provera
9. Spermicide (alone)

Section IV

Pediatric Diseases

15 Hematologic Disorders

NUTRITIONAL ANEMIAS

IRON DEFICIENCY ANEMIA

What is it?

A decreased hemoglobin (Hgb) below 95% for age that is caused by lack of iron (Fe); it is the most common anemia

What is the cause?

Usually secondary to inadequate iron in diet or chronic blood loss (e.g., from peptic ulcer, Meckel diverticulum, polyp, hemangioma, inflammatory bowel disease)

What is the physiologic effect?

Decreased production of heme proteins involved in oxygen transport (Hgb), electron transport (cytochromes), and oxidative metabolism (NADH)

What are the signs and symptoms?

1. Pallor, fatigue, shortness of breath.
2. Pagophagia (ingestion of nonfood substances, such as ice, paper, dirt/clay) or pica (ingestion of lead-containing substances)
3. Spoon-shape nails (koilonychia)
4. Enlarged spleen
If not severe, iron deficiency anemia is suggested by routine lab screenings.

What does a CBC show?

Hypochromic, microcytic RBCs; decreased reticulocytes; decreased mean corpuscular volume (MCV); decreased mean corpuscular hemoglobin (MCH)

What are the effects on indices of iron storage and transport?

Decreased iron, ferritin, and transferrin saturation; increased total iron-binding capacity (TIBC)

Why are free erythrocyte protoporphyrins (FEP) increased?

Low iron level limits the production of Hgb. FEP are heme precursors that accumulate as a result.

What investigations may be done to detect occult blood loss?

Stool guaiac, urinalysis, a careful menstrual history

How may iron deficiency anemia be diagnosed if other tests and investigations are equivocal?

By the child's response to a trial of iron administration

What is the treatment?

1. Oral therapy with elemental Fe (3 mg/kg/day for 3–4 months); reticulocyte response should be seen in 1–2 weeks
2. Determine and correct the etiology of Fe deficiency

What are the complications?

Oral administration of iron can stain teeth and cause nausea, abdominal pain, and constipation. However, if deficiency is not corrected, psychomotor and cognitive functions may become impaired.

FOLATE DEFICIENCY ANEMIA

What is it?

Decreased Hgb caused by folate deficiency

What is the physiologic effect?

Inactivation of folate-dependent enzymes with decrease in 1-carbon transfer reactions

What are the etiologies?

1. Dietary deficiency is the most common etiology
2. Increased folate demands: hemolytic anemia, sickle cell disease, pregnancy
3. Thalassemias
4. HIV
5. Malabsorption
6. Certain drugs, such as antiepileptics, trimethoprim-sulfa, alcohol
7. Disorder of metabolism

What are the signs and symptoms?	Pallor, fatigue, shortness of breath; infants may fail to gain weight and suffer chronic diarrhea
What are laboratory findings?	1. CBC shows decreased Hgb and increased MCV 2. Hypersegmented neutrophils 3. Low reticulocyte count 4. Low serum folate 5. Elevated serum LDH 6. Nucleated RBCs with megaloblastic morphology
What is the treatment?	Oral supplementation with folate; increased reticulocytes peak at 1 week and Hgb is normal in 6–8 weeks; duration of therapy is based on etiology

VITAMIN B_{12} DEFICIENCY (PERNICIOUS ANEMIA)

What is it?	Decreased Hgb cause by vitamin B_{12} deficiency
What is the physiologic effect?	Deficit of methylcobalamin (coenzyme B_{12}), which is a required cofactor in conversion of homocysteine to methionine (via methionine synthetase); methionine is critical in formulation of tetrahydrofolates.
What are the etiologies?	1. Dietary deficiency (e.g., seen in vegans) 2. Decreased absorption in GI tract (e.g., in children who have had their terminal ileum removed) 3. Defects in B_{12} transport or metabolism
What are characteristic laboratory findings?	Increased MCV, multilobed neutrophils, decreased serum B_{12}, increased serum methylmalonic acid and homocysteine
What are the signs and symptoms?	Nausea, diarrhea, abdominal pain, glossitis; neurologic sequelae include subacute degeneration of spinal cord, decreased vibratory and position sense, pyramidal signs, and peripheral neuropathy; cerebral symptoms and depression may be present

What are findings on bone marrow aspirate?

Megaloblastic changes

What does the Schilling test evaluate?

The Schilling test uses vitamin B_{12} incorporated with ^{57}Co to test for B_{12} absorption. The labelled B_{12} is given orally and is followed by a large IV dose of unlabelled B_{12}. If the labelled B_{12} is absorbed, it will be displaced by the unlabelled B_{12} and excreted in the urine. If this phase suggests that labelled B_{12} was not absorbed, another oral dose of labelled B_{12} is given simultaneously with intrinsic factor (IF). If labelled B_{12} is then later excreted, the insufficient or poorly functioning IF is the cause for B_{12} deficiency. If labelled B_{12} is still not excreted, a primary malabsorption condition exists.

What is the treatment?

For deficiency without malabsorption or an IF defect, oral vitamin B_{12} is sufficient. A malabsorption or IF defect usually requires vitamin B_{12} injections for life.

How is response monitored?

The child should be monitored for response manifested by clinical improvement, increased reticulocytes, decreased MCV, and decreased methylmalonic acid.

What are complications?

Rapid correction of severely anemic patients can be associated with thrombosis, embolism, and hypokalemia. Neurologic symptoms usually improve slowly and may not completely resolve.

HEMOGLOBINOPATHIES

THALASSEMIA

What is it?

Inherited anemia caused by gene mutations that affect the synthesis of human Hgb chains, most commonly α and β chains; clinical syndromes vary in severity

Who is affected?

α-Thalassemia is more common in people of Asian and African origin; β-thalassemia is more common in people of Mediterranean and African origin.

What is the pathophysiology?

Decreased or absent synthesis of α or β chains leads to increased amounts of rare Hgb compared with normal Hgb. Severe forms of thalassemia lead to hemolysis and ineffective RBC production in the bone marrow.

What is different about the α-globin genes?

Normally, there are **four** α-globin genes (two on each homologous chromosome). Therefore, there are different combinations of α-globin gene abnormalities.

What are the four types of α-thalassemia?

Silent carrier. $\frac{1}{4}$ genes affected: hematologically normal; electrophoresis normal

Thal trait. $\frac{2}{4}$ genes affected: mild anemia, decreased MCV, presence of target cells, electrophoresis normal

Hgb H disease. $\frac{3}{4}$ genes affected: moderate hemolytic anemia, decreased MCV, presence of target cells, splenomegaly, electrophoresis reveals Hgb A and H (β_4)

Hydrops fetalis. $\frac{4}{4}$ genes affected: fetal death, electrophoresis reveals Hgb H and Barts (γ_4)

What are the four types of β-thalassemia?

β-thalassemia is more heterogeneous. Severity is based on the specific mutation in a gene rather than the number of genes affected.

1. **Silent carrier:** hematologically normal, electrophoresis normal

2. **Thal trait:** mild anemia, decreased MCV and MCH, presence of target cells, electrophoresis reveals increased Hgb A_2 and F

3. **Thal intermedia:** severe anemia without transfusion requirement, decreased MCV and MCH, presence

of target cells, electrophoresis reveals increased Hgb A_2 and F.

4. **Thal major:** severe anemia with transfusion requirement, decreased MCV and MCH, presence of target cells, growth retardation, bone deformity, hepatosplenomegaly, electrophoresis reveals increased Hgb A_2 and F

What are common diagnostic studies?

CBC, Hgb electrophoresis, measurement of α- and β-chain biosynthesis

What is the treatment for:

Mild syndromes?

Folic acid supplementation, avoidance of oxidant drugs, transfusion if necessary

Severe syndromes?

Folic acid supplementation, transfusion protocol with chelation of Fe, splenectomy if hypersplenism develops, bone marrow transplantation

What are common complications?

Cholelithiasis, increased susceptibility to infection, bone marrow hyperplasias with bone deformity, Cooley's facies, "hair-on-end" skull radiograph; liver, endocrine, and cardiac abnormalities associated with Fe overload

SICKLE CELL DISEASE

What is it?

Hemoglobinopathy in which α chains are normal, but β chains are abnormal because valine is substituted for glutamic acid at position 6

Who is most commonly affected?

People of Central African, Mediterranean, and Indian descent, but sickle cell disease can be seen in any population

What is the pathophysiologic effect?

Hgb S forms polymers within red cells, causing sickling of the cells when Hgb is deoxygenated. This sickling causes sludging and obstruction in vessels with subsequent tissue hypoxia.

What are five common types of sickle cell disease?

Sickle trait: Hgb AS; not associated with increased morbidity and mortality

Sickle disease: Hgb SS; clinically variable in severity from mild to debilitating

Sickle SC disease: Hgb SC; mild chronic hemolytic anemia with variability in complications from vaso-occlusion; splenomegaly

Sickle β-thalassemia: two forms, $β^+$ and $β^0$; Hgb A is produced in the former, not the latter; sickle $β^0$-thalassemia (i.e., no Hgb A produced) is clinically similar to Hgb SS; splenomegaly

Sickle α-thalassemia: variable clinical picture

What diagnostic studies are used, and what do they show?

1. CBC: decreased Hgb, normal MCV if not thalassemic
2. Blood smear: sickled forms, target cells, Howell-Jolly bodies
3. Hgb electrophoresis:
   Sickle disease: 80%–100% Hgb S, 0%–20% Hgb F
   Sickle SC disease: 50% Hgb S, 50% Hgb C
   Sickle β-thalassemia: 75%–100% Hgb S, 0%–20% Hgb F, 3%–6% Hgb A_2
   Sickle α-thalassemia: 80%–100% Hgb S, 0%–20% Hgb F

What are the clinical presentations?

1. Pain from vaso-occlusion in the bone, hand and foot ("hand–foot syndrome"), abdomen, and chest; patient may also experience CVA and/or priapism
2. Splenic sequestration
3. Aplastic crisis
4. Infection is caused by decreased opsonins and splenic function and **is the most common cause of death in children with sickle cell disease.** Common organisms include pneumococci, *H. influenzae*, *Salmonella*, and *Mycoplasma*.

What is the treatment for:
Vaso-occlusive crisis?   Hydration, pain medications

For chest syndrome? O_2, pain medications, antibiotics, simple transfusion versus exchange

For CVA?   Exchange transfusion with chronic transfusion protocol to keep Hgb S < 30%

For aplastic crisis?   Supportive care, transfusion if necessary

For splenic sequestration?   Emergent transfusion with subsequent splenectomy

For infection?   Appropriate antibiotics, penicillin prophylaxis, pneumococcal vaccine

What are common progressive complications?
Cardiovascular?   Cardiomegaly and cardiomyopathy secondary to Fe overload and chronic anemia

Pulmonary?   Progressive disease with infarcts and infections

Hepatic?   Cholecystitis, hepatitis, glomerular and tubular fibrosis

Renal?   Hematuria, hyposthenuria

Ophthalmologic?   Retinopathy

Skeletal?   Codfish vertebrae, aseptic necrosis

HEMOLYTIC ANEMIAS

GLUCOSE-6-PHOSPHATE DEHYDROGENASE (G6PD) DEFICIENCY

What is G6PD?   G6PD is a dehydrogenase involved in the pentose phosphate pathway, which is important in NADPH production.

What causes its deficiency?   Mutation in G6PD gene; the condition is X-linked recessive

What is the physiologic effect of G6PD deficiency?	In the RBC deficient of G6PD, oxidative stress depletes NADPH and GSH with subsequent oxidation of Hgb, causing cell membrane damage and hemolysis
What are the signs and symptoms?	An asymptomatic child with G6PD deficiency usually has normal hematologic parameters, but when faced with oxidative stress, the child will have jaundice, hemoglobinuria, splenomegaly, and anemia.
What are some oxidative triggers?	Fava beans, bacterial infections, certain drugs (e.g., sulfas, antimalarials, analgesics)
What diagnostic study is used?	Measurement of G6PD activity in RBCs of reticulocyte-poor blood
What is the treatment?	Usually supportive; with severe hemolysis, transfusion is occasionally necessary

SPHEROCYTOSIS

What is it?	Autosomal dominant congenital hemolytic anemia with spherical RBCs
What is the pathophysiologic effect?	Loss of membrane surface area due to deficiencies in some RBC proteins (e.g., spectrin, ankyrin) leads to spherically shaped, less deformable cells, which become subject to lysis and trapping in the spleen.
What are the signs and symptoms?	May be mild or severe and include anemia, hemoglobinuria, jaundice, and splenomegaly; hemolysis increases with infections.
What diagnostic studies are used?	1. CBC: Hgb is decreased 2. Blood smear, which shows increased spheres and reticulocytes 3. Osmotic fragility test

What is the treatment?

Supportive usually, if the clinical course is mild

Splenectomy, +/- cholecystectomy if severe anemia, recurrent significant hemolysis, or cholecystitis exist; splenectomy is usually delayed until after age 6 if possible.

What are some common complications?

Aplastic crisis, cholecystitis, transfusion dependence

APLASTIC ANEMIA

What is it?

Pancytopenia secondary to decreased production of blood cells because of destruction of stem cells in bone marrow or because of abnormal bone marrow environment; may be inherited or acquired

How is it classified?

1. Severe: granulocyte count < 500, platelet count < 20K, reticulocyte count < 1% after correction for Hgb; hypocellular bone marrow biopsy
2. Mild or moderate: mild-to-moderate cytopenia; normal or increased bone marrow cellularity

What are some causes?

Acquired: drugs, radiation, viral infections, PNH, preleukemia

Inherited: Fanconi anemia, congenital dyskeratosis, Schwachman-Diamond syndrome, myelodysplasia

What are the signs and symptoms?

Fatigue, pallor, and increased bleeding and infections

What diagnostic studies are used?

1. CBC, which shows pancytopenia and decreased reticulocytes
2. Bone marrow biopsy, which shows hypocellularity
3. Consider viral titres, screening for paroxysmal nocturnal hemoglobinuria (PNH), and DNA breakage studies for Fanconi anemia

What is the treatment?	Bone marrow transplant; immunosuppressive therapy (e.g., antithymocyte globulin, cyclosporine, steroids); hematopoietic growth factors; supportive care with antibiotics and transfusion therapy
What is the prognosis?	Prognosis in severe aplastics is poor without bone marrow transplant. If related matched donor available, transplant is primary therapy. **Pretransplant transfusions should be avoided as much as possible.**

GAUCHER DISEASE

What is it?	Inherited storage disease with deficiency of enzyme **glucocerebroside β-glucosidase**
How is it inherited?	As an autosomal recessive disorder
What is the physiologic effect?	Accumulation of glucocerebroside in reticuloendothelial (Gaucher) cells
What are the three types?	1. **Chronic non-neuronopathic (adult form):** clinical course variable and may include anemia, thrombocytopenia with marrow infiltration, bleeding tendency, hepatosplenomegaly, and aseptic necrosis of bones 2. **Acute neuronopathic (infantile form):** severe, with presentation in infancy; CNS infiltration with neuro defects and hepatosplenomegaly; death usually occurs by 2 years of age. 3. **Subacute neuronopathic (juvenile form):** neurologic defects occur later in course of disease and may increase after splenectomy
In what ethnic group is the adult form commonly found?	Ashkenazi Jews

What do diagnostic studies show?	1. Bone marrow biopsy shows Gaucher cells 2. Decreased lysosomal β glucocerebrosidase in leukocytes or cultured skin fibroblasts 3. Increased acid phosphatase and angiotensin-converting enzyme
What is the treatment for non-neuronopathic Gaucher disease?	1. Enzyme replacement therapy 2. Bone marrow transplant 3. Splenectomy if hypersplenism exists, but this may increase other symptoms; splenectomy is now only rarely performed

POLYCYTHEMIA

What is it?	RBC count, Hgb level, and total RBC volume all exceed the upper limits of normal. In postpubertal children, it is distinguished by a Hgb > 16 g/dl and a total RBC mass > 35 ml/kg.
What is the appropriate term for high Hgb with a concurrent decrease in plasma volume (e.g., as occurs in acute dehydration and burns)?	Hemoconcentration
What is polycythemia rubra vera?	This is a primary myeloproliferative polycythemia.
What are the diagnostic criteria?	1. Increased total RBC volume, Hgb, and hematocrit 2. Arterial oxygen saturation ≥ 92% 3. Splenomegaly
What are laboratory findings?	Thrombocytosis, leucocytosis, increased leucocyte alkaline phosphatase, increased vitamin B_{12} or unsaturated B_{12}-binding capacity
What is the treatment?	Phlebotomy, chemotherapy
What are the long-term risks?	Myelofibrosis or acute leukemia

What is the prognosis?	Poor
What is secondary polycythemia?	Polycythemia due to other inciting causes
What are these causes?	1. Hypoxia 2. Hemoglobinopathies 3. Neonatal conditions, such as twin-twin or maternal hemorrhage, infants of diabetic mothers, intrauterine growth retardation, neonatal thyroid toxicosis, adrenal hypoplasia, trisomy 21 4. Benign and malignant tumors that secrete erythropoietin 5. Excess presence of anabolic steroids caused by either adrenal disease or excessive administration of anabolic steroids 6. Familial

GRANULOCYTE DISORDERS

What is leukocyte adhesion deficiency (LAD)?	It is a deficiency of a β_2 integrin. The condition is autosomal recessive and results in deficiency of leukocyte adhesion to offending agents.
What are the clinical manifestations?	Leukocytosis, delayed umbilical cord separation, and bacterial infections
What is Chédiak-Higashi syndrome?	An autosomal recessive disorder affecting granule-bearing cells. Granulocytes and melanocytes are characteristically affected.
How are granulocytes affected?	There are defects in chemotaxis, degranulation, and bactericidal activity.
What are the clinical manifestations?	Oculocutaneous albinism, large neutrophil granules, recurrent bacterial infections
What is chronic granulomatous disease (CGD)?	A genetically heterogeneous condition that results in a defect in "respiratory burst" in leukocytes

What is the respiratory burst?

It is a reaction catalyzed by NADPH that forms hydrogen peroxide and hydroxyl radicals, which are thought to play a key role in microbial killing.

What are the clinical manifestations?

Recurrent bacterial and fungal infections

What is the treatment?

There is no cure. Trimethoprim-sulfamethoxazole prophylaxis may limit infections. γ-Interferon or bone marrow transplant may help some patients.

What is the definition of neutropenia?

Absolute neutrophil count (ANC) <1000

What is cyclic neutropenia?

The neutrophil count cycles between a normal and low ANC

What is autoimmune neutropenia?

It is a condition resulting from the presence of antineutrophil antibodies. It is usually found in infants with no predisposing cause. Antibodies against neutrophils are also seen in neonates following transplacental transfer of maternal IgG (alloimmune neonatal neutropenia; ANN) or in neonates whose mothers have an autoimmune disease (**neonatal maternal autoimmune neutropenia**).

Can infection induce neutropenia?

Yes

What types of infection most commonly cause this?

Viral infections; however, bacterial, mycobacterial, and rickettsial infections may also cause neutropenia

What is Kostmann syndrome?

This is a rare autosomal recessive condition associated with neutropenia at birth.

What is the cause of this disease?

Unknown

What are the clinical manifestations?

Severe, often fatal, infections

What is Schwachman-Diamond syndrome?

An autosomal recessive condition characterized by neutropenia and pancreatic insufficiency; chemotaxis is also defective in these neutrophils

What are the clinical manifestations?

Pancreatic insufficiency, potential growth failure, dry skin, eczema, and ichthyosiform lesions

For which malignancy are these patients at risk?

Leukemia

What are treatment options for neutropenia conditions?

1. First and foremost, judicious use of antibiotics may be required to either treat or prevent serious infection.
2. Steroids may be used in autoimmune neutropenia.
3. Granulocyte colony-stimulating factor (G-CSF) may be used in some neutropenic conditions.
4. γ-Interferon may be useful in CGD.
5. Bone marrow transplant may be used in Chédiak-Higashi syndrome, CGD, Wiskott-Aldrich syndrome, and LAD.

PLATELET DISORDERS

CONGENITAL PLATELET DISORDERS

What is Wiskott-Aldrich syndrome?

Thrombocytopenia, purpura, eczema, and an increased susceptibility to infection due to impaired humoral immune responses and chemotaxis of neutrophils

What is the cause?

This syndrome is transmitted as an X-linked recessive trait.

What causes the thrombocytopenia?

Uncertain—probably an intrinsic platelet abnormality or defective formation or release of platelets; however, the number of megakaryocytes is normal

What are treatment options?

1. Splenectomy improves platelet count; however, there is an increased risk of postsplenectomy sepsis. Patients must receive prophylactic penicillin.
2. Administration of transfer factor
3. Bone marrow transplantation

What are the long-term risks of Wiskott-Aldrich syndrome?

5% of patients develop lymphoreticular malignancies

What is TAR syndrome?

Thrombocytopenia associated with **A**plasia of the **R**adii and thumbs; there may also be cardiac and renal anomalies

What are clinical manifestations of thrombocytopenia?

Hemorrhage, which may be evident even in the first days of life (e.g., during circumcision)

What are laboratory findings?

Thrombocytopenia; normal Hgb, and possibly leukocytosis

What findings are on bone marrow aspirate?

Megakaryocyte count is normal, but the nuclear morphology may be abnormal.

What is Fanconi anemia?

It is an aplastic anemia characterized by pancytopenia with associated skeletal, solid organ, and skin abnormalities.

What is the cause?

It is an autosomal recessive inherited condition.

What are its clinical manifestations?

Usually pancytopenia at 3 to 4 years of age, which can lead to bleeding and infection; other manifestations include hyperpigmentation and café au lait spots, skeletal abnormalities, (especially absent or hypoplastic thumbs), short stature, and other anomalies; skeletal findings may be subtle in some patients

What are four major risks of Fanconi syndrome?

1. Hematologic malignancy
2. Infections
3. Bleeding
4. Solid organ (especially liver) failure

What are bone marrow findings?

Aplasia (similar to that seen in acquired aplastic anemia)

What are treatment options?

1. Steroids and androgens may help, but relapse occurs in 50% of patients.
2. G-CSF may be a potential treatment.
3. Bone marrow transplant

What is the prognosis? Poor; the median survival age is 16 years

What is Bernard-Soulier syndrome? It is a condition involving a platelet adhesion defect.

What is the cause? It is an autosomal recessive inherited trait.

What are laboratory findings? Moderate thrombocytopenia with large platelets

What are clinical manifestations? Bleeding of various tissues

What is the treatment? Administration of platelets during bleeding episodes

What is Kasabach-Merritt syndrome? It is a condition of platelet trapping and consumptive coagulopathy associated with congenital hemangioma, usually of the liver.

What is the pathophysiology? Trapping and destruction of platelets within the extensive vascular bed of the hemangioma

What are peripheral blood smear findings? Thrombocytopenia with RBC fragments

What are bone marrow findings? Normal megakaryocytes

What are clinical manifestations? Spontaneous hemorrhage

What are treatment options?
1. Steroids
2. α-Interferon
3. Occlusion of hepatic artery supply if the hemangioma is in the liver
4. Resection or compression of hemangioma, although this might result in uncontrollable hemorrhage
5. Radiation to the hemangioma

What is hemolytic-uremic syndrome (HUS)? Acute hemolytic anemia, thrombocytopenia, and renal failure

What is the cause?

It is thought to be caused by a variety of bacteria. One of the most commonly identified pathogens is *E. coli* **0157:47.**

What are clinical symptoms?

Usually there is a prodrome of gastroenteritis or diarrhea with subsequent development of bloody diarrhea. Decreased urine output with renal insufficiency may ensue. There may also be an associated inflammatory colitis. Finally, neurologic symptoms may develop.

What are the treatments?

Generally supportive care. Renal failure may need to be managed with dialysis. Platelets may be given if bleeding becomes life-threatening. Plasma infusion or exchange, or intravenous immunoglobulin may be of some help. Occasionally colon resection may be needed if the inflammatory colitis proceeds to a life-threatening state.

What is the prognosis?

90%–95% of patients with HUS survive, of which the vast majority recover normal renal function.

What is thrombotic thrombocytopenic purpura (TTP)?

It is a condition characterized by thrombocytopenia and hemolytic anemia.

What are clinical manifestations?

Hemorrhage; neurologic sequelae may include aphasia, blindness, and convulsions due to embolism and thrombosis of small blood vessels of the brain

What are treatment options?

1. Plasmapheresis and plasma infusions are effective in 60%–70% of cases. Platelets and blood may be administered as needed.
2. Steroids
3. If condition is refractory to the above therapies, splenectomy may used

What are some common drugs that may cause drug-induced thrombocytopenias in children?	Tegretol, dilantin, sulfadomides, trimethoprim-sulfmethoxazole (Bactrim), chloramphenicol

IDIOPATHIC THROMBOCYTOPENIC PURPURA (ITP)

What is it?	Development of platelet antibodies with subsequent destruction of platelets
What is the peak age for ITP?	2–4 years
In whom is it most commonly seen?	Previously healthy children often after viral illness; can be associated with autoimmune disease and HIV
What are characteristic laboratory and diagnostic findings?	1. Platelet count < 50,000/mm^3 2. Sparse, large platelets on blood smear 3. Bone marrow aspirate shows an increased number of megakaryocytes, usually of immature forms 4. Anti-platelet immunoglobulins are present.
What are treatment options?	1. If not severe (platelet count > 20,000), observation 2. If severe, steroids, intravenous immunoglobulin, and possible splenectomy (if chronic) 3. Platelet transfusions are usually not useful but are used in conjunction with other therapy with serious bleeds or surgery.
What are complications?	Severe GI or CNS hemorrhage, hematuria
What is the prognosis?	Majority of childhood disease is benign and self-limited; 10%–15% develop chronic ITP.

COAGULATION DEFECTS

HEMOPHILIAS A AND B

What is hemophilia A, or classical hemophilia?	Factor VIII deficiency

What is hemophilia B, or Christmas disease?

Factor IX deficiency

What is the pathophysiology of these conditions?

Both are X-linked recessive disorders with decreased production of factor VIII or IX. There is a moderately high spontaneous mutation rate.

How is the severity of hemophilia A classified?

By the percent of factor VIII present:
Severe < 1%
Moderate 1%–5%
Mild > 5%

What is the physiologic result?

Inability to generate normal fibrin

What are the signs and symptoms?

Bleeding, including neonatal bleeding (especially with circumcision) or intracranial hemorrhage; easy bruising and bleeding with mild trauma; and oral, muscular, or joint bleeding

How is the diagnosis made?

1. Family history
2. Prolonged PTT; bleeding time is usually normal, except in very severe cases
3. Decreased factor VIII or IX level

What is the treatment?

Replacement therapy with factor: recombinant factor VIII now available; factor IX not recombinant; DDAVP may be useful in patients with mild hemophilia

How much does 1 unit/kg of factor VIII raise the patient's plasma factor VIII?

1 unit/kg of factor VIII will give 2% rise in plasma factor VIII.

1 unit/kg of factor IX?

1 unit/kg factor IX will give 1% rise in plasma factor IX.

How much factor is appropriate for:
    Mild-to-moderate hemorrhage?

Achieve factor level of **30%–40%.**

    Major surgery or life threatening bleed?

Achieve **100%** and maintain for **7–14 days.**

Oral bleed?	May also use antifibrinolytics (e.g., aminocaproic acid)
What are complications of these deficiencies?	1. Damage from repeated joint bleeds 2. Serious hemorrhage 3. Development of factor inhibitors (usually seen in factor VIII deficiency) 4. Infections (e.g., HIV, hepatitis) from factor replacement

VON WILLEBRAND DISEASE

What is it?	Autosomal dominant disorder of von Willebrand factor (vWF) protein production; several variants known based on laboratory tests and platelet count; in the most severe case, there is an undetectable level of vWF and a decreased level of factor VIII
What is the physiologic result?	Inability of platelets to adhere to damaged endothelium
How common is von Willebrand disease?	It is the most common inherited bleeding disorder.
What are the signs and symptoms?	Easy bruising and bleeding with or without trauma; history of recurrent epistaxis or menorrhagia; clinical severity may vary; some affected persons may be asymptomatic
How is the diagnosis made?	1. Bleeding time prolonged; PTT may be increased 2. A decrease in von Willebrand antigen, ristocetin cofactor, and factor VIII levels 3. Platelet count may be decreased in certain variants 4. Normal-to-abnormal vWF multimers 5. Testing often has to be repeated to assure diagnosis
What is the treatment?	1. DDAVP can be used to increase vWF in some types. 2. Cryoprecipitate or certain factor VIII concentrates (e.g., Humate-P) can be used in DDAVP-failure patients, in

severe bleed, or in major surgery. Patients with oral bleeds may also benefit from antifibrinolytics (e.g., α aminocaproic acid).

DISSEMINATED INTRAVASCULAR COAGULOPATHY (DIC)

What is it?

Consumptive coagulopathy that activates the plasma coagulation system and depletes clotting and antithrombotic factors as well as platelets

What is the physiologic effect?

Cycle of intravascular thrombosis and fibrinolysis, particularly in small vessels

What are common etiologies?

Sepsis, malignancy (especially promyelocytic leukemia), obstetric complications, extensive tissue damage from trauma, burns, hypoxia, snake bites

What are signs and symptoms?

Bleeding or clotting, embolic signs, oozing from vascular access or phlebotomy sites

What are the diagnostic findings?

Decreased platelet levels, prolonged PT and PTT, decreased fibrinogen, increased fibrin split products

What is the treatment?

1. Successful treatment is possible only with correction of underlying etiology.
2. Symptomatic treatment includes transfusion with platelets, FFP, and cryoprecipitate.
3. Heparin may be used at times if thrombosis is a prevalent symptom.

What are the complications?

Severe bleeding or thrombosis in the GI, pulmonary, and CNS systems

NEONATAL ALLOIMMUNE THROMBOCYTOPENIA

What is it?

Infants born with severe thrombocytopenia secondary to having different platelet antigens from mother, with subsequent platelet destruction by maternal antiplatelet antibodies; similar to Rh sensitization in blood groups

Is there a high risk of bleeding?

Yes. It may occur prenatally.

How is it diagnosed?

Platelet typing of mother and father

What is the treatment?

1. Transfusion with irradiated maternal platelets
2. Steroids pre- or postnatally
3. Possible IV immunoglobulin

INTRODUCTION TO PEDIATRIC CARDIOLOGY

GENERAL CONSIDERATIONS

What percent of pediatric cardiology patients have a congenital heart defect (CHD)?	90%; 10% have acquired heart disease (e.g., myocarditis, cardiomyopathy, hypertension)
What are the most common types of heart conditions that cause clinical problems in newborns?	Cyanotic or severe obstructive lesions
What symptomatology alerts pediatricians to heart defects in infants and school-age children?	Murmurs, of which a vast majority are "innocent" or functional; atrial septal defect (ASD) and ventricular septal defect (VSD) are the most common causes of organic murmurs
In preadolescents and adolescents?	Chest pain (usually noncardiac in origin), palpitations, and hypertension
What is congestive heart failure (CHF)?	It is a clinical syndrome in which the heart is unable to pump adequately to support the circulation. Pulmonary insufficiency may result from excessive blood backing up in the pulmonary bed. Failure to thrive occurs because of the inability to take in enough calories to grow normally.
Is CHF a diagnosis?	No

CYANOTIC CONGENITAL HEART DEFECTS

TRUNCUS ARTERIOSUS

What is it?	A CHD consisting of a single vessel arising from the heart that branches to

form the aorta and pulmonary arteries
(PAs)

What are the four types?

Type I: a common PA arises from the
truncus and divides into left and right
PAs

Type II: separate right and left PAs arise
from the posterior aspect of the
truncus

Type III: separate right and left PAs
arise from the lateral aspects of the
truncus

Type IV: pulmonary blood flow
originates from aortopulmonary
collateral arteries

**What are associated
defects?**

VSD, semilunar valve abnormalities

**In what syndrome is
truncus arteriosus seen?**

DiGeorge syndrome

**How does truncus
arteriosus present?**

1. Most common presentation is CHF
   caused by either excessive pulmonary
   blood flow or truncal valve
   insufficiency.
2. Less common presentation is cyanosis
   from stenosis of the PA origin.

**What are the signs and
symptoms?**

Tachypnea, tachycardia, holosystolic
murmur with loud single S_2

**What are the radiographic
findings?**

Cardiomegaly, increased pulmonary
vascular markings; one third of patients
have right aortic arch

**What other diagnostic
studies are used?**

1. ECG: shows biventricular
   hypertrophy
2. Echocardiography
3. Cardiac catheterization before
   surgical repair

What is the treatment?

Medical: management of CHF with
diuretics and afterload reduction

Surgical:
1. Establish continuity from right
   ventricle (RV) to PA with conduit
2. VSD closure

What are the complications of surgical repair?	Conduit failure Truncal valve insufficiency
What are the outcomes?	1. Surgically untreated cases usually result in death in early childhood (< 1 year of age). Survivors who have not undergone surgical repair usually develop pulmonary vascular obstructive disease. 2. Results of surgical therapy are continually improving, with early survival now at 80%–90%; long-term survival data are not yet available.

TRANSPOSITION OF THE GREAT ARTERIES

What is it?	CHD in which the aorta arises from the RV, and the PA arises from the left ventricle (LV)
What are some associated defects?	VSD, pulmonary stenosis, ASD, patent ductus arteriosus, coarctation of the aorta
Transposition of the great arteries represents what percent of all CHDs?	10%–it is the second most common CHD after VSD
What is the physiologic result?	Cyanosis; oxygenated blood remains in pulmonary circulation and deoxygenated blood in the systemic circulation (called *parallel* rather than normal *series* circuit); blood mixes through a PDA, patent foramen ovale, and a VSD if present
What are the signs and symptoms?	1. Cyanosis in the newborn period 2. With a large VSD, there may be minimal cyanosis, but there will be CHF 3. No murmur in the absence of VSD
What are the radiographic findings?	Classically described as an "egg on its side," with normal heart size and narrow mediastinum

What other diagnostic studies are used?

1. ECG, which is usually normal at birth
2. Echocardiography
3. Cardiac catheterization: can perform balloon atrial septostomy (Rashkind procedure) if needed for better mixing of oxygenated and deoxygenated blood; this is a temporizing measure

What is the treatment?

Medical: prostaglandin infusion to maintain patency of ductus arteriosus until septostomy or surgery

Surgical:
1. Pre-1980: Mustard or Senning procedure (atrial baffle), either of which may still be used in infants with severe pulmonary stenosis
2. Post-1980: Jatene procedure (arterial switch)

When should surgical repair be performed?

Infants without VSD should be repaired within 2 weeks to avoid weakness of LV muscle. If a VSD is present, then atrial septostomy and pulmonary banding may be performed first if needed; final repair can be performed after the 2-week period (however, the earlier, the better).

What are the complications of atrial baffle repair?

Atrial dysrhythmias are common. Other complications include superior vena cava (SVC) obstruction, baffle leak, tricuspid valve insufficiency, and RV failure.

Of arterial switch?

May have early myocardial ischemia caused by the manipulation necessary to reimplant the coronary arteries; 20% have postoperative supravalvular pulmonary stenosis

What is the outcome of atrial baffle?

Early survival is about 85%. However, long-term sequelae are significant and include atrial arrhythmias, sick sinus syndrome, RV failure, and sudden death.

Of arterial switch?

Good–90% to 95% survival at 1 year

TRICUSPID ATRESIA

What is it?

A CHD characterized by agenesis of the tricuspid valve

What are common associated defects?

ASD, small RV, malposition of great arteries, VSD, pulmonary stenosis

Tricuspid atresia represents what percent of all CHDs?

2%–it is the third most common CHD (after VSD and transposition of the great arteries)

What is the physiologic result?

Cyanosis that is mild to severe, depending on the size of the VSD and degree of pulmonary stenosis; all patients have right-to-left shunt at atrial level; if transposition of the great arteries is present, CHF develops early due to pulmonary overload

What are the signs and symptoms?

1. Cyanosis in the newborn period
2. There may be excessive pulmonary blood flow and CHF (especially with associated transposition of the great arteries)
3. Murmur from VSD (holosystolic) or from pulmonary stenosis (systolic ejection)

What are the radiographic findings?

Mild cardiomegaly; pulmonary segment is usually small in those infants with cyanosis

What diagnostic studies are used?

1. ECG shows tall, notched P waves consistent with right atrial enlargement, and left axis deviation consistent with left ventricular hypertrophy (LVH)
2. Echocardiography
3. Cardiac catheterization: enlargement of atrial communication can be accomplished if needed

What is the treatment?

Surgical treatment:
1. Palliative SVC-to-PA (Glenn) shunt in infancy
2. A modified Fontan procedure in childhood (all systemic venous return directed to PA); this is also known as

the caval-pulmonary isolation procedure; ASD or patent foramen ovale is closed at this time

What are the complications of surgical repair?

1. Shunts may clot or develop stenosis
2. Pleural and pericardial effusions
3. Supraventricular arrhythmias
4. Left ventricular dysfunction may be a late outcome

What is the outcome?

Post-Fontan procedure: resolved cyanosis, exercise capacity reduced, 10-year survival is about 65%

TETRALOGY OF FALLOT

What is it?

A CHD characterized by:
1. VSD
2. Pulmonary stenosis
3. Aortic override
4. Right ventricular hypertrophy (RVH)

What is the physiologic result?

VSD allows interventricular shunting, usually right-to-left. Degree of right-to-left shunting depends on degree of pulmonary outflow obstruction. Exercise worsens shunting.

What are the signs and symptoms?

1. Cyanosis: worsens with activity or may be spontaneous (i.e., tetralogy, or "tet spell")
2. Child assumes squatting position to relieve cyanosis, which is believed to increase systemic pressure and therefore relieve right-to-left shunt
3. Normal S_1, soft S_2, systolic ejection murmur

How may a cyanotic spell be managed?

Before surgical repair, use O_2. Morphine and/or propranolol may help.

What are the radiographic findings?

Boot-shaped heart ("coeur en sabot"), which is cause by hypertrophied RV and absence of prominent PAs

What other diagnostic studies are used?

1. ECG: shows right axis deviation and evidence for RV hypertrophy
2. Echocardiography: Doppler is helpful to assess flow to PAs
3. Cardiac catheterization: look for degree of stenosis of pulmonary outflow, multiple septal defects, and coronary artery abnormalities

What is the treatment?

Primarily surgical:
1. Systemic-to-pulmonary shunt will temporize until child is bigger and stronger (usually by toddler age). Blalock-Taussig shunt employs end-to-side subclavian-to-pulmonary artery shunt; an H graft may also be used between these two vessels.
2. Definitive repair of defect involves closing VSD and widening pulmonary outflow tract

What are the complications of definitive surgical repair?

Residual VSD

Arrhythmias, particularly ventricular ectopy

Subacute bacterial endocarditis (patient should always receive prophylactic antibiotics when appropriate)

What is the outcome?

Ninety percent of patients who undergo definitive repair survive well into adulthood (but slightly less than the average person). Working capacity, maximum heart rate, and cardiac output are generally less than that in the average person.

DOUBLE-OUTLET RIGHT VENTRICLE

What is it?

CHD in which both the aorta and PA arise from the RV; this condition may be seen as part of a continuum with tetralogy of Fallot

What are some associated defects?

VSD (the "outlet" for left ventricle blood) and various malpositions of the PA and aorta

It represents what percent of all CHDs?

1%

What is the physiologic result?

It ranges from VSD physiology (left-to-right shunt with increased flow to lungs) to tetralogy of Fallot physiology (right-to-left with decreased flow to lungs), depending on the size of VSD, the position of the PA and aorta, and the amount of pulmonary stenosis.

What are the signs and symptoms?

Vary with type of physiology:
1. Cyanosis is present if pulmonary blood flow is decreased.
2. CHF is present if pulmonary blood flow is increased.

What are the radiographic findings?

They are similar to those seen with tetralogy of Fallot. However, there may be fullness of PAs with pulmonary edema if there is no pulmonary stenosis.

What diagnostic studies are used?

1. ECG: right axis deviation and evidence for RVH are the most common findings
2. Echocardiography: distinguishes type of VSD and relationship to PA and aorta
3. Cardiac catheterization before surgical repair

What is the treatment?

The goal is to establish LV-to-aorta continuity and RV-to-PA continuity if possible
1. Decreased pulmonary blood flow: systemic-to-pulmonary shunt is placed in infancy, followed by VSD closure and right ventricular outflow tract reconstruction in childhood
2. Excessive pulmonary blood flow: pulmonary artery band (Damon-Muller procedure) in infancy, and VSD repair later in childhood

What are the major complications of surgical repair?

Residual VSD, outflow obstruction

What is the outcome?	Good results in those with VSD physiology and simple repair

EISENMENGER SYNDROME

What is it?	The result of a CHD that allows right-to-left shunt in response to marked elevation of the pulmonary vascular resistance; this term is commonly used to describe such a shunt in VSD with pulmonary hypertension; Eisenmenger syndrome is also sometimes used to describe idiopathic primary pulmonary hypertension in which the pulmonary pressure is markedly elevated in the absence of any structural cardiac lesion
What is the physiologic result?	High pulmonary vascular resistance elevates PA pressure and deoxygenated blood enters the systemic circulation
What are the signs and symptoms?	Cyanosis and poor exercise tolerance; sudden death may occur
What are the radiographic findings?	Decreased pulmonary vascular markings Heart size usually normal
What other diagnostic studies are used?	1. Cardiac catheterization is used for diagnosis and to determine if operable 2. ECG: RVH as well as characteristics of the particular CHD causing the syndrome 3. Echocardiography: Right-sided pre-injection period:ejection time ratio is increased secondary to pulmonary vascular resistance Early closure of pulmonic valve 4. Catheterization: bidirectional shunt at ventricular defect with equal systolic pressures in systemic and pulmonary circulations
What is the treatment?	Medical: calcium channel blockers or prostacyclins; benefits are short term Surgical: heart–lung transplantation offers improvement in symptoms, but long-term outcome limited

What is the outcome?	Poor prognosis

HYPOPLASTIC LEFT HEART SYNDROME

What is it?	CHD characterized by underdevelopment of the left heart (i.e., mitral valve, LV, aortic valve, and ascending aorta)
Hypoplastic left heart syndrome represents what percent of all CHDs?	7%
What is the physiologic result?	Systemic circulation depends on right-to-left flow at ductus arteriosus; almost uniformly fatal within first weeks of life
What are the signs and symptoms?	1. Cyanosis within hours of birth 2. Circulatory collapse with poor perfusion 3. Soft systolic murmur
What are the radiographic findings?	Usually mild cardiomegaly at first and then rapidly becomes more marked with an increase in pulmonary vascularity
What diagnostic studies are used?	1. ECG: RVH is commonly seen 2. Echocardiogram for diagnosis
What is the medical treatment?	Prostaglandin infusion until surgical intervention or "passive euthanasia'

What is the surgical treatment?	1. Norwood procedure, which is a three-stage procedure:
	    Stage I: atrial septostomy, ligation of distal main PA with connection of proximal PA to aorta; synthetic shunt from aorta to distal main PA
	    Stage II: connection of SVC to PAs
	    Stage III: connection of inferior vena cava (IVC) to PAs
	    (After stages II and III, systemic venous return enters pulmonary veins directly.)
	2. Orthotopic heart transplant

What are the complications of surgical repair?	1. Norwood multistage procedure ultimately requires Fontan procedure 2. Transplantation complications include infection, rejection, coronary artery disease, and malignancy
What are the outcomes?	Uniformly fatal if surgically untreated; staged surgical survival limited, with mortality after stage I alone > 25%; transplant offers best outcomes

TOTAL ANOMALOUS PULMONARY VENOUS RETURN

What is it?	A CHD in which the pulmonary veins do not connect to the left atrium (LA)
Where do the anomalous pulmonary veins drain?	The pulmonary veins connect to the heart in three major areas: 1. **Supracardiac**–connect to vertical vein or SVC 2. **Cardiac**–connect to coronary sinus 3. **Subcardiac**–connect to IVC below the diaphragm; obstruction of pulmonary venous return is most common in this group
What is the physiologic result?	**Unobstructed flow:** comparable to ASD with left-to-right shunt [enlarged right atrium (RA) and RV] **Obstructed flow:** decreased filling of LA and LV, cyanosis, and decreased cardiac output
What are the signs and symptoms?	Unobstructed flow may present with tachypnea and murmur. Obstructed flow may present with cyanosis and circulatory collapse.
What are the radiographic findings?	Cardiomegaly with increased vascular markings Classic "snowman" shape to heart secondary to vertical vein; large SVC and enlarged right atrium
What other diagnostic studies are used?	1. ECG: RVH is commonly seen 2. Echocardiography 3. Cardiac catheterization is used for definitive confirmation of drainage pattern

What is the treatment?	Surgical: connect pulmonary venous confluence to left atrium and close patent foramen ovale/ASD, so as to separate the pulmonary venous system from the systemic venous system
What are the complications of repair?	Continued obstruction of pulmonary venous return to LA, persistent pulmonary hypertension
What is the outcome?	Infants with severe pulmonary venous obstruction have the worst outcome and face a 30%–35% early and late mortality following surgery. If there is no obstruction, surgical results are excellent.

PULMONARY ATRESIA WITH INTACT VENTRICULAR SEPTUM

What is it?	A CHD consisting of an underdeveloped right ventricle and an imperforate pulmonary valve
It represents what percent of CHD?	1%
What are the physiologic results?	Severe cyanosis as newborn; all have right-to-left shunt at atrial level; pulmonary blood flow supplied by patent ductus arteriosus
What are the signs and symptoms?	Cyanosis Circulatory collapse if patent ductus arteriosus closes
What are the radiographic findings?	Normal-size heart with decreased pulmonary lung markings (dark lung fields) if patent ductus arteriosus is small or closed
What other diagnostic studies are used?	1. ECG: may show LVH 2. Echocardiography 3. Cardiac catheterization to plan management

What is the treatment?	Medical: prostaglandin infusion until surgery
	Surgical:
	1. Palliative shunt
	2. Right ventricular outflow patch
	3. Transplant
	4. RV–PA homograft
	5. Fontan procedure (beyond infancy)
What are the complications of repair?	Palliative shunts may clot or develop stenosis and RV may fail to grow
What are the outcomes?	High mortality for all procedures; long-term survival limited

ACYANOTIC CONGENITAL HEART DEFECTS

ATRIAL SEPTAL DEFECT

What is it?	CHD consisting of a hole in the septum between the right and left atria
What are the three types?	1. Secundum ASD (most common)
	2. Primum ASD (associated with other endocardial cushion defects)
	3. Sinus venosus ASD (rare)
ASD represents what percent of all CHDs?	5%–10%
Is ASD more common in males or females?	Females, by 2 to 1
What is the physiologic result?	Left-to-right shunt with volume overload of RA, RV, and PA
What are the symptoms?	Usually asymptomatic in children; may ultimately cause right heart congestion, but this would not occur until the third to fifth decades of life in untreated patients
What are the physical signs?	1. Nonspecific systolic ejection murmur from increased pulmonary flow
	2. Widely (or fixed) split of S_2
	3. May have diastolic rumble of increased flow across tricuspid valve

What are the radiographic findings?	Cardiomegaly due to enlargement of RA and RV; prominent PA segment
What diagnostic studies are used?	1. ECG: may have RVH 2. Echocardiography 3. Cardiac catheterization if primum or sinus venosus defect
What is the treatment?	Surgical closure
What are the complications of surgical repair?	10% may have atrial dysrhythmia
What is the outcome?	Very good—most studies suggest best outcome if repaired before adolescence

VENTRICULAR SEPTAL DEFECT

What is it?	CHD consisting of a hole in the septum between the right and left ventricles
What are the four types?	Type I–supracristal (subpulmonary) Type II–perimembranous Type III–inlet (atrioventricular canal type) Type IV–muscular
VSD represents what percent of CHDs?	20%–it is the most common CHD
What is the physiologic result?	Left-to-right shunt with increased volume of blood circulated to the lungs
What determines the volume of the shunt?	Size of the hole and the resistance in the lungs
What are the signs and symptoms of a small VSD?	No symptoms, with loud holosystolic murmur
Of moderate-to-large VSD?	Signs of pulmonary congestion (e.g., tachypnea, poor feeding) with holosystolic murmur and diastolic rumble
What are the radiographic findings of small VSD?	Normal

Of moderate-to-large VSD?	Cardiomegaly with increase in vascular markings
What other diagnostic studies are used?	1. ECG: may show LVH 2. Echocardiography 3. Cardiac catheterization to plan for surgery
What is the treatment for a small VSD?	Possibly none; at least 50% close spontaneously
Moderate VSD?	May require diuretics until surgical repair; child will usually be allowed to grow as much as possible, with repair sometimes delayed until the early toddler years
Large VSD?	Requires patch closure, which is usually done at 3–12 months of age
What are common complications of surgical repair?	Residual VSD
What is the outcome?	Good survival with few sequelae

PATENT DUCTUS ARTERIOSUS

What is it?	Persistent patency of the ductus arteriosus
It represents what percent of all CHDs?	5%–10%
What group of infants is at risk for patent ductus arteriosus?	Premature infants–as many as 75% of infants of 28 to 30 weeks gestation have a patent ductus arteriosus
Is it more common in males or females?	Females
What is the physiologic result?	Left-to-right shunt from aorta into PA With a large patent ductus arteriosus, LA and LV enlargement may occur, leading to CHF Rare association with pulmonary hypertension (Eisenmenger syndrome)

What are the signs and symptoms?	1. Usually asymptomatic in older children 2. Small infants may have signs of pulmonary congestion 3. Continuous murmur in the second intercostal space, bounding pulses
What are the radiographic findings?	May show cardiomegaly due to LA and LV enlargement
What other diagnostic studies are used?	1. ECG: may show LVH 2. Echocardiogram with color flow Doppler to demonstrate defect 3. Catheterization is only needed if another associated defect is suspected or if there is pulmonary hypertension
What is the treatment?	Few close after infancy. They usually require division and ligation or interventional catheterization to close it. A symptomatic defect in a premature baby may sometimes close with indomethacin treatment; however, this may only work temporarily and thus only serves as a bridge to surgical repair.
What are the complications of repair?	Residual shunt
What is the outcome?	Excellent prognosis

PULMONARY VALVE STENOSIS

What is it?	Congenital obstruction of the right ventricular outflow tract; valve or subvalve (infundibulum) obstructions are most common
Pulmonary stenosis represents what percent of all CHDs?	5%
What is the physiologic result?	High right ventricular pressure; if severe, can produce cyanosis by right-to-left shunt at atrial level (patent foramen ovale or ASD)

What are the signs and symptoms?	1. Mild-to-moderate stenosis: no symptoms 2. Severe stenosis: cyanosis, reduced exercise capacity 3. Systolic ejection murmur, may have click
What are the radiographic findings?	Most are normal, but some may have a prominent main PA segment
What other diagnostic studies are used?	1. ECG: may be normal or may show RAD, RVH 2. Echocardiography; Doppler assesses severity of obstruction 3. Cardiac catheterization if obstruction severe; balloon valvuloplasty for therapy if severe
What is the treatment?	1. Mild-to-moderate stenosis: none 2. Severe valve stenosis: valvuloplasty by catheterization or by open operation 3. Severe infundibular stenosis (double-chambered RV): operative removal of obstructing muscle bundles
What are the complications of repair?	Complications are few—some children may have pulmonary insufficiency
What is the outcome?	Mild-to-moderate stenosis: normal cardiac function Severe stenosis: good surgical and catheterization results

COARCTATION OF THE AORTA

What is it?	A CHD consisting of a narrowed area of the aortic arch at the level of the ductus arteriosus (or ligamentum)
It represents what percent of all CHDs?	8%
Is it more common in males or females?	Males, by a 2–5 to 1 ratio

What is the physiologic result?

1. Obstruction to systemic cardiac output
2. Upper body hypertension
3. LVH
4. Collateral vessels develop to distribute blood to lower body

What are the signs and symptoms?

Mild obstruction: no symptoms
Moderate-to-severe obstruction: CHF

What are findings on examination of pulses?

Pulses are diminished in lower extremities and there is a time delay (lag) between brachial and femoral pulse waves.

What are the radiographic findings?

1. Classic finding is a **reverse "3" sign** of dilated ascending artery, coarctation segment, and descending aorta
2. **Rib notching** from dilated intercostal vessels

What other diagnostic studies are used?

1. Physical exam: feel pulses and take blood pressure in all extremities
2. ECG may be normal; infants may have RVH and older children may have LVH
3. Echocardiography may be diagnostic
4. Catheterization: "gold standard" for diagnosis

What is the treatment?

Medical: management of CHF until surgical repair
Surgical options include:
1. Subclavian flap angioplasty
2. Resection of coarct segment with end-to-end anastomosis
3. Graft placement
4. Interventional catheterization with balloon dilatation

What are the complications of repair?

Recoarctation from scarring
Residual gradient (native arch is small)
Paradoxical hypertension in 25%
Postcoarctectomy syndrome: abdominal pain and bleeding postsurgery

What are some associated cardiac anomalies?	50% also have bicuspid aortic valve; also commonly associated with VSD and less often with mitral valve disease (which affects outcome)
What is the outcome?	Generally good, but follow-up is necessary to monitor for restenosis, hypertension, endocarditis, and aneurysm formation

BACTERIAL ENDOCARDITIS

What is it?	An inflammatory process caused by a bacterial infection of a valve, endocardium, or blood vessel; process can be subacute or fulminant, depending on bacterial agent
What are the most common etiologic agents?	*Streptococcus viridans* and *Staphylococcus aureus*, accounting for about 80% of cases
What is the physiologic result?	May have acute valvular dysfunction; CHF
What are the signs and symptoms?	Fever Peripheral embolization Nonspecific symptoms (e.g., myalgia, arthralgia, malaise) New or changing heart murmur
What diagnostic studies are used?	1. Blood cultures 2. Measure acute phase reactants (suggestive, not diagnostic) 3. Echocardiogram–diagnostic when large intracardiac vegetation is present, but usually not diagnostic
What is the treatment?	1. Antibiotic treatment of identified pathogen; generally at least 4 weeks intravenously 2. Surgical valve replacement for intractable heart failure
How can it be prevented?	Antibiotic prophylaxis is recommended at the time of surgical or dental procedures in children with any CHD or conditions at risk for endocarditis.

What are the outcomes?	Streptococcal endocarditis generally has a good outcome; staphylococcal and fungal endocarditis have high morbidity and mortality rates.

ACUTE RHEUMATIC FEVER

What is it?	Rare inflammatory complication following infection with Group A β-hemolytic streptococcus (usually pharyngitis); multiple organ systems may be affected by the inflammatory vasculitis; it is the most common cause of acquired heart disease in children
What is the physiologic result?	Inflammation may cause carditis (acutely) and valvular dysfunction (chronically).
What are the most common results of acute rheumatic fever carditis?	Mitral and aortic valve insufficiency

What are Jones criteria?

Major:
  Polyarthritis
  Carditis
  Chorea
  Erythema marginatum
  Subcutaneous nodules
Minor:
  Arthralgia
  Fever
  Laboratory evidence of inflammation [elevated erythrocyte sedimentation rate (ESR) or C-reactive protein (CRP)]
  Prolonged PR interval

What is required for diagnosis?	Two major Jones criteria, or one major and two minor Jones criteria with evidence of previous streptococcal infection

What diagnostic studies are used?

1. Throat culture
2. ASO titer, Anti DNase B titer
3. ESR, CRP
4. ECG
5. Echocardiogram to evaluate evidence of carditis (atrial insufficiency, mitral regurgitation)

What is the treatment?	Treat streptococcal pharyngitis Treat inflammation with high dosage of aspirin for 4–8 weeks or steroids for 2–3 weeks Treat CHF if present
What long-term treatment is required?	After initial treatment, patients should remain on chronic (i.e., lifelong) penicillin therapy to prevent future acute rheumatic fever (secondary prevention). Patients should also receive subacute bacterial endocarditis prophylaxis when appropriate.
What are the outcomes?	Generally very good; rarely, severe carditis may cause severe valvular dysfunction that requires valve replacement.

MYOCARDITIS

What is it?	An infection of the heart muscle
What causes it?	Eighty percent of cases are **viral.** Bacterial agents are the second most common cause. Most common viruses isolated are coxsackie, influenza, and ECHO.
What is the physiologic result?	Inflammation of cardiac muscle with cellular infiltrate
What are the signs and symptoms?	Fever, tachycardia and dysrhythmia, heart failure
What diagnostic studies are used?	Viral cultures and myocardial biopsy
What is the treatment?	Supportive care; use of steroids is controversial
What are the outcomes?	Generally good with improvement of CHF; however, myocarditis may proceed to development of dilated cardiomyopathy

CARDIOMYOPATHY

Hypertrophic Cardiomyopathy

What is it?
Cardiac disease characterized by markedly thickened LV

What is the etiology?
Altered cardiac myosin; certain gene defects are associated with severe disease and sudden death

What is the physiologic result?
Impaired filling secondary to thick (stiff) heart; there may also be significant left ventricular outflow obstruction

What are the signs and symptoms?
Sudden death may be first indication of disease
Systolic ejection murmur if there is significant outflow obstruction
Dysrhythmia
Exercise limitation

What diagnostic studies are used?
1. ECG: which may reflect LVH and T-wave abnormalities
2. Echocardiogram

What is the medical treatment?
Some patients improve when treated with β-blockers or calcium channel blockers. However, agents that reduce ventricular preload or afterload or stimulate cardiac contraction may worsen outflow obstruction. Therefore, diuretics, vasodilators, and digoxin are usually contraindicated.

What is the surgical treatment?
Some centers advocate:
1. Myotomy, or for severe outflow obstruction, myectomy
2. Mitral valve replacement
3. Pacemaker placement

What is the outcome?
Variable–most patients are diagnosed as adults and remain stable with low rate of sudden death. The prognosis is worse for those diagnosed as children or those in a family with high rate of sudden death.

Dilated Cardiomyopathy

What is it?	Cardiac disease characterized by dilated, poorly contractile LV
What causes cardiomyopathy?	Cause is generally unknown, but is most likely secondary to myocarditis
What is the physiologic result?	CHF
What are the signs and symptoms?	1. Pulmonary congestion 2. Hepatomegaly 3. Murmur: absent or soft S_3 present
What are the radiographic findings?	Cardiomegaly Increased pulmonary vascular markings
What other diagnostic studies are used?	1. ECG: nonspecific findings 2. Echocardiogram demonstrates dilated chamber with decreased function
What is the treatment?	Medical: digitalis, diuretics, afterload reduction Surgical: orthotopic transplantation
What is the outcome?	Poor prognosis if diagnosed at older than 2 years of age

ARRYTHMIAS

What is an arrhythmia?	Heart rhythm other than regular sinus rhythm
What is sinus arrhythmia?	Marked variation of the sinus rate with breathing; it is normal and expected in children

Common Atrial Arrhythmias

What is sinus tachycardia?	Sinus rate greater than normal for age
What is sinus bradycardia?	Sinus rate less than lower limits of normal for age
When is a pacemaker needed?	When rate is very slow (i.e., < 30 beats/min) or cardiac output is compromised

What are premature atrial contractions (PACs)?	The QRS complex occurs early, without compensatory pause. P waves may change morphology.
Is treatment needed?	No
What is wandering atrial pacemaker?	P wave and PR intervals change; QRS complex is normal
Is treatment necessary?	Normal variant; no treatment necessary
What is atrial tachycardia (supraventricular tachycardia)?	Narrow QRS tachycardia; rate generally > 200 beats/min
What usually causes it?	Mostly idiopathic; 10%–20% may have Wolff-Parkinson-White syndrome (pre-excitation may occur via accessory pathway that bypasses the AV nodes)
Is it likely to resolve on its own?	The younger the patient, the more likely it is to resolve and not require long-term treatment.
What is the treatment?	Vagal stimulation; medical therapy with digoxin or β blockade; pharmacologic (adenosine) or electroshock cardioversion if unstable; ablation of accessory pathways available in some centers for older children
When do atrial fibrillation or flutter occur in children?	Occur rarely in pediatric patient, mostly postoperatively

Ventricular Arrhythmias

What are common ventricular arrhythmias?	1. Premature ventricular contractions: isolated wide QRS beats that all have the same morphology (shape); can occur in 5% of normal children 2. All other ventricular arrhythmias are rare and require evaluation
What is wide QRS tachycardia?	Considered ventricular tachycardia until proven otherwise

What is the differential diagnosis?	Electrolyte disturbance, drug toxicity (think digoxin), myocarditis, and myocardial ischemia

MITRAL VALVE PROLAPSE

What is it?	Condition in which the posterior mitral leaflet has excessive movement after closure; commonly overdiagnosed in healthy children
With what conditions may it be associated?	Connective tissue diseases, such as Marfan syndrome
Is it more common in males or females?	Females
What is the physiologic result?	Normal physiology; occasionally children present with nonexertional chest pain
What are the signs and symptoms?	1. Midsystolic click 2. Late systolic murmur of mitral insufficiency may be present (louder with standing) 3. Mitral valve prolapse has been associated with anxiety, palpitations, and chest pain
What are the radiographic findings?	Normal
What other diagnostic studies are used?	1. ECG: may have repolarization abnormalities or dysrhythmia 2. Echocardiogram: for diagnosis and to assess for mitral insufficiency
What is the treatment?	Antibiotic prophylaxis during surgical or dental procedures to prevent endocarditis if mitral regurgitation is present; treatment with β-blockers may decrease chest pain and palpitations
What are the outcomes?	It has been associated with endocarditis, dysrhythmia, and sudden death in adults. In childhood, it appears to be benign in the absence of connective tissue disease.

AORTIC STENOSIS

What is it?	CHD in which there is obstruction of left ventricular output caused by a narrow aortic valve
What are the three types?	Valvular, subvalvular and supravalvular; valvular stenosis is most common and secondary to bicuspid or unicuspid valve
It represents what percent of all CHDs?	5%
Is it more common in males or females?	Males
What is the physiologic result?	1. Obstruction causes increased LV pressure and muscle hypertrophy 2. Ascending aorta dilated 3. If aortic stenosis is severe, it may develop "failure" or LV dilation 4. Stenotic aortic valves also frequently insufficient (aortic insufficiency)
What are the symptoms?	Mild-to-moderate AS: none Severe AS: congestive heart failure, exercise intolerance, chest pain, syncope
Physical signs?	Harsh systolic ejection murmur heard best at right upper sternal border with radiation to neck; high-pitched diastolic blowing murmur along left sternal border if aortic insufficiency is present
What are the radiographic findings?	May show cardiomegaly with dilated ascending aorta
What other diagnostic studies are used?	1. ECG: classically shows LVH; severe aortic stenosis has LVH criteria with negative T waves in lateral precordial leads (LVH with strain) 2. Echocardiography assesses valve anatomy and gradient by Doppler 3. Cardiac catheterization: "gold standard" for determining severity and valve area

What is the treatment?	Mild-to-moderate defect: none
	Severe defect: interventional catheterization or surgical valvuloplasty
	Goal is to try and reduce aortic stenosis gradient without producing aortic insufficiency
	Mechanical valve replacement is delayed as long as possible to avoid multiple operations (growing child) and anticoagulation complications
What are the complications of repair?	Residual stenosis; valvular insufficiency
What are the outcomes?	Severe aortic stenosis diagnosed in infancy has poor prognosis and requires multiple procedures throughout childhood with fairly high morbidity. Bicuspid aortic valve may be the most common CHD; it is generally not stenotic in childhood (systolic ejection click on PE) but is the most common cause of aortic stenosis in adulthood.

ATRIOVENTRICULAR CANAL (AVC) DEFECT

What is it?	A CHD derived from failure of endocardial cushion development
What are the two types?	1. Complete: inlet VSD, primum ASD, and common atrioventricular valve
	2. Partial: primum ASD and cleft mitral valve
With which genetic defect is AVC defect commonly associated?	Trisomy 21
AVC defect represents what percent of CHD?	2%
What is physiologic result of complete AVC defect?	Left-to-right shunt at combined atrial–ventricular septal defect with pulmonary congestion and elevation of pulmonary artery pressures

Of partial AVC defect? Left-to-right shunt with ASD physiology

What are the signs and symptoms of complete AVC defect? Usually failure to thrive and CHF caused by pulmonary overcirculation; murmur often soft and nonspecific

Of partial AVC defect? Usually asymptomatic; systolic murmur of increased pulmonary flow and holosystolic murmur of mitral insufficiency

What are the radiographic findings? Cardiomegaly with increased vascular markings

What other diagnostic studies are used?
1. ECG: classically demonstrates superior QRS axis (QRS positive in lead I and negative in lead AVF)
2. Echocardiography for diagnosis
3. Cardiac catheterization for hemodynamic data before intracardiac repair

What is the treatment?
Medical: manage CHF until surgical correction
Surgical:
1. Complete AVC: patch closure of ASD, VSD, and construction of a tricuspid valve and mitral valve from common AV valve tissue
2. Partial AVC: patch closure of ASD and repair of cleft in mitral valve

What are the most common complications of complete AVC defect? Mitral insufficiency or mitral stenosis from reconstruction; if severe, it may require mechanical valve replacement

Of partial AVC defect? Residual mitral insufficiency

What are the outcomes?
Residual defects are common following surgical repair.
If AVC defect is associated with trisomy 21, life expectancy is reduced to 40–50 years of age.
Fifty percent of children with trisomy 21 have congenital heart defects–VSD and ASD are most common, followed by AVC defect and tetralogy of Fallot.

Respiratory and Thoracic Disorders

CONGENITAL DIAPHRAGMATIC HERNIA (CDH)

What is it?
A congenital defect in the diaphragm due to failure of the pleuroperitoneal canal to close at 8 weeks' gestation

What is a Bochdalek hernia?
A type of hernia most commonly referred to when speaking of CDH; it is a posterolateral defect; 15% have an intact sac

What is a Morgagni hernia?
An anterior, parasternal defect; it is usually smaller than a Bochdalek, tends to have an intact sac, and does not have the pulmonary and systemic ramifications of a Bochdalek hernia

Which is more common?
Bochdalek

What is the incidence?
About 1 in 4,000 live births

What percent of Bochdalek hernias are on the left?
85%

What is the distribution of males and females?
1:1 male-to-female ratio

What are the anatomic ramifications of Bochdalek hernia?
The abdominal contents remain in the chest. The lung on the involved side is small and hypoplastic, but the lung on the opposite side may also have evidence of hypoplasia. The abdominal cavity may be smaller than normal. There is **malrotation of the bowel.**

Of Morgagni hernia?
The viscera may be in the hernia. Chest structures are not significantly affected.

What are the physiologic ramifications of a Bochdalek hernia?

Bochdalek CDH was once believed to be a surgical emergency.
It is now understood that pulmonary vascular hyperreactivity (and therefore pulmonary hypertension) and pulmonary hypoplasia are the major complications.

Of Morgagni hernia?

Usually none, unless the hernia is very large

What are signs and symptoms of a Bochdalek hernia?

Respiratory distress usually immediately at birth; the infant's chest appears expanded, with scaphoid abdomen; occasionally, a child may survive undetected in the perinatal stage, but then present days to weeks later with GI difficulties

Of Morgagni hernia?

May be asymptomatic; or, child may have mild respiratory symptoms or GI difficulties

What are prenatal ultrasound findings of Bochdalek hernia?

A multicystic appearance in the involved chest; there may be polyhydramnios

What are perinatal radiographic findings in a Bochdalek hernia?

Chest radiograph shows viscera in chest. NG tube is often seen curling into the involved chest field if the stomach is herniated into chest.

Why are radiographic findings in a Morgagni hernia more subtle?

Because the defect is anterior

TREATMENT

What constitutes the initial management of a Bochdalek hernia?

Intubation, oxygenation, ventilation, sedation, paralysis

What are the ventilation goals?

Infant requires 100% O_2 and hyperventilation with a conventional or high oscillatory ventilator to keep postductal pH in 7.50–7.60 range and Pco_2 in 25-30 mm Hg range to avoid pulmonary shunting. These infants are extremely tenuous and even very small changes in ventilation or oxygenation parameters may send the infant into a lethal respiratory spiral.

What are some commonly used vasodilators?

Tozalozine, prostacyclin, and currently nitric oxide; the latter is promising, but none are the panacea

What may be necessary if conventional therapy fails?

ECMO

What is ECMO?

Extra Corporeal Membrane Oxygenation; essentially, it is a lung bypass machine

What is the primary goal of ECMO?

To allow the lung to grow and the pulmonary hypertension to subside

What is involved in surgical correction?

Surgical correction is performed via subcostal (or occasionally chest) incision with closure of the diaphragm after reduction of the viscera. A patch may be needed to close the diaphragm and/or abdomen.

When should surgical repair be performed?

Most surgeons still undertake repair within 48 hours of initial diagnosis. Repair may be undertaken prior to, during, or after ECMO if ECMO is needed. Opinions are divided about the appropriate timing for surgical correction in general.

What is the "honeymoon period"?

After surgical correction, the baby improves briefly, but then declines again.

What is treatment for a Morgagni hernia?

Treatment is surgical closure of the defect with routine supportive pre and post-operative care. This is usually done through a transverse substernal incision.

PROGNOSIS

What is the outcome for Bochdalek hernia?

50%–75% survive, depending on the medical/surgical center.
Some infants may have long-term respiratory deficiency, GI reflux, or CNS sequelae from hypoxia.

What percentage of infants with CDH placed on ECMO survive?   ~60%

What is the prognosis for Morgagni hernias?   Excellent

EMPHYSEMA

What is it?

An enlargement of the airspaces distal to the terminal bronchioles due to either dilatation or destruction of the surrounding walls

What is the pathophysiology?

1. **Hyperexpansion of distal airspace** to fill space left by loss of adjacent lung volume from resection or atelectasis (**"compensatory emphysema"**)
2. **Obstruction of gas egress** by foreign body, mass (e.g., adenopathy), or mucosal edema (e.g., asthma)
3. **Destruction of airspace walls**, typically from presence of proteases in excess of proteinase-inhibitor activity either because of a deficiency in inhibitor concentration/activity (as in **α-1-antitrypsin deficiency**) or an excess of protease concentration/activity (as in **cystic fibrosis**, **bronchopulmonary dysplasia**, or **cigarette smoking**)

What are the signs and symptoms?

They vary with underlying etiology. A child may be asymptomatic (e.g., compensatory emphysema following lobectomy). Alternatively, symptoms may include cough and dyspnea, due to either massive focal enlargement with restriction of adjacent normal lung or to the underlying etiology (e.g., α-1-antitrypsin deficiency). There may be decreased breath sounds and/or an inspiratory phase lag over the involved region.

How is it diagnosed?

Radiograph, although delineation of etiology may require other measures; obstructive emphysema can be distinguished from the other forms by obtaining images (plain or fluoroscopic) during expiration, because the increase in lung volume will persist; decubitus positioning may be used for this purpose

What does a radiograph show?

Area of **hyperlucency** and **decreased lung (vascular) markings**; may have associated contiguous areas of opacity (either primary or compressive atelectasis) and/or mediastinal shift

By contrast, in asthma, the hyperlucency is generalized with compression of the mediastinum and flattening of the diaphragm.

What are four etiologies?

1. **Congenital** (usually restricted to one lobe)
2. **Partial airway obstruction,** such as:
   Foreign body
   Extrinsic compression (e.g., mediastinal tumor, adenopathy, vascular ring)
   Tumor or polyp (rare in children)
3. **Atelectasis/iatrogenic** (e.g., postlobectomy or postpneumonectomy)
4. **Inflammatory/underlying medical disease,** such as:
   Cystic fibrosis
   α-1-antitrypsin deficiency (rarely causes lung disease before late adolescence)
   Bronchopulmonary dysplasia
   Asthma

Treatment?

Depends on etiology:
1. Congenital: remove involved lobe
2. Obstruction: remove foreign body or relieve obstruction
3. All other causes: good pulmonary toilet with management of underlying condition

LOBAR EMPHYSEMA

What is it?	Overdistention of a histologically normal lung lobe
What are the causes?	Traditionally, it is thought to be caused by poorly developed cartilage of the involved bronchus, creating a "ball-valve" effect; may also be acquired
What are the symptoms?	Mild-to-moderate tachypnea and failure to thrive
How is it diagnosed?	Chest radiograph and possibly CT scan
Treatment?	Usually resection of involved lobe; acquired forms may resolve spontaneously

LUNG CYSTS

What are they?	Simple cysts of the lung that most commonly reflect injury to the lung
What are three common causes of injury to the lung?	1. Trauma 2. Mechanical ventilation, particularly in premature infants 3. Cysts caused by disease processes, such as infection or cystic fibrosis

PNEUMONIA/PNEUMONITIS

What is it?	It is an inflammatory (pneumonitis) and/or infectious (pneumonia), exudative process involving the distal airspace. The term is also applied to processes involving the lung interstitium ("interstitial pneumonia/pneumonitis"). It should be distinguished from processes involving the trachea (tracheitis), bronchi (bronchitis), and distal airways (bronchiolitis).
What is the incidence?	It varies with age. Risk is roughly 5% per year in the preschool age group. It is also increased in institutional settings (e.g., dorms, military).

What are the signs and symptoms?

They vary with age and etiologic organism:
1. Commonly associated with cough, fever, and chills, but child also may have chest pain, vomiting, diarrhea, abdominal pain (can mimic gallbladder disease or **appendicitis!**)
2. On physical exam: **tachypnea,** evidence of increased work of breathing (e.g., nasal flaring, retractions).

What do percussion, auscultation, and oximetry show?

Percussion may demonstrate an area of dullness, either from consolidation or associated pleural effusion. **Auscultation** may reveal areas of decreased breath sounds and inspiratory crackles/rales; however, auscultation may reveal normal breath sounds, especially in small infants. **Oximetry** usually reveals mild-to-severe desaturation, depending on severity of process.

How is it diagnosed?

Diagnosis can be made clinically, although radiograph should be used for confirmation in immunocompromised and severely ill children and children with a history of repeated episodes.

How is the etiologic agent determined?

By blood or sputum culture, although in mild cases in an otherwise healthy child this is probably unnecessary; identification is more urgent in the immunocompromised child, thus bronchoscopy or biopsy for diagnosis may be warranted

What are the etiologies?

They vary with age and immune status. In all groups, however, **viral pathogens are most common**. Typical bacterial etiologies are as follows:

Newborn: Group B strep, gram-negative bacilli, *Chlamydia*

1 month–6 years: *Streptococcus pneumoniae, Haemophilus influenzae*

Adolescents: *Mycoplasma, S. pneumoniae*

Hospitalized or immunocompromised children: gram-negative rods (e.g., *Pseudomonas, Klebsiella, E. coli, Serratia*), fungi (*Candida*), and nonbacterial agents (*Pneumocystis*, CMV, EBV).

If aspiration is a possibility, consider anaerobes as well. **Geographic or exposure considerations** may dictate consideration of other agents, such as fungi (coccidiomycosis, blastomycosis, histoplasmosis) or TB.

Treatment?

Most healthy children can be treated as outpatients with **oral antibiotics** (e.g., amoxicillin ± clavulanate, erythromycin, cephalosporin) and **antipyretics**. Generally, cough suppressants are avoided, but they may be acceptable at bedtime to facilitate sleep. Severely ill children (i.e., those with high fever, dehydration, intractable cough, hypoxemia) may to be admitted to a hospital for IV antibiotics and supportive therapy (e.g., IV fluids, oxygen, chest PT). **Any immunocompromised child should be admitted.**

What are some complications?

Pleural effusion, empyema, pulmonary abscess, respiratory failure, bronchiectasis (more common with recurrent episodes, but may occur acutely and be reversible)

AIRWAY FOREIGN BODY

Where do foreign bodies lodge?

Usually below the carina; in toddlers, foreign bodies lodge with equal incidence in either mainstem; in older children, they usually lodge in the right mainstem

What are the symptoms?

Coughing, gagging, choking, wheezing; an asymptomatic interlude may follow

What are the radiographic findings?	1. Either hyper- or hypoinflation of affected lung may occur. 2. Foreign body will be visible if radio-opaque.
Treatment?	Removal via rigid bronchoscopy, preferably with the patient breathing spontaneously under anesthesia
What are the sequelae if the foreign body is not removed?	Pneumonitis/pneumonia Abscess Bronchiectasis Pulmonary hemorrhage Erosion and perforation

CYSTIC FIBROSIS (CF)

What causes CF?	A defect in the cystic fibrosis transmembrane regulator protein
How is CF transmitted?	Autosomal recessive trait; 1 in 20 Caucasians carry the gene
How common is CF?	About 1 in 2,000 Caucasian births; also found in other populations
What is the pathophysiology?	Abnormal, thickened secretions in a variety of organs that cause inspissation and mucous buildup
How does it present?	1. Meconium ileus in the neonate 2. Recurrent bronchitis/pneumonia 3. Malabsorption with failure to thrive 4. Male infertility (also, about 5%–10% of males will have an absent vas deferens)
How common is meconium ileus in CF?	**10%** of CF infants have meconium ileus; **99%** of infants with meconium ileus have CF.
How is CF diagnosed?	Usually via an elevated sweat chloride concentration; DNA testing for specific mutations may also be used
What is the most common gene mutation in Caucasians?	ΔF508, although there is a wide variety of other mutations

Treatment?	Nutritional support
	Pancreatic enzymes
	Chest physical therapy
	Antibiotics
	Bronchodilators
	Lung transplant is now being attempted
	Gene therapy is in experimental stages
What is the outcome?	With appropriate therapy, many patients live into adulthood. End-stage event is usually respiratory failure.

TRACHEOMALACIA

What is it?	Suboptimal integrity of the tracheal wall and cartilage rings that leads to partial collapse of the trachea upon inspiration
Who gets this?	Neonates; it reflects incomplete maturation of the tracheal structures
What are some associated conditions?	It can be a primary condition or exacerbated by other conditions, such as esophageal atresia or vascular rings.
What are the signs and symptoms?	Infant may present with inspiratory stridor. If severe, infant may have "dying spells," which are periods of prolonged apnea resulting in cyanosis and requiring stimulation for resolution.
How is it diagnosed?	**Fluoroscopic** exam of the airway may reveal collapsing nature of the trachea. **Bronchoscopy** will reveal collapse of the airway or some point of compression.
Treatment?	If condition is primary, it is usually self-resolving. If associated with exacerbating process, then that process needs to be corrected (e.g., division of vascular ring). Occasionally, aortopexy is done to enhance opening of the trachea.

PNEUMOTHORAX

| **What is it?** | Separation of the visceral pleura from the parietal pleura, resulting in the presence of air in the pleural space |

What are the most common causes in infants?	Barotrauma, hyaline membrane disease, bronchopulmonary dysplasia
In older children?	Trauma, rupture of apical bleb, cystic fibrosis, severe coughing, asthma
What are the symptoms?	Mild-to-severe respiratory distress; a small pneumothorax may be asymptomatic
What is a tension pneumothorax?	Air collection in the pleural space under pressure, creating a shift in the mediastinum, compression of the opposite lung, and hemodynamic compromise. **THIS IS A LIFE-THREATENING CONDITION!**
How is pneumothorax diagnosed?	Chest radiograph. Occasionally, the supine trauma victim will have pneumothorax discovered during a CT scan, because the air is anterior in this situation.
Treatment?	A small, asymptomatic, pneumothorax may be allowed to resolve spontaneously. Most commonly, chest tube placement is required until air leak seals. If pneumothorax is associated with trauma, it is best to place a chest tube, regardless of the size of the pneumothorax.
How is recurrent pneumothorax treated?	Instillation of a sclerosing agent, such as talc or tetracycline, via a chest tube or thoracoscopy Resection of apical bleb or other site of parenchymal leak via thoracoscopy or thoracotomy
How is tension pneumothorax treated?	**Immediate placement of a chest tube.** If a tube is not available, a large bore angiocatheter or needle should be placed in the **second intercostal space** anteriorly for decompression.

CHYLOTHORAX

What is it?	An accumulation of lymph fluid (chyle) in the thorax; it can be congenital or acquired
What are the common congenital causes?	Either **abnormalities of the thoracic duct** or **birth trauma**

What are six common causes of acquired chylothorax?

1. Trauma
2. Operative injury (especially during cardiothoracic procedures)
3. Neoplasm
4. Thrombosis of subclavian vein or superior vena cava
5. Lymphangiomatosis
6. Severe coughing

What are the symptoms?	Respiratory insufficiency or distress if collection is large enough
How is it diagnosed?	Chylothorax appears as a radio-opaque fluid collection on chest radiograph. Diagnosis is confirmed by thoracentesis and analysis of the fluid.

What are five typical characteristics of chyle?

1. Appearance may be milky or straw colored
2. Lymphocyte predominance
3. Protein content ≥ 5 g/dl
4. Fat content ≥ 400 mg/dl
5. Triglyceride level ≥ 110 mg/100 ml

Initial treatment?

1. Thoracentesis with change to a low fat diet or parenteral nutrition
2. Chest tube drainage or repeated thoracentesis as necessary

What are three surgical options that may be used for refractory cases?

1. Right thoracotomy with ligation of thoracic duct
2. Thoracoscopy of affected side with clipping of leak and/or application of fibrin glue
3. Pleuroperitoneal shunt placement

ASTHMA

What is it?

A chronic lung disease defined as reversible narrowing or obstruction of large and middle airways due to hyperresponsiveness to various immunologic and nonimmunologic stimuli

What is the prevalence?

It is the most common chronic disease in childhood. Its prevalence in the United States is **5%–7%**.

What is believed to be the pathophysiology of asthma?

Airway hyperresponsiveness is the central feature of asthma, resulting in bronchial smooth muscle constriction, mucus hypersecretion, and mucosal inflammation. Asthmatic lungs are believed to be more sensitive to challenges by allergens, physical stimuli (e.g., cold air, exercise) and environmental triggers (e.g., viruses).

What are the mediators of asthma?

Mediators are released by **eosinophils, mast cells,** and **alveolar macrophages**. The mediators include **histamine, eosinophil granular products, leukotrienes, prostaglandins,** and **thromboxanes**.

What are extrinsic and intrinsic asthma?

Extrinsic asthma is caused by allergens. Common allergens are pollens, dust mites, and animal dander.
Intrinsic asthma is nonallergic or non-IgE mediated; common triggers include cold air, odors, smoke, and viruses.

What are the signs and symptoms?

Mild: wheezing or coughing at night or with exercise
Moderate: wheezing at rest
Advanced: increased respiratory rate, retractions, cyanosis, decreased or absent inspiratory breath sounds, increased accessory muscle use due to the need to maintain lungs in a hyperinflated state, marked expiratory wheezing, pulsus paradoxus, agitation

What are the typical findings on chest radiograph?

1. Pulmonary hyperinflation with flattening of the diaphragm
2. Increased AP diameter
3. Increased lung markings due to inflammation changes
4. Atelectasis

In exacerbations of asthma, what would you expect the blood pH to be?

Initially a **respiratory alkalosis** exists due to hyperventilation. As respiratory effort worsens, CO_2 retention occurs and **respiratory acidosis** can develop. Finally, a **metabolic acidosis** can develop secondary to increased lactic acid and ketosis due to increased muscular effort and poor oxygen intake.

What is the differential diagnosis of wheezing?

Common diagnoses: bronchial asthma; foreign body; cystic fibrosis; infection, especially upper respiratory infection; laryngotracheomalacia; bronchiolitis; and bronchopulmonary dysplasia
Uncommon diagnoses: vascular rings, laryngeal webs, enlarged lymph node, and bronchostenosis

What are four goals of treatment of asthma?

1. To maintain normal activity levels
2. To prevent symptoms, such as cough or nighttime shortness of breath
3. To prevent recurrent exacerbations
4. To avoid adverse effects from medication

What are the two major classes of pharmacotherapeutic agents?

1. **Bronchodilators:** β-adrenergic agonists, theophylline, anticholinergic agents
2. **Anti-inflammatory agents:** cromolyn sodium, nedocromil sodium, corticosteroids (oral or inhaled)

What are signs of theophylline overdose?

Early signs are insomnia, headache, nausea, and vomiting. High theophylline levels may cause seizure, coma, and death.

What factors can affect theophylline metabolism?

Age, immunizations, smoking, other medications, and infection

What are other treatment modalities besides medications?	Environmental control, patient education, and immunotherapy
What is exercise-induced asthma?	Airway narrowing that occurs minutes (5-10) after vigorous activity
How can it be prevented?	Treating patient with β_2-agonist or cromolyn before exercise

PECTUS DEFORMITY

PECTUS EXCAVATUM

What is pectus excavatum?	Also known as "funnel chest," this condition manifests as a significant depression of the sternum.
What is the etiology?	It is believed to be caused by an overgrowth of the cartilage connecting the sternum to the ribs.
What are the significant anatomic and physiologic effects?	The heart is shifted to the left, and in severe deformities, the lungs are compressed. Children may manifest symptoms of asthma or dyspnea on exertion. However, many children are asymptomatic.
What are common associated conditions?	Scoliosis Marfan syndrome Club foot Syndactylism Klippel-Feil syndrome Mitral valve prolapse
What are two indications for surgery?	1. Significant respiratory insufficiency 2. Cosmetic correction; children with uncorrected pectus deformity are often ridiculed by their peers and may be self-conscious
How is repair accomplished?	The offending cartilages are removed while the surrounding perichondrium is preserved. The sternum is then elevated by any of a number of different methods and secured. Often, a metal strut is placed substernally for support and is removed 3–6 months later. New cartilage grows back within the perichondrium in the appropriate position.

What is the outcome?	Uniformally the cosmetic and the physiologic results are quite good. Patients may return to full activity after 3–6 months.

PECTUS CARINATUM

What is pectus carinatum?	A condition in which the sternum protrudes; it is also a result of overgrowth of costal cartilages
What are associated conditions?	Congenital heart disease Marfanoid habitus Scoliosis Kyphosis Muscular/skeletal defects Asthma
Are these types of associated conditions more common in pectus carinatum or pectus excavatum?	Pectus carinatum
How is repair accomplished?	Similar to pectus excavatum, with depression and stabilization of the sternum

ESOPHAGEAL DUPLICATION CYST

What is it?	Congenital cyst arising from an abnormality in foregut development
What is the location?	Mediastinum; it may share a common wall with the esophagus
What is the histology?	Squamous epithelial lining, but may have ciliated mucosa with some cartilage in the wall
How does it present?	Respiratory distress, or it may be an incidental finding on radiograph
What are the radiographic findings?	Solid-appearing mediastinal mass
How is it diagnosed?	Chest radiograph, CT scan

Treatment?	Surgical excision via thoracotomy or thoracoscopy; if there is a common wall with the esophagus, cyst mucosa should be stripped from the common wall

BRONCHOGENIC CYST

What is it?	Congenital cyst arising from cells that become isolated during bronchial development
What are the two locations?	**Central:** near the hilum or mediastinum; usually solitary **Peripheral:** may be multiple
How does it present?	May be found incidentally on radiograph, or may cause respiratory distress
What are the radiographic findings of central and peripheral cysts?	**Central:** solid-appearing mass, or cystic lesion with air-fluid level **Peripheral:** multi-loculated appearance that may be confused with cystic adenomatoid malformation or even diaphragmatic hernia
How is it diagnosed?	Chest radiograph, CT scan
Treatment?	**Central:** surgical excision of cyst **Peripheral:** wedge resection or resection of involved lung lobe

PULMONARY SEQUESTRATION

What is it?	Mass of abnormal lung tissue receiving an abnormal (i.e., systemic) blood supply, with no communication with the tracheobronchial tree
What are two types?	1. **Intralobar** (90%): lies within the lobe of a lung; arterial supply is systemic; venous drainage may be systemic or pulmonary 2. **Extralobar** (10%): has its own pleura; may have immature parenchyma or an associated cystic adenomatous malformation; arterial supply and venous drainage may be systemic or pulmonary

What are the symptoms?	Usually asymptomatic at birth; serial bouts of pneumonia follow after 1 to 2 years
How is it diagnosed?	Chest radiograph, CT scan
Treatment?	Surgical excision; must be aware of systemic arterial supply, especially through the diaphragm
What are three associated anomalies?	1. Congenital heart defects 2. Congenital adenomatoid malformation 3. Arteriovenous malformation with shunting

CYSTIC ADENOMATOID MALFORMATION (CAM)

What is CAM?	Congenital cystic changes of the lung
What are the types?	I: Large, irregular cysts II: Smaller, more closely arranged cysts III: Dense, small cysts; may resemble fetal lung
What is the histology?	Cuboidal and low columnar epithelium; few mucogenic cells
How do they arise?	Excessive proliferation of bronchioles at the expense of alveoli
What are the symptoms?	May be an asymptomatic finding on radiograph **Respiratory distress** in infants if cysts are large (usually type II or III) Older children or adults may present with **infection**
How is it diagnosed?	Usually made by chest radiograph and CT scan; a CAM may sometimes be detected on prenatal ultrasound
Treatment?	Excision of affected lobe or lobes

EPIGLOTTITIS

What is it?

Rapidly progressive bacterial infection, causing acute inflammation and edema of the epiglottis and adjacent structures (aryepiglottic folds, arytenoids); also known as supraglottitis

Why is it important?

It is **life threatening**! Affected children may have sudden and complete airway obstruction.

Average age at presentation?

2–6 years of age; peak incidence is $3\frac{1}{2}$ years of age; however, infants, older children and adults are rarely affected

Is there seasonal incidence?

No

What are the causative agents?

Haemophilus influenzae type **B** is the primary cause. It is rarely caused by pneumococci, staphylococci, streptococci.

What is the classic presentation?

Previously well child with sudden onset of symptoms; 4–12-hour history of sore throat, high fever, dysphagia, irritability, or lethargy; symptoms continue to progress rapidly

What are the classic signs?

Child is febrile, toxic, and anxious appearing, with inspiratory stridor and in respiratory distress. Child often is leaning forward with an open mouth, drooling. Child usually is aphonic, but may have a muffled "hot potato" voice if speaking. Child prefers to sit in the tripod position.

What is the tripod position?

A sitting position in which the arms are extended in front of the body, supporting the trunk; neck is hyperextended with the chin protruding

Why does the child sit in this position?

It maximizes the size of the supraglottic airway.

Differential Dx?

See Croup (pg 219)

What is involved in the initial evaluation and management?

Quickly proceed with the epiglottitis protocol that has been established at your medical facility. This may involve:
1. Keeping the patient calm, with parents
2. Administering 100% O_2, without further agitating the child (parents can hold the child)
3. Assembling at bedside: CPR equipment, including resuscitation bag and mask, intubation equipment, and instruments for emergency thyroidotomy
4. Calling senior pediatrics, anesthesia, and otolaryngology staff to bedside
5. Taking patient (with parents) to OR for induction of anesthesia (if needed), placement of IVs, direct laryngoscopy, intubation, blood and epiglottis cultures (equipment and expertise for an emergency tracheostomy should be present)
6. Admitting to ICU—remember that not every child with epiglottitis will have the classic signs and symptoms. **It is better to initiate a "false" epiglottitis drill than to miss this disease.**

What laboratory and diagnostic studies are ordered?

Only after the epiglottitis protocol has been performed and the patient has a secure airway:
1. Blood cultures, which usually are positive for *H. influenzae* type B
2. WBC, which may be moderately increased with a left shift
3. Lateral neck radiographs, which show a thickened epiglottis ("thumb sign") and a distended hypopharynx

What should you NOT do when evaluating the patient?

Do *not* agitate the child. Do *not* make the child lie supine. Do *not* try to visualize the pharynx or epiglottis with a tongue blade.

No labs, needle sticks, or radiographs should be used before establishing epiglottis protocol. (**All of these things can lead to airway obstruction and/or cardiopulmonary arrest.**)

How is diagnosis confirmed?

Diagnosis is confirmed later by seeing an edematous cherry-red epiglottis on endoscopy.

What is the treatment?

Maintain adequate (usually artificial) airway until inflammation and edema resolve; often 36–72 hours

Parenteral antibiotics directed against *H. influenzae*, assuming this is the cause; classically, ampicillin and chloramphenicol have been used, but now a third-generation cephalosporin (e.g., cefotaxime or ceftriazone) is also an option; treat for 7–10 days

Rifampin prophylaxis to treat carrier state and prevent further spread of disease

When is rifampin prophylaxis used?

When:
1. *H. influenzae* is the etiologic agent
2. Patient has nonimmunized or immunocompromised household contacts < 4 years of age
3. Patient has day care (> 25 hours/week) contacts < 2 years of age

Who needs it?

All household and day care contacts (if they include children) and the patient, immediately before discharge

Is the *H. influenzae* (HIB) vaccine decreasing the incidence of childhood epiglottitis?

Yes

CROUP

What is it?

Viral infection of the upper and lower respiratory tract that causes subglottic inflammation (laryngotracheobronchitis)

What are the classic features?

Stridor and barking cough

What is the usual age at presentation?

3 months to 3 years of age; peak incidence at 2 years of age

What is the epidemiology?

Males > females
Peak occurrence in fall and winter (epidemics); also occurs in spring

What are the causative agents?

Parainfluenza virus, especially type 1, is the primary cause. Others include influenza virus, respiratory syncytial virus, adenovirus, *Mycoplasma pneumoniae*, and measles virus.

What are the symptoms and history?

It is often preceded by several days of upper respiratory symptoms, followed by hoarseness and a deepening, nonproductive cough that sounds similar to barking or is "seal-like." Symptoms may fluctuate, occurring on and off over several days and **worsening at night**. Stridor and mild dyspnea may occur and usually resolve in a few hours. However, respiratory distress can become severe.

What is the usual presentation?

Varies—children may be alert and comfortable, with only mild URI symptoms and an intermittent barking cough or they can present with agitation, hypoxia, stridor, and respiratory distress (tachypnea, nasal flaring, retractions); most cases are mild

What is the differential Dx?

1. **Infection:** epiglottitis, bacterial tracheitis, peritonsillar abscess, retropharyngeal abscess, diphtheria
2. **Foreign body/aspiration**
3. **Angioneurotic edema/anaphylaxis**
4. **Neoplasm**
5. **Trauma:** burns/thermal injury, blunt trauma

How is the diagnosis made?

Clinically—**try not to agitate the child, particularly if the symptoms are severe** (see Epiglottitis, pg 216)

What diagnostic studies are used?

Perform studies *only* if patient is not in significant respiratory distress:
1. Anterior-posterior neck radiographs may show a "pencil tip" or **"steeple sign"** of the subglottic trachea. Do *not* use a radiograph to make definitive management decisions in a patient with an unstable airway.
2. Lab studies (e.g., CBC) usually not helpful

Why do some children improve spontaneously?

Because of natural fluctuations in the disease

Exposure to cold night air is thought to help, but this is largely anecdotal.

What is the treatment for mild cases?

1. Humidification: not clearly proved useful but still the first line of treatment; can be via cool mist humidifier, warm vaporizer, or steam from a bathroom shower
2. Cool night air

What is the treatment for severe cases?

For more severe symptoms requiring hospitalization:
1. **Airway support**, including O_2 and intubation if necessary; pulse oximetry is helpful, but clinical assessment and close observation are of paramount importance
2. **Humidification**: cool mist or croup tent
3. **Racemic epinephrine** may cause rapid improvement in symptoms. If used, patient must be hospitalized because of **rebound phenomenon**—stridor and respiratory distress may abruptly return when effect of epinephrine wears off, usually within 2 hours.
4. **Corticosteroids** (dexamethasone): on admission

Do most cases of croup need hospitalization?	No. Most cases of croup can be managed at home. Symptoms typically resolve within a few days.
What is spasmodic croup?	A benign condition with recurrent episodes of stridor and barking cough; may be associated with viral illnesses; typically resolves spontaneously and is rarely associated with severe respiratory distress

PIERRE ROBIN MALFORMATION

What is it?	Congenital micrognathia
What may be associated findings?	Cleft palate and glossoptosis
What are the symptoms?	Respiratory distress may occur when the infant is supine. Feeding difficulties also may arise, especially with palate and tongue abnormalities.
What is the treatment?	1. For the micrognathia per se, proper positioning (prone) and possibly a nasopharyngeal tube usually allow appropriate respiration. The mandible grows faster than the child and is usually no longer a problem by 3 months of age. Rarely, suturing the tip of the tongue to the lower lip is needed to support a patent airway. 2. Surgical intervention will be necessary for palate abnormalities. A tracheostomy may be needed until repairs are completed. If feeding is very difficult, a gastrostomy tube may be needed.

CHOANAL ATRESIA

What is it?	Congenital persistence of a bony membrane across the nasopharyngeal passage
What are the symptoms?	Respiratory difficulty at birth, because infants prefer nasal breathing

How is it diagnosed?	Inability to pass a suction catheter into the pharynx via the nasal passages May be confirmed by contrast nasopharyngography
What is the treatment?	Initial treatment: maintenance of the oral airway until the infant can breath on its own Resection of the bony septum and placement of stents until the passage epithelializes

VOCAL CORD PARALYSIS

What is it?	Paralysis of one or both cords, which may be either congenital or acquired
What are four common causes of acquired vocal cord paralysis?	1. Birth trauma 2. Patent ductus arteriosus ligation 3. Increased intracranial pressure 4. Intracranial hemorrhage
Is unilateral or bilateral paralysis more common?	Unilateral
What are the symptoms?	May be minimal if paralysis is unilateral; however, bilateral paralysis may cause inspiratory and expiratory stridor, or frank respiratory distress
How is it diagnosed?	**Laryngoscopy** with the infant under light anesthesia allows visualization of cord movement, or lack thereof, during spontaneous breathing.
What is the treatment?	Most cases of paralysis resolve spontaneously after 4–6 weeks. However, tracheostomy may be needed to alleviate severe symptoms resulting from bilateral paralysis.

LARYNGEAL WEB

What is it?	Congenital abnormality of the glottic region resulting in a web-like lesion; webs present in varying sizes and thicknesses

What are the symptoms?	Range from mild inspiratory/expiratory stridor to frank distress
What is the treatment?	A thin web may be lysed with cautery or a laser. A thicker web may require more extensive reconstruction. Tracheostomy is necessary for treatment of a thick web.
What is laryngeal atresia?	Complete nonformation of the laryngeal area, which is incompatible with life unless there is a large trachea-esophageal fistula

BRANCHIAL CLEFT REMNANTS

What are they?	Remnants of branchial arches that are embryologic sources of head and neck structures
What forms may they take?	Cysts, sinuses, fistulae
What are the locations of the commonly found remnants?	**First branchial remnant:** lies anterior to the ear and may extend to the eustachian tube **Second branchial remnant:** begins in the midneck, anterior to the sternocleidomastoid muscle, and may extend up through the carotid bifurcation to the pharynx **Third branchial remnant:** begins superior to the medial portion of the clavicle and passes lateral to the carotid bifurcation, up toward the pharynx
What is the presentation?	Draining area, dimple, or mass at one of the three branchial remnant sites; infection may occur as first sign
What is the treatment?	Surgical excision; more than one incision may be needed for extensive lesions

THYROGLOSSAL DUCT REMNANT

What is it?	Remnant of embryologic path that the thyroid takes from the foramen cecum to its final position

What forms may it take?	Cyst (75%) Sinus (25%)
What is the presentation?	The child usually has an asymptomatic mass in the anterior midline of the neck. It may present as an infected, draining site. The mass moves upward with swallowing.
What is the treatment?	Surgical excision with a Sistrunk procedure: the cyst or sinus is excised widely along its tract to the base of the tongue; excision includes the middle third of the hyoid bone
Are thyroid function tests necessary?	If thyroid tissue is found in the excised tissue
Why?	It may represent the only thyroid tissue the child has, necessitating thyroid hormone replacement.

SUBGLOTTIC STENOSIS

What is it?	Narrowing of the subglottic region, which may be either **congenital** or **acquired**
How is it acquired?	Usually sequelae of a previously placed endotracheal tube that was too large or inappropriately secured
What are the symptoms?	Inspiratory or expiratory stridor; inflammation of any kind may cause frank distress
What is the treatment?	**Congenital:** usually supportive; infant will outgrow **Acquired:** if severe, may require tracheostomy, then appropriate surgical procedure (laryngotracheoplasty or anterior cricoid split)

19

Gastrointestinal Disorders

SHORT-GUT (SHORT-BOWEL) SYNDROME

What is it?

A clinical syndrome of nutrient malabsorption and excessive intestinal fluid and electrolyte losses that occurs following massive small intestinal loss or resection

What are the three most common causes in children?

1. Malrotation with midgut volvulus
2. Small intestinal atresia(s)
3. Necrotizing enterocolitis

Together, these three diagnoses account for nearly 90% of cases of childhood short-gut syndrome.

How much small intestine does an infant have?

A full-term infant has approximately **250 cm** of small intestine, whereas an adult has between 600 and 800 cm of small intestine. The diameter of the small intestine also increases from 1.5 cm during infancy to 3.5 cm during adulthood.

How much intestine does a child need to lose before developing short-gut syndrome?

There is no absolute amount of intestinal loss that defines short-gut syndrome. As much as 75% of the small intestine may be lost without serious long-term problems, provided the duodenum, terminal ileum, and ileocecal valve are spared. In contrast, the loss of 25% of the small intestine coupled with the loss of the terminal ileum and the ileocecal valve may cause significant difficulties.

What is the primary symptom?

Diarrhea

What are the clinical results?

Growth failure, protein-calorie malnutrition, recurrent dehydration, and a variety of nutritional deficits

Does it matter which part of the bowel is lost?

Yes. Loss of much of the jejunum may cause few long-term symptoms because the ileum "adapts." In contrast, the jejunum is less adaptable and thus unable to develop some of the more specialized functions of the distal small intestine when there is loss of the ileum.

What does the loss of the terminal ileum or ileocecal valve cause?

Usually, vitamin B_{12} deficiency and bile salt malabsorption; loss of the ileocecal valve predisposes the child to bacterial contamination of the small bowel as well as poor regulation of flow of intestinal contents

What is the treatment?

Therapy is often divided into two phases:
1. During the **acute phase**, which usually lasts several weeks after surgery, the child often suffers from massive secretory diarrhea. Attention must be paid to fluid and electrolyte status. H_2 receptor antagonists may help decrease intestinal secretion. Parenteral nutrition should be commenced as soon as possible to prevent catabolism.
2. After the child has stabilized, the goal of **chronic therapy** is to support normal growth and development while maximizing intestinal adaptation. Maximal intestinal adaptation following massive small bowel resection may not occur until 6–12 months after surgery. Calories are provided totally or in part from TPN during this time period.

Is enteral nutrition beneficial?

Yes. It stimulates bowel growth and adaptation. The optimal nutrient composition is controversial. The initial feedings usually constitute an elemental formula provided as a constant infusion through a nasogastric or gastrostomy tube.

How are attempts at enteral feeding regulated?

The volume and concentration of the formula are adjusted in response to stool volume and clinical symptoms, such as feeding residuals, vomiting, and abdominal bloating.

What is the prognosis?

With improvements in surgical technique and parenteral nutrition, long-term survival for patients is good. Current evidence indicates that children with more than 20 cm of small intestine and an ileocecal valve are ultimately capable of enteral nutrition alone.

NECROTIZING ENTEROCOLITIS (NEC)

What is it?

An acute fulminating, inflammatory disease of the intestine associated with focal or diffuse ulceration and necrosis of the small bowel, colon, and rarely the stomach

What are common complications of NEC?

NEC is the most common cause of gastrointestinal perforation and acquired short-gut syndrome among hospitalized premature infants.

Which infants are most susceptible to NEC?

NEC is predominantly a disease of premature infants. The overall incidence varies from 3% – 5% of all neonatal intensive care unit admissions. Full-term infants rarely acquire NEC—when they do, the disease primarily involves the colon.

What causes NEC?

The pathogenesis is multifactorial. It likely represents a final common pathway for an immature intestine's response to injury rather than a distinct disease. Factors implicated include:
1. Ischemia–reperfusion injury of the intestine
2. Enteral alimentation
3. Infectious and inflammatory agents
4. An immature immune system
5. Immature intestinal mucosa

What are the signs and symptoms?

1. **Early gastrointestinal signs** and symptoms are nonspecific and may include vomiting or delayed gastric emptying, increased gastric residual volume, hematemesis, bright red blood from the rectum, diminished or absent bowel sounds, abdominal distension with or without tenderness, and diarrhea.
2. The infant may also experience a number of **nonspecific nongastrointestinal symptoms** consistent with bacterial sepsis, including apnea, respiratory distress, bradycardia, lethargy, temperature instability, cyanosis, mottling, systemic acidosis, and hyper- or hypoglycemia.
3. As the **disease progresses**, the infant may develop septicemia, disseminated intravascular coagulation, hypotension, ascites, and intestinal perforation with peritonitis.

How is NEC diagnosed?

The diagnosis of NEC is largely a clinical one. Confirmation can be provided by the radiographic presence of pneumatosis intestinalis (i.e., accumulation of gas within the intestinal wall), portal venous gas, or pneumoperitoneum.

What is the differential Dx?

Sepsis with ileus
Malrotation with midgut volvulus
Pseudomembranous colitis
Hirschsprung disease
Intussusception
Gastric stress ulcer
Hemorrhagic disease of the newborn
Swallowed maternal blood

What is the treatment?

1. Enteral feedings should be discontinued, and nasogastric suction and intravenous fluids started.
2. Parenteral antibiotics should be administered.
3. Abdominal radiographs should be performed every 6 hours to detect

early perforation and to follow the radiographic course of the disease.

Do most cases resolve with medical treatment?

Yes

What are absolute indications for surgery?

Clinical deterioration unresponsive to medical therapy or evidence of intestinal perforation warrant immediate surgical intervention.

What does surgery usually involve?

It usually involves resection of the perforated and/or necrotic bowel, an end stoma, and mucous fistula. The bowel may be reconnected when the infant is fully recovered. Alternatively, placement of an abdominal drain alone may ameliorate systemic symptoms until a more definitive procedure can be performed.

When can feeding be reintroduced?

In uncomplicated cases, enteral feedings are gradually reintroduced 7–10 days after medical therapy.

What are long-term complications of NEC?

Short-gut syndrome if significant bowel resection is needed
Bowel stricture develops in 18%–25% of cases, with **two thirds involving the left colon**. Infants who recover with medical therapy only should receive an UGI with follow-through 6 weeks after recovery to look for strictures.

CELIAC SPRUE (GLUTEN ENTEROPATHY)

What is it?

An acquired form of malabsorption; in susceptible hosts, the ingestion of gluten (e.g., wheat gluten and other similar proteins) causes immunologically mediated damage to the small intestinal mucosa

At what age does it present?

Children present from 12 to 18 months of age.

What does the onset of symptoms correspond with?

The introduction of wheat products into the child's diet

What are the signs and symptoms?

1. The child will often have diarrhea, a protuberant abdomen, and wasted extremities. Height and weight are often less than the third percentile for the child's age.
2. Less common signs and symptoms are intermittent vomiting, irritability, abdominal pain, peripheral edema, long eyelashes, clubbing, and rectal prolapse.
3. A small number of children may present with isolated growth failure and an absence of gastrointestinal symptoms.

What is the differential Dx?

The differential Dx includes other causes of intestinal malabsorption. The **most common cause of chronic malabsorption in childhood is cystic fibrosis.** Other causes include milk protein enteropathy, chronic giardiasis, Shwachman-Diamond syndrome, isolated pancreatic enzyme deficiencies, intestinal lymphangiectasia, abetalipoproteinemia, and chronic infections associated with immunodeficiency disorders.

What are some associated laboratory findings?

Most laboratory abnormalities in celiac sprue are caused by chronic malabsorption:
1. Iron deficiency anemia
2. Deficiencies of fat soluble vitamins (some children may present with a prolonged prothrombin time because of vitamin K deficiency)
3. Abnormal 72-hour fecal fat excretion and D-xylose absorption
4. IgA deficiency

How is it diagnosed?

1. Small intestinal biopsy, revealing villous atrophy with hyperplasia of the crypts and abnormal surface epithelium while the child is eating a gluten-containing diet

2. A full clinical remission after complete withdrawal of gluten from the diet

What is the treatment?

The cornerstone of therapy is a **strict gluten-free diet,** in which wheat, oats, rye, and barley are excluded from the diet and substituted with rice and corn. Parents must be instructed to carefully read all food labels, because wheat by-products are added to many foods. In severe cases, a short course of corticosteroids may be beneficial.

How long do patients have to stay on a gluten-free diet?

Celiac sprue is a lifelong disorder

What is a risk to affected individuals who continue to eat gluten?

Greatly increased risk of developing small bowel lymphoma

PEPTIC ULCER DISEASE (PUD)

What is it?

The disruption of the gastric or duodenal mucosal barrier by a combination of pepsin and gastric acid

Do children get ulcers?

Yes

What is the incidence?

The overall incidence in children is unknown. However, it has been estimated that 3–4 in 10,000 pediatric inpatients have PUD.

Do babies make enough acid to develop ulcers?

Yes—by 48 hours of life most infants have a gastric pH between 1 and 3, and by 3 years of age gastric acid secretion approximates adult values.

What are the signs and symptoms?

The most common symptom is abdominal pain, often most severe at night. Children older than 6–7 years of age generally complain of classic epigastric pain. However, surprisingly few young children complain of upper abdominal pain. More often, young children complain of generalized or periumbilical pain, and occasionally right lower quadrant pain. Less common symptoms include vomiting, hematemesis, or melena.

Is perforated ulcer common in children?

No

What is in the differential Dx?

The differential diagnosis is extensive and includes functional abdominal pain, irritable bowel syndrome, gastroesophageal reflux, cholelithiasis, pancreatitis, urinary tract infection or obstruction, lower lobe pneumonia, Crohn disease, ovarian cysts, appendicitis, and constipation.

How is PUD diagnosed?

The most reliable diagnosis occurs via flexible **fiberoptic endoscopy**. The sensitivity and specificity of double-contrast radiographic studies are only 60%–70%.

What are treatment options?

1. Antacids neutralize acid
2. H_2 receptor antagonists or proton-pump inhibitors inhibit acid secretion
3. Sucralfate or bismuth compounds provide a protective mucosal barrier

These therapies may be used individually or in combination.

How effective is medical treatment?

The most frequently prescribed therapy is a 6- to 8-week course of an H_2 receptor antagonist, which is effective in 85%–95% of cases.

What is the role of *Helicobacter pylori* in childhood PUD?

Unclear—it is estimated that 15% of children undergoing diagnostic endoscopy have evidence of *H. pylori* infection, but rates vary widely from 5%–75%. Nevertheless, children with documented *H. pylori* infection should probably be treated to eradicate the organism.

INTUSSUSCEPTION

What is it?

An intussusception occurs when a segment of intestine with its associated mesentery (the intussusceptum) telescopes into an adjacent segment of intestine (the intussuscipiens).

Age at presentation?

More than 50% of recognized cases occur between 3–12 months of age, and more than 75% occur before 2 years of age.

Is there a sex predilection?

Boys are affected three times more often than girls.

What segments of intestine are most commonly involved?

Most cases are ileocolic, with the intussusception starting immediately proximal to the ileocecal valve and telescoping into the cecum. Colocolic, ileoileal, and ileoileocolic intussusceptions are much less common.

What are the causes?

More than 90% of cases are idiopathic and do not have an identifiable "anatomic lead point." Some researchers have hypothesized that various viral illnesses cause hypertrophy of Peyer patches in the terminal ileum, which serve as a lead point for the intussusception.

What is the most commonly *identified* lead point?

Meckel diverticulum

Are there any disorders that seem to predispose a child to intussusception?

Children with **cystic fibrosis** are at significantly greater risk for developing intussusception, and their symptoms may be atypical. Other disorders associated with intussusception include Henoch-Schönlein purpura, Meckel diverticulum, juvenile inflammatory polyps, and *Ascaris lumbricoides* infestation.

What are the signs and symptoms?

Intussusception is characterized by the sudden onset of episodic crampy abdominal pain. There is often vomiting associated with the pain. Between episodes of pain, the child may be asymptomatic. Passage of stool and flatus is diminished. Passage of dark blood per rectum ("currant-jelly stools") suggests venous congestion and mucosal sloughing. As the symptoms progress, the child may become increasingly lethargic or somnolent. **Only 10%–15% of affected children have the classic triad: abdominal pain, a palpable sausage-shaped abdominal mass, and currant-jelly stools.**

How is it diagnosed?

Because the presentation is extremely variable, clinicians must maintain a high index of suspicion. Laboratory findings are nonspecific and may include an elevated WBC and electrolyte abnormalities consistent with dehydration. Upright and supine abdominal radiographs may be normal or may demonstrate a nonspecific bowel gas pattern or a pattern suggesting an abdominal mass, intestinal obstruction with air-fluid levels, or rarely, free air consistent with intestinal perforation. Ultimately, the **diagnosis is usually established with an air or barium enema, which may also be therapeutic.**

What is the treatment?

Standard procedure for diagnosis and treatment of an intussusception is either an air or a barium enema. However, the child should receive **IV hydration and antibiotics before the enema.** Evidence of peritonitis or a general toxic state may be relative contraindications to the enema. A surgeon should be immediately available when an enema is performed in case the enema is unsuccessful or perforation occurs.

How often is an enema successful?

In about 80% of cases; however, the success rate is significantly reduced if symptoms have been present > 48 hours

What is the risk of perforation?

Approximately 1%

What is the incidence of recurrence after enema?

Approximately 10%—most recurrences occur within 48 hours of the initial episode

What are indications for surgery?

When radiographic reduction fails or in children who have signs and/or symptoms suggesting peritonitis or intestinal perforation. Occasionally, the intussuscepted section must be resected because of the bowel cannot be reduced during surgery, or because the intussuscepted portion is necrotic.

ANORECTAL MALFORMATIONS

What is imperforate anus?

A spectrum of anomalies caused by an arrest of anorectal development during the cloacal stage between 4–12 weeks gestation

How does it manifest in boys?

There is no anal opening and in most cases (90%) there is a fistula between the rectum and the urinary tract. This fistula may communicate with the urethra, the prostatic urethra, or the bladder.

How does it manifest in girls?

No opening in the anal region, but about 80% have a fistula into the vagina

How are high, intermediate, and low anomalies defined?

1. High anomalies occur when the rectal atresia is above the levator sling.
2. Intermediate lesions exist when the atresia occurs at the level of the levator sling.
3. Low anomalies occur when the atresia is below the levator sling.

On radiographs, the levator sling is determined by identifying the pubococcygeal line (which represents the upper portion of the levator sling) and the line between the ischial tuberosities (which represents the lower aspect of the levator sling).

Why is the level of the anomaly important?

The higher the anomaly, the less well formed are the sphincter mechanisms and the neurogenic innervation of these mechanisms. High anomalies are also more likely to present with rectourinary fistulas in boys and high vaginal fistulas in girls.

Are boys or girls more prone to high anomalies?

Boys

Are other anomalies common when imperforate anus is recognized?

Yes, including:
Duodenal atresia
Esophageal atresia
Vertebral anomalies
Renal anomalies
Down syndrome
Congenital heart disease
Limb anomalies
Imperforate anus represents one manifestation of the **VACTERL** association.

How is this condition managed?

1. In boys, initial end colostomy with distal stoma formation is usually needed. The extent of the anomaly is then assessed with a contrast study through the distal stoma into the atretic rectum. A VCUG is also needed to test for a possible rectourinary fistula. Other studies are required to look for the common associated anomalies. These will include appropriate limb and vertebral radiographs, abdominal ultrasound, and echocardiography.
2. In girls, if there is an external opening into the fourchette of the vagina or immediately posterior to this, it can be dilated for the passage of stool. Assessment for other associated anomalies is needed as described above.

How is definitive treatment undertaken?

Usually the posterior sagittal anoplasty (popularized by Peña) is used to reconstruct the anus. In girls, it may performed during the neonatal stage when there is an external opening. More commonly, imperforate anus repair should take place between 2–6 months of age.

What are the outcomes?

Satisfactory continence is usually obtainable in infants with low-lying lesions. Continence decreases to about

50%–75% in intermediate and high lesions.

What are cloacal malformations?

A condition in girls that represents a common opening of the vagina and rectum, or the urethra, vagina, and rectum

What is the treatment?

Assessment is performed in a manner similar to that for imperforate anus. Ultimately, all three pathways must be reconstructed, usually from the posterior approach.

What is cloacal exstrophy?

A severe malformation that results in an imperforate anus with exstrophy of the bladder and with a plate of distal bowel connected to the midline of the bladder. This bowel plate has an opening from the proximal bowel and then an opening to a distal blind end of the bowel. Openings to a duplicated appendix are also seen. There is also widening of the pubis symphysis and usually an associated omphalocele.

Does it occur in both boys and girls?

Yes. However, the female gender is usually assigned and the testes are removed if present, because reconstruction of an adequate phallus is extremely difficult.

What is the treatment?

The two halves of the exstrophic bladder are separated from the middle bowel plate. The bladder is then reconstructed. The bowel is tubularized and brought to the abdominal wall as an end colostomy. The omphalocele is closed. The widened pubis symphysis is approximated. Reconstruction of the vagina and the urethra usually is performed at a later procedure.

ULCERATIVE COLITIS

What is it?

An inflammatory bowel condition that involves rectal and colonic mucosa; the rectum is usually involved first and the disease progresses proximally in a contiguous manner

What are the characteristics of the mucosa?

Crypt abscesses form leading to mucosal ulcerations, pseudopolyps, and ultimately a denuding of the mucosa.

What is the etiology?

It is uncertain, but an autoimmune process with a genetic predisposition is currently the most popular theory. About 15% of patients have a family member with inflammatory bowel disease.

What are associated conditions?

Ankylosing spondylitis and **uveitis** are associated. Other associated conditions include growth retardation, anemia, osteoporosis, nephrolithiasis, arthralgia, skin lesions (e.g., erythema nodosum, pyoderma gangrenosum), liver lesions (e.g., sclerosing cholangitis, fatty infiltration of liver), and aphthous stomatitis.

What is the age of onset?

It usually is recognized during adolescence or the third decade, but occasionally earlier.

What are the signs and symptoms?

Can be insidious—crampy abdominal pain can progress to diarrhea containing blood or pus. If unchecked, a toxic colitis can ensue. Occasionally, the toxic, fulminant form of ulcerative colitis is the initial presentation.

How is it diagnosed?

By endoscopy and biopsy of colonic mucosa

What is toxic megacolon?

A fulminant presentation of ulcerative colitis characterized by colonic dilatation, a low motility state, probable bacterial overgrowth. Patients are severely ill with septic manifestations. Supportive therapy is needed with IV fluids, antibiotics, and bowel rest.

How is ulcerative colitis treated?

Medical: Initial treatment includes sulfasalazine, steroids, and steroid enemas. Metronidazole may also be helpful. Antidiarrheal medicines should be used with care, because toxic megacolon may result. Medical therapy is not curative.

Surgical: Ultimately, virtually all patients need surgery. The curative procedure is a total proctocolectomy. Patients may choose to have a permanent end ileostomy or undergo an ileoanal pull-through. The ileum may be pulled through straight or after the formation of a J- or S-shaped pouch.

What are the outcomes?

Surgical removal of the colon and rectum is curative. The pull-through procedure causes an increased amount of bowel movements, but with appropriate training and medical support, patients may experience as low as 4–8 bowel movements daily.

How is the large bowel at risk if not removed?

Colon cancer risk can be 3%–5% in the first decade of the disease, and as high as 20% in each subsequent decade.

CROHN DISEASE

What is it?

An inflammatory bowel condition that is transmural and marked by bowel wall thickening, ulcerations of mucosa, and "skip lesions" (i.e., lesions separated by normal portions of bowel); characteristic granulomas appear in 60% of patients

Which parts of the gastrointestinal tract may be affected?

Any part! Crohn disease tends to involve the distal small bowel and colorectal regions most frequently.

What is the epidemiology?

There is no difference in incidence of the disease in boys and girls; however, it is five times more common in whites than in blacks.

In what age group does Crohn disease usually present?

Adolescents and young adults

What are the signs and symptoms?

It can be insidious at onset. Typical symptoms include weight loss, abdominal pain, diarrhea, and fever. A perianal ulcer or abscess may be the initial manifestation. There may be occasional rectal bleeding, but this is much less frequent than in ulcerative colitis.

Are there extraintestinal manifestations?

Possibly—they include growth retardation, lack of sexual maturation, skin lesions, liver lesions, uveitis, and anemia

What is the treatment?

1. Usually, attempts are made to modify diet to include high-caloric, high-protein, low-roughage, low-fat intake.
2. Medical therapy includes sulfasalazine, azathioprine, cyclosporine, and steroids.

What are indications for surgery?

1. Failure of medical therapy to treat symptoms
2. Intestinal obstruction
3. Abdominal abscess
4. Enteric fistulae or fistulae to genitourinary tract
5. Perirectal fistula or abscess
6. Perforation of bowel (rare)

What is the surgical strategy?

It must be designed to treat the specific problem. It usually requires resection of the offending bowel or drainage of perirectal abscesses. However, only the bowel producing the symptoms should be removed. Surgery is a palliative, not a curative, procedure.

Can Crohn disease be cured?

There is currently no known cure.

ANTIBIOTIC-RELATED COLITIS (PSEUDOMEMBRANOUS COLITIS)

What is antibiotic related colitis?	A condition in which the normal intestinal flora is altered because of the use of antibiotic medicine
What are the signs and symptoms?	Generally, an increase in diarrheal stools; stools may be bloody in severe cases.
What is the most common identified pathogen?	*Clostridium difficile*
How is it identified?	By a stool culture or by identification of the toxin in the stool; sheets of WBCs are seen in the stool.
What is the treatment?	Generally, discontinuing the antibiotic allows recovery of normal stool flora and function. If *C. difficile* is identified, then Vancomycin or Flagyl (either po or IV) may be used for a cure.

HENOCH-SCHÖNLEIN PURPURA (HSP)

What is it?	HSP is a systemic vasculitis syndrome, perhaps the most common form of acute vasculitis affecting children.
At what age is HSP common?	Peak incidence occurs at 4–5 years of age, but is reported in patients ranging from 6 months of age to adulthood.
Are boys or girls more commonly affected?	Boys are affected slightly more frequently than girls.
Are there temporal or geographic predilections to HSP?	HSP occurs throughout the year, but there is an increased incidence in the **spring** and **fall**. Most cases are sporadic; however, temporal and geographic clusters of HSP are not uncommon.
What is the pathognomonic physical finding in HSP?	Virtually all patients have a characteristic skin rash: **palpable purpuric lesions** measuring 2–10 mm in diameter. Patients may also present with coalescent ecchymoses and pinpoint petechiae. Typically, the purpura are concentrated on the buttocks and lower extremities, but are not confined to those areas. New lesions appear in

crops, then fade over several days. In one third of all patients, other symptoms precede the onset of the rash, thus making it difficult to establish the diagnosis.

What are common orthopedic manifestations?

Painful joint swelling occurs in approximately 80% of patients (ankles, knees, and the dorsum of hands and feet). The arthralgia is self-limited and usually abates with bed rest.

What are common GI manifestations?

Colicky abdominal pain, often accompanied by vomiting, occurs in 75% of patients. Occult or gross gastrointestinal bleeding is present in 40% of patients. **Intussusception** has been reported in 3%–5% of patients. Bowel infarction, perforation, and massive gastrointestinal bleeding are rare but life-threatening complications. Gastrointestinal involvement before the appearance of the rash may mimic a surgical abdomen (appendicitis) or inflammatory bowel disease.

What are common renal manifestations?

Nephritis occurs in 50% of patients. Unlike joint or gastrointestinal involvement, nephritis virtually never precedes the onset of the rash. Nephritis may be delayed for a number of weeks after the appearance of other symptoms. However, if nephritis is going to occur, it usually becomes apparent within 3 months. Nephritis is manifested by microscopic or gross hematuria. Proteinuria is present in two thirds of patients, and 25% of patients will be hypertensive.

What are some of the less common complications?

Because HSP is a systemic vasculitis, any organ system may be affected. Other complications include CNS complications, intracranial bleeding, seizures, hemiparesis, coma, pancreatitis, hydrops of the gallbladder, orchitis, pulmonary hemorrhage, ocular involvement, and carditis.

How long does HSP last?

The average duration of acute HSP is 2–4 weeks.

What is the risk of recurrence?

Up to 50% of patients will have one or more recurrences.

Who is most likely to have a recurrence?

Patients with nephritis

What is the usual nature of recurrence?

Recurrences tend to mimic the original episode, but they are usually milder and of shorter duration.

What are the characteristic histologic features of HSP?

HSP is a leukocytoclastic vasculitis affecting small vessels. Biopsies of purpuric lesions show polymorphonuclear leukocyte infiltration in and around dermal capillaries. Immunofluorescent studies demonstrate granular deposits of IgA in the walls of dermal vessels.

What characterizes the histologic changes in the kidney?

They range from minimal change to focal or diffuse mesangial proliferation. The characteristic finding of immunofluorescence is diffuse mesangial IgA deposits.

How is HSP diagnosed?

On clinical grounds—there is no diagnostic laboratory test for HSP. Laboratory studies help to exclude other conditions that resemble HSP.

What typical laboratory values should be obtained?

1. CBC, platelets
2. Urinalysis, BUN, Cr
3. Timed urine collection for protein excretion and GFR

What are characteristic serologic findings?

50% of patients show increased serum IgA. ANA, RF, and ANCA are negative.

What is the etiology?

Unknown—the epidemiology of HSP suggests an infectious etiology, and a variety of organisms have been implicated

What does HSP most likely represent?

An unusual immune response to a variety of infectious or environmental insults. It is clear that IgA plays a pivotal role in the immunopathogenesis of HSP.

What is the pathophysiology of HSP?

Patients with HSP often have IgA-containing circulating immune complexes. Deposition of these immune complexes in vessel walls results in inflammatory vasculitis and accounts for the histologic and clinical features of HSP.

What is the treatment?

The mainstay of therapy is supportive care.

Why must hypertension be treated?

It must be treated aggressively to prevent intracranial bleeding.

Which drugs should be particularly avoided?

Salicylates and other drugs that interfere with platelet function should be avoided in patients with active gastrointestinal bleeding.

Are steroids helpful?

Corticosteroids are beneficial in alleviating joint and abdominal pain, but there is no evidence that corticosteroids affect the cutaneous purpura or hasten the resolution of the disease. Corticosteroids have no benefit in treating established nephritis.

What is the prognosis?

The prognosis is excellent for most patients.

Which manifestation is most prone to chronic problems?

Nephritis

What percent of patients develop end-stage renal failure?

< 5%

Who is at the highest risk for developing renal failure?

Patients with gross hematuria, massive proteinuria, and hypertension during the acute phase of the illness are at highest risk for the development of end-stage renal disease.

INTESTINAL TRANSPORT DEFECTS

What are they?

Isolated abnormalities of the absorption and/or secretion (i.e., transport) of specific ions or nutrients across the intestinal mucosa

How common are transport defects?

There are several defects that occur quite commonly. Cystic fibrosis is probably the most common transport defect and is related to the abnormal secretion of chloride across many different tissues, including the intestinal mucosa.

What is the general symptom?

In most cases **chronic diarrhea** presents. However, symptoms of each defect are best explained by understanding which ion or nutrient cannot be absorbed and/or transported.

What is congenital chloridorrhea?

The chloride–bicarbonate exchange mechanism in the ileum and colon is dysfunctional, causing excessive chloride secretion with resultant secretory diarrhea and hypokalemic metabolic alkalosis.

What is congenital glucose–galactose malabsorption?

The active transport of glucose and galactose across the intestinal mucosa is defective, thus the ingestion of any glucose or galactose causes osmotic diarrhea. Affected infants have severe diarrhea with profound growth failure.

What is X-linked hypophosphatemic rickets?

The renal and intestinal phosphate transport protein is defective, causing inadequate intestinal phosphate absorption, excessive urinary phosphate loss, and severe rickets.

What is the treatment?

There are no specific treatments for most transport defects. Instead, the patient's symptoms and the metabolic abnormalities caused by the specific transport defect are treated.

APPENDICITIS

What is it?	Inflammation/infection of the appendix caused by occlusion of its lumen
What may cause obstruction?	Stool (fecalith); inflamed or swollen lymphoid follicles; pinworm; or carcinoid tumors

What is the symptomatology?

1. Abdominal pain: starts as generalized pain caused by irritation of visceral pain fibers; pain migrates to right lower quadrant as worsening appendicitis causes local irritation of peritoneum
2. Nausea and vomiting: usually follows onset of pain
3. Fever: usually, but not always present
4. Anorexia

What are findings on physical examination?

Localized guarding and referred pain to the right lower quadrant; diffuse tenderness if ruptured

Diminished bowel sounds

Pain upon iliopsoas extension

Possible mass or tenderness anteriorly on rectal exam

Possible palpable mass in right lower quadrant if rupture is contained

What do diagnostic studies show?

1. WBC: elevated with left shift; usually 11,000–18,000 if unruptured, but may be higher if ruptured
2. Urinalysis: a few (3–5) WBCs may be present secondary to local irritation of ureter or bladder
3. Abdominal radiograph: usually normal, but may show:
   Fecalith
   Ileus or sentinel loop
   Loss of fat stripe in right lower quadrant
   Slight concavity of spine to right
   Air/fluid level in right lower quadrant suggestive of abscess
4. Ultrasound: may show thickened appendix or mass consistent with an abscess

5. Barium enema: nonfilling of appendix with irregularity of cecum
6. CT scan: best for delineating complex abscess

What is the treatment for uncomplicated appendicitis?

Surgical removal of appendix with perioperative antibiotic coverage is usually adequate

For ruptured appendix?

Surgical removal of appendix and longer coverage with antibiotics (5–10 days)

For complex abscess?

May require initial drainage with later removal of appendix

What disease process may be present in an infant with appendicitis?

Hirschsprung disease

PANCREATITIS

What are the most common causes of pancreatitis in children?

Trauma
Cholelithiasis
Cystic fibrosis
Congenital anomalies, such as choledochal cyst or pancreas divisum

What are the signs and symptoms?

Patients experience midepigastric pain with vomiting. Tenderness is usually present in the midepigastrum. A palpable mass may be present if there is extensive inflammation of the pancreas or pseudocyst formation.

What diagnostic studies are used?

1. **Ultrasound** and **CT scan** are usually the best initial imaging studies.
2. Analysis of serum amylase and lipase as well as urine clearance of amylase are helpful.
3. Endoscopic retrograde cholangiopancreatography (ERCP) may be necessary to delineate ductal anatomy, although this is usually performed when the pancreatitis has subsided and a cause is still unknown.

What is the treatment?	IV fluids and cessation of oral intake; meperidine is usually the medicine of choice for pain management
Is surgical treatment needed?	In the vast majority of cases, pancreatitis will resolve with medical treatment.
When is surgery indicated?	1. Occasionally, a pseudocyst will form, which often resolves within 3–4 weeks. However, if it persists beyond this, external drainage via a percutaneously placed catheter, or internal drainage via cyst-gastrostomy, cyst-duodostomy, or cyst-jejunostomy may be needed.
	2. Chronic pancreatitis with pancreatic ductal dilatation may require a pancreaticojejunostomy (Peustow procedure).
	3. Occasionally, extreme hemorrhagic pancreatitis may require debridement of the pancreas.
	4. Trauma to the pancreas may disrupt the main pancreatic duct, thus requiring distal pancreatectomy with spleen preservation.

HEMOLYTIC-UREMIC SYNDROME (HUS)

What is it?	It is a clinical syndrome of microangiopathic hemolytic anemia, thrombocytopenia, and acute renal failure. HUS is the **most common cause of acute renal failure in children**.
What causes HUS?	Two thirds of cases are preceded by an infection with verotoxin-producing *Escherichia coli* **0157:H7**. However, HUS may occur following infection with other bacterial pathogens, including *Shigella, Campylobacter, Salmonella,* and *Yersinia.*
What is the pathogenesis of HUS?	A variety of different bacterial toxins induce endothelial damage, which in turn initiates intravascular platelet activation, causing a diffuse small-vessel

thrombosis throughout numerous organ systems.

What are the signs and symptoms?

95% of HUS cases are preceded by gastroenteritis, and in nearly 75% of cases, the associated diarrhea is bloody.

Diffuse abdominal pain and vomiting are common.

Resolution of the gastrointestinal symptoms is associated with the abrupt onset of pallor, easy bruisability and/or petechiae, and oliguria secondary to acute renal insufficiency. (The decreased urine output is often attributed to dehydration; children may be treated with IV fluids, causing edema and hypertension secondary to fluid overload.) Affected children often are extremely irritable or encephalopathic.

Seizures are not uncommon.

How is HUS diagnosed?

Because HUS is a syndrome, it is diagnosed on clinical grounds.

What are common laboratory findings?

1. Thrombocytopenia
2. Anemia
3. Elevated Bun and Cr
4. Elevated LFTs (50% of patients)
5. Elevated serum amylase and lipase (25% of patients)
6. RBC and WBC on stool smear
7. Positive stool cultures for *E. Coli* 0157:H7, *Campylobacter*, *Shigella*, or *Salmonella* in some cases

What are radiographic and colonoscopic findings?

Barium enema generally demonstrates intestinal ischemia with thumb printing, mucosal irregularity, and ulcerations. Colonoscopic findings are nonspecific; hyperemic mucosal edema and friability. Barium enema and colonoscopy are not routinely performed unless the diagnosis is uncertain.

What is the treatment?

Purely supportive: Patients with severe gastrointestinal symptoms are put at bowel rest and parenteral nutrition is started. When clinically indicated, red cell transfusions and diuretics are administered and fluid intake restricted. Progressive renal insufficiency may necessitate initiation of peritoneal dialysis or hemodialysis.

What percent of children recover renal function?

95% of affected children recover renal function within 2–3 weeks.

What are possible long term complications?

Chronic renal insufficiency
Intestinal fistulae or strictures
Stroke with CNS deficits
Chronic exocrine pancreatic insufficiency

CONSTIPATION

What is it?

A symptom, not a disease–it is the **painful** passage of large and/or hard bowel movements or the inability to expel a bowel movement

What are normal childhood bowel habits?

Infant: average stool frequency is 4 per day; 95% of children have from 1 stool every other day to 4 stools per day
6 months to 2 years: average stool frequency is 2 per day; 95% of children have from 1 stool every other day to 4 stools per day
Older than 2 years: average stool frequency is 1 per day; 95% of children have from 1 stool every third day to 3 stools per day

What is the relation between constipation and frequency of bowel movements?

The frequency of defecation is influenced by diet and social custom. Constipation refers to the character of the stool and the symptoms associated with defecation rather than the frequency of defecation.

How common is constipation in children?

During the first 5 years of age, as many as **20%** of children will be brought to medical attention because of constipation. **Constipation is the single most common reason children are referred to a pediatric gastroenterologist.**

What are the symptoms?

1. Pain associated with the passage of bowel movements
2. Large and/or hard bowel movements
3. Infrequent bowel movements

Many children will also experience intermittent crampy abdominal pain, abdominal distension, or a decreased appetite.

What are the physical signs?

A distended abdomen with palpable stool in the colon.

On rectal exam, anal fissures may be present, and the rectum is generally enlarged and filled with stool. Chronic constipation is the most common cause of rectal prolapse in children.

Why do children develop constipation?

In otherwise healthy children, more than 99% of cases do not have a clearly identifiable etiology and are called *functional constipation*. In most children, the constipation develops after the passage of several large or hard bowel movements with associated pain. This often occurs following weaning, a change in diet, school entry, a bout of gastroenteritis, or during toilet training.

What is the treatment?

The primary goal is to eliminate the pain associated with defecation. This generally means softening the stools.

1. In young children, fruit juices or dark Karo syrup is effective. Alternatively, osmotic cathartics, such as magnesium hydroxide (milk of magnesia) or lactulose, are safe and effective.
2. In older children with chronic constipation, dietary measures are often inadequate and laxatives must be administered. These include magnesium hydroxide (milk of magnesia), mineral oil, lactulose, senna derivatives, and dioctyl sodium sulfosuccinate (Colace).

3. In the most severe and chronic cases, it is often necessary to administer several enemas to evacuate the colon before oral cathartics are effective. Rarely, manual disimpaction under anesthesia is required.

What are the risks of laxative use?

In an otherwise healthy child, the use of any over-the-counter laxative is safe. The major side effects of laxative overdosage are diarrhea, nausea and vomiting, and abdominal cramps. Despite rumors to the contrary, the long-term use of laxatives is not associated with dependency or "cathartic colon."

How are functional constipation and Hirschsprung disease differentiated?

In most cases they can be differentiated on the basis of the history and physical examination. Functional constipation is far more common than Hirschsprung disease.

ENCOPRESIS

What is it?

Fecal incontinence, or soiling

How common is encopresis in children?

Among children older than 4 years of age, between 1%–3% will be incontinent of stool more than once weekly.

What causes encopresis?

The majority of childhood encopresis is caused by prolonged constipation with resulting overflow incontinence.

What are some of the other causes of fecal incontinence in children?

In rare circumstances, it is the presenting symptom of an underlying neurologic deficit, such as very low meningomyelocele or tethered spinal cord

Is encopresis primarily a psychological problem?

Although many children with chronic encopresis have psychological and behavioral difficulties, many of these problems are a result, rather than the cause, of their fecal soiling.

What is a typical history like?

In almost all affected children there is at least a remote history of constipation. Soiling generally begins as small streaks of stool in the underwear. As the problem progresses, the volume and frequency of the soiling increases, and eventually the child is passing formed or semiformed stools in his underwear. The child denies any sense of the need to defecate prior to the accidents. If soiling occurs several times daily, it is often confused with diarrhea.

What is commonly found on physical examination?

1. A protuberant abdomen is present with stool palpable throughout the colon.
2. On exam, the rectal sphincter is often lax and the rectum is large and filled with soft stool.
3. An abdominal radiograph shows abundant stool throughout the colon.

What is the treatment?

It basically is the same as that for severe, chronic constipation–the colon must be completely evacuated with enemas, oral cathartics, or by manual disimpaction. When the colon is completely empty, laxatives are started in doses sufficient to produce one or two soft stools daily. The child should be encouraged to sit on the toilet for 5–10 minutes after breakfast and dinner. Some children may benefit from biofeedback therapy.

HIRSCHSPRUNG DISEASE

What is it?

Aganglionosis of the rectum or colon, causing a functional obstruction; the aganglionosis extends from the rectum proximally in a contiguous manner to some level, usually the upper rectum or colon

What is the transition zone?

It is the point where aganglionic bowel meets ganglionic bowel. It can be anywhere, but is usually in the rectosigmoid region. Occasionally the entire colon may be aganglionic, resulting in total colonic Hirschsprung disease.

What are the signs and symptoms?

They may be insidious. Initial manifestation may be failure to pass meconium within the first 24 hours of life (95% of patients). Subsequently, increasing difficulty with bowel movements ensues, leading to severe constipation, overflow diarrhea, and sometimes enterocolitis and sepsis.

What are associated conditions?

Down syndrome
Waardenburg syndrome
Cartilage-hair hypoplasia
Neonatal appendicitis

How is it diagnosed?

1. **Contrast enema** is used to search for the transition zone. The ganglionic portion will be dilated. This may not be evident early in the course.
2. Definitive diagnosis is made by **absence of ganglionic cells** and increased acetylcholinesterase staining on a rectal biopsy specimen. Cholinergic and adrenergic nerve endings also may be evident.

What is the treatment?

When diagnosed, a leveling colostomy (i.e., a colostomy immediately proximal to the level of the transition zone) is performed. Later, a colon pull-through procedure (Swenson, Soave, Duhamel) may be performed. In selected patients, the pull-through can be performed at the initial operation.

What are the outcomes?

With appropriate surgical care, 85% of patients will have normal bowel function. Others may have functional motility difficulties despite presence of ganglion cells.

MALROTATION

What is it?

Failure of the gut to make its normal 270° counterclockwise rotation during in utero development

What are the anatomic results?

1. Unrotation of gut of varying degrees with the ligament of Treitz to the right of or at the midline, and a mobile cecum
2. Ladd's bands
3. Narrow mesenteric pedicle

What are Ladd's bands?

Peritoneal attachments of the now mobile ascending colon to the right abdominal wall; they may stretch across the duodenum, causing obstruction

What is the most dangerous aspect of malrotation?

The narrow pedicle may cause volvulus and subsequent loss of part or all of the bowel. This may be lethal!

At what age does malrotation present?

Any age! However, about 80% of patients with malrotation who have symptoms do so within the first 2 months of life.

What are some associated anomalies?

Duodenal and intestinal atresia
Hirschsprung disease
Mesenteric cysts

What are some conditions in which malrotation is always found?

Diaphragmatic hernia
Gastroschisis
Omphalocele

What are the symptoms?

1. Vomiting, usually of bilious material **(Vomiting of bilious material in an infant is diagnosed as malrotation with volvulus until proven otherwise!)**
2. Intermittent abdominal pain
3. Systemic collapse if volvulus has progressed to frank bowel necrosis

What are the signs?

1. Patient may have a distended abdomen
2. Usually no peritoneal irritation unless bowel injury is present
3. Dehydration and weight loss.

How is it diagnosed?

An upper GI is the definitive diagnostic study. A barium enema may show malposition of cecum, but the position may appear normal even if the cecum is mobile.

What is the treatment?

Surgical correction with the **Ladd procedure.** The duodenum is mobilized and straightened, Ladd's bands are divided, the colon is mobilized to the left with the cecum situated near the sigmoid colon, and an appendectomy is performed.

What is done if volvulus is present?

The bowel is turned counterclockwise on its mesentery until the volvulus is relieved. If there is necrotic bowel, this is resected, and anastomosis or stomas are performed as appropriate. If the viability of the bowel is uncertain at the end of the procedure, the abdomen is closed and re-explored in 12–24 hours.

What is the outcome?

The outcome is usually very good. However, if volvulus is serious, an extensive loss of bowel may result in short-gut syndrome.

CONGENITAL DUODENAL OBSTRUCTION

What is it?

An obstruction of the duodenum secondary to failure of the recanalization process of the fetal duodenum; it occurs during the eighth to tenth week of development

What are the most common types of congenital duodenal obstruction?

Duodenal atresia
Duodenal stenosis
Duodenal web

What is annular pancreas?

A failure in the proper rotation of the pancreas may cause an annular pancreas, which also causes duodenal obstruction. Some researchers theorize that annular pancreas is an anatomic phenomenon secondary to one of the primary duodenal conditions noted above.

Where is the obstruction usually located?

Usually in the first or second part of the duodenum; it may involve the entrance of the common bile duct

What are the signs and symptoms?

1. Vomiting, which may be bilious
2. Abdomen may be distended secondary to distended stomach and duodenum

What are prenatal findings?

An ultrasound may show presence of polyhydramnios and a dilated duodenum.

What is the characteristic radiographic finding?

"**Double-bubble**" sign of dilated stomach and duodenum

How is a definitive diagnosis made?

A contrast study shows total or partial duodenal obstruction with a rounded dilated duodenum (as opposed to the beak-like appearance found in malrotation with volvulus)

What are some associated anomalies?

One third of affected infants have Down syndrome. Other anomalies include intestinal atresia, malrotation, imperforate anus, cardiac anomalies, and other anomalies of VACTERL association.

How is it treated preoperatively?

Nasogastric drainage with rehydration. Surgical correction may be done semi-electively unless malrotation is suspected, which makes repair more urgent.

What are three surgical options?

1. Duodenoduodenostomy (most common)
2. Vertical duodenotomy through an involved web or stenosis with transverse duodenoplasty
3. Duodenojejunostomy

Malrotation or other atresia must be sought at operation.

What is the outcome?

Uniformly the outcome is good, although it may be days to weeks until the duodenum recovers enough to tolerate full enteral feedings.

INTESTINAL ATRESIA

What is it?	A congenital condition in which the lumen of the bowel is interrupted
Where may an intestinal atresia occur?	Anywhere from the jejunum to the rectum; atresias may be multiple
How are they classified?	**Type I:** The mucosa is interrupted by a web, but the proximal dilated loop of bowel and decompressed distal loop are still connected at the serosal level. **Type II:** The proximal dilated bowel and distal decompressed bowel are connected by a fibrous atretic cord. **Type IIIa:** The proximal and distal portions of bowel are separated as is the mesentery to these two portions of bowel. **Type IIIb:** The distal atretic bowel is spiraled around a segmental artery in an apple-peel form. **Type IV:** Multiple atresias
How do they occur?	They are believed to be the result of a vascular accident in utero.
How do they present?	Newborns generally develop a distended abdomen soon after birth, if it is not already present at birth. Bilious vomiting ensues, or if a nasogastric tube has already been placed, voluminous bilious output is present. Infants may pass meconium because atresias occasionally develop after meconium has passed to the distal bowel in utero. Rarely, the proximal portion of bowel may perforate in utero.
What is the differential Dx?	Malrotation with volvulus Bowel duplication Internal hernia Adynamic ileus with sepsis Meconium ileus Hirschsprung disease

How is it diagnosed?	A contrast enema is performed in the newborn when evidence of bowel obstruction occurs. A microcolon will be visualized without connection to the proximal dilated bowel.
What is the treatment?	Surgical correction is necessary. For jejunal, ileal, or proximal colonic atresia, a resection of the dilated portion of the proximal bowel and the atretic portion of the distal bowel is needed, followed by an end-to-end anastomosis. Any of a variety of maneuvers may be used to equalize the caliber of the proximal and distal ends of the bowel. For distal colonic atresia, an end colostomy is performed first, and later an anastomosis is performed.
What is the outcome?	The current survival rate is 90%–100%.

ESOPHAGEAL ATRESIA/TRACHEOESOPHAGEAL FISTULA (TEF)

What is it?	A spectrum of anomalies consisting of discontinuity of the esophagus and/or fistula, or fistulae between the esophagus and the trachea
What are the five types?	**Type A:** esophageal atresia without fistula **Type B:** esophageal atresia with fistula between upper portion of esophagus and trachea **Type C:** esophageal atresia with fistula between lower portion of esophagus and trachea **Type D:** esophageal atresia with a fistula between the upper portion of esophagus and trachea and a fistula between the lower portion of esophagus and trachea **Type E:** esophagus in continuity with isolated fistula between esophagus and trachea
Which type is most common?	Type C (85%)

What is the incidence?

1 in 3000 births, with an equal incidence between boys and girls

Prematurity is common

What is the VACTERL association?

A constellation of anomalies that commonly occur together, either entirely or in part:

Vertebral

Anorectal (imperforate anus)

Cardiac

Tracheal

Esophageal

Renal/genitourinary

Limb/lumbar

Infants need to be screened for all of these anomalies when any one of them is present.

What other anomalies are commonly associated with TEF?

Duodenal atresia and bowel atresias

What are the symptoms of TEF?

Types A, B, C, D: excessive drooling; feeding induces choking, coughing, regurgitation, and cyanosis

Type E: presentation usually delayed; feeding induces coughing and choking; repeated episodes of pneumonia

What are chest/abdomen radiographic findings?

Type A: dilated upper esophageal pouch with gasless abdomen

Type C: dilated upper esophageal pouch with normal bowel pattern

Types B, D, E: may be normal

How is it diagnosed?

Types A, B, C, D:
1. Inability to pass suction catheter beyond upper esophagus
2. Presence of gas in bowel indicates fistula or fistulae between esophagus and trachea
3. Instillation of thin barium into esophageal pouch confirms discontinuity of esophagus and determines if there is a fistula between upper pouch and trachea

Type E: barium swallow; may need to instill barium into esophagus with patient in Trendelenburg position to demonstrate fistula

What is the treatment?

Type A:
1. Placement of gastrostomy tube
2. Esophagostomy with later colon interposition, jejunal interposition, or gastric tube formation
3. No esophagostomy with subsequent constant drainage of the upper pouch with a Replogle tube, and attempt at primary closure at around 12 weeks of age after the esophagus has had time to grow; if anastomosis is not possible, one of the options from number 2 above must be performed

Types B, C, D:
1. Thoracotomy via fourth intercostal space
2. Extra pleural approach
3. Division of fistula(e) with anastomosis of esophagus

Type E: division of fistula via right cervical incision

What are the possible complications?

Infection, stricture of esophagus, leak of esophageal anastomosis, recurrence of fistula

PYLORIC STENOSIS

What is it?

Hypertrophy of the pyloric muscle, causing gastric outlet obstruction

What is the incidence?

~1 in 500–1000
Male-to-female ration is 4:1
It often occurs in the firstborn male. There is a higher incidence in children of affected parents.

What is the etiology?

Unknown; suggested processes include decreased number of ganglion cells, hypergastrinemia, edema secondary to feeding, and a decrease in nitric oxide synthase

What is the most common symptom?	Progressive, projectile, **non-bilious** vomiting that occurs after feeding (**The infant is then very hungry again.**)
What are the physical signs?	1. Abdominal protuberance secondary to gastric distention 2. Gastric waves visible through abdominal wall 3. Palpable pylorus deep in epigastrium (**"olive sign"**) 4. Dehydration sometimes present
What metabolic abnormalities are noted?	1. Dehydration 2. Hypokalemic, hypochloremic metabolic alkalosis 3. Hypoglycemia Rehydration and correction of electrolytes are necessary before surgery. Potassium and glucose need to be included in resuscitative fluid.
How is it diagnosed?	By an ultrasound or upper GI series. In the latter, the "string sign" (i.e., a string of barium passing through pylorus) is seen.
How is it treated?	Ramstedt pyloromyotomy
What is the outcome?	Uniformly excellent; babies begin feeding 4–6 hours after surgery

INTESTINAL POLYPS

What are they?	Tumors that protrude into the lumen of the bowel
What are the most common polyps in children?	**Juvenile inflammatory polyps**
What are juvenile inflammatory polyps?	They are mucosal lesions consisting of dilated and tortuous mucous-filled glands, with a prominent inflammatory infiltrate in the lamina propria. The glands are composed of well-differentiated, mucous-secreting cells.

What size are they?	Grossly, the polyps are erythematous pedunculated masses between 0.5–3 cm in diameter. They are often quite friable and bleed when manipulated with a colonoscope.
Where in the bowel are they most commonly found?	Although juvenile inflammatory polyps may develop anywhere in the large intestine, nearly two thirds are located in the **distal colon** beyond the splenic flexure.
Are polyps solitary or multiple?	More than half of affected children have more than one polyp.
Are juvenile inflammatory polyps considered precancerous?	No
What are the signs and symptoms?	Intermittent painless **rectal bleeding** in children 1–10 years of age is the most common clinical presentation. The blood is generally bright red and either streaked on or intermixed with the stool.
What are some less common presentations?	1. Intermittent abdominal pain 2. Vomiting 3. Colocolonic intussusception 4. Prolapse of the polyp through the anal canal
How common are juvenile inflammatory polyps?	Juvenile inflammatory polyps are the most commonly identified cause of **painless** rectal bleeding in children between 1–10 years of age.
How are they diagnosed?	Flexible colonoscopy is employed for diagnostic and therapeutic purposes. When a polyp is identified during colonoscopy, polypectomy is usually safely performed with snare electrocautery.
Must all polyps be removed?	Most juvenile inflammatory polyps ultimately outgrow their vascular supply, become necrotic, and autoamputate. In some children, the diagnosis is first suspected when the child passes a polyp in the stool. Given the absence of

malignant potential and the relative lack of symptoms caused by most of these polyps, colonoscopic intervention is not always warranted.

What other types of polyps may develop in children?

There are several rare autosomal dominant polyposis syndromes that may present during childhood, including Peutz-Jeghers syndrome, familial polyposis coli, Cowden syndrome, and Gardner syndrome.

Can these polyps become malignant?

Yes

BEZOAR

What is it?

A mass of ingested material, usually hair and vegetable matter, that has congealed and settled in the stomach

What is the cause?

It usually results from children (more commonly boys) eating their own hair. (Often, emotionally disturbed children will do this; however they do not always form bezoars.)

What are the symptoms?

Nausea, vomiting, early satiety, inability to eat, weight loss

What are the physical signs?

Mass in epigastrium or left upper quadrant

How is it diagnosed?

Usually with an upper GI series

What is the treatment?

Removal of the bezoar is performed via open gastrotomy. Meat tenderizer or removal with endoscopy may be used for small bezoars. **Note:** Any underlying emotional disorders should be evaluated and treated.

PICA

What is it?

Persistent eating of significant amounts of non-nutritive substances

Does pica always indicate a serious problem?

Not always—during the first 2 years of life, mouthing and eating a wide variety of objects is normal exploratory behavior. In many older children and adults, the chewing and eating of non-nutritive substances (e.g.,fingernails, pencils, ice cubes) represents a habit rather than a serious medical problem.

What are the causes?

The pathophysiology is not understood. Pica is most commonly observed in children with developmental disabilities, autism, or mental retardation.

What are the complications of pica?

Complications are related to the substances ingested. The most serious complications of pica are intestinal obstruction and lead poisoning. Remember: Pica is a symptom, not a disease, and its presence may indicate an underlying disorder.

MECKEL DIVERTICULUM

What is a Meckel diverticulum?

It is a true diverticulum because it contains all layers of bowel. It is a remnant of the embryonic vitelline or omphalomesenteric duct.

What is the incidence?

2% of the population

Where is it located?

Along the antimesenteric border of the ileum, usually within 2 feet of the ileocecal valve in an adult

What types of ectopic tissue may be present?

Pancreatic or gastric ectopic mucosa may be present in 25% of the cases.

What are the symptoms?

Most Meckel diverticula are asymptomatic throughout life. However, if symptoms do occur, they may include profuse rectal bleeding (most common symptom), abdominal pain caused by inflammation, and obstruction caused by intussusception.

What causes bleeding from Meckel diverticulum?	Erosion of mucosa opposite the diverticulum caused by production of acid from ectopic gastric mucosa
How is it diagnosed?	A diagnosis can usually be made with a technetium-99M pertechnetate scan, which images gastric mucosa
What is the treatment?	Surgical excision of the diverticulum with primary bowel closure; removal may be performed via a wedge of the bowel containing the diverticulum or a total resection of the bowel segment with end-to-end anastomosis
What is a Littre hernia?	An umbilical or inguinal hernia containing a Meckel diverticulum

PERIANAL AND PERIRECTAL ABSCESS

What is a perianal abscess?	An infected collection located in the subcutaneous area of the perianal region
Who is most commonly infected in the pediatric population?	Infants
What is the most common cause?	An infected diaper rash
What are the signs and symptoms?	A firm red fluctuant area in the perianal region is commonly found; the infant may have a fever and may be irritable
What is the treatment?	Usually, lancing the area for adequate drainage is appropriate treatment. Antibiotics may be necessary to resolve the surrounding cellulitis.
What is a perirectal abscess?	An infected collection that extends up within the intersphincteric region
What are the signs and symptoms?	This condition may present with fever and pain. However, external signs may be minimal initially because the infection is more recessed from the perianal region.

Who is most commonly affected in the pediatric population?

Infants—in these cases the abscess usually results from stool gathering within a violated anal crypt

What is the treatment?

Lancing for adequate drainage is the first stage of treatment. Antibiotics are necessary for perirectal abscesses.

Can these recur?

Yes. If they do recur, it is likely that a fistula has formed.

How are these treated?

Definitive treatment is provided by placing a probe through the skin opening to the open anal crypt. Then, the overlying skin and muscle are divided and the fistula is curetted.

What conditions can predispose older children to perianal and perirectal abscess?

Crohn disease
Leukemia
Immunodeficiency disorders

20

Liver and Hepatobiliary Disorders

CHOLELITHIASIS (GALLSTONES)

What are the three types of gallstones?

1. Cholesterol
2. Pigment
3. Mixed type stones

Which stones are most common in children?

Despite an increased incidence of pigmented stones in children, **cholesterol stones** are still the most common type.

What causes cholesterol stones?

An imbalance in the concentration of **lecithin, bile salts,** and **cholesterol** within bile

What are three causes of pigmented stones?

1. Breakdown products from blood in hemolytic diseases, such as hereditary spherocytosis, thalassemia, pyruvate kinase deficiency, hexokinase deficiency, autoimmune hemolytic anemia, and hemolysis after open-heart surgery
2. Abnormal absorption of bile after ileal resection
3. Cholestasis resulting from total parenteral nutrition

What is the incidence of gallstones in children?

2 per 1000 children

What are risk factors for gallstones in neonates and infants?

Prematurity
Ileal resection
Cystic fibrosis
TPN
Prolonged fasting

What are predisposing conditions in older children?

Generally, the presence of a hemolytic disorder; cholesterol gallstones tend to be idiopathic

How do gallstones present clinically?

Biliary colic: this represents intermittent right upper quadrant pain, associated with eating, which results from obstruction of the cystic duct by a stone

Cholecystitis: inflammation of the gallbladder secondary to cystic duct obstruction from a stone

Common bile duct obstruction: may cause jaundice, acholic stools, dark urine, and **cholangitis**

What is the most useful imaging study?

Ultrasound is best for detecting stones within the gallbladder as well as any evidence of extrahepatic ductal dilatation, which suggests the presence of an obstructing gallstone within the common bile duct.

What are five useful laboratory values?

1. **Serum bilirubin** may be elevated in hemolytic disorders or if the common bile duct is obstructed. There may be mild elevation during cholecystitis.
2. **Alkaline phosphatase.** An elevated value may represent common bile duct obstruction.
3. **Hepatocellular enzymes** may be elevated in cases of cholestasis.
4. **γ-Glutamyl transferase** may be elevated in the presence of an obstructing common bile duct stone.
5. **Elevated serum amylase** may indicate the presence of associated pancreatitis and/or common bile duct obstruction.

What are two types of treatment?

1. Surgical resection of the gallbladder with an intraoperative cholangiogram is usually performed. If common duct stones are present, they are removed via a common bile duct exploration, through the cystic duct, or via ERCP.
2. Expectant management. In an infant or child who develops sludge or gallstones from TPN cholestasis, and who is otherwise asymptomatic, stones may be expected to resolve after the TPN has been discontinued.

HEPATITIS

What is hepatitis?	Inflammation of the liver (hepatocytes)
Are all types of hepatitis infectious?	No
What are causes of hepatitis other than viruses?	Trauma Metabolic diseases, such as **galactosemia** and **α-1-antitrypsin deficiency** Reye syndrome Vascular obstruction Chemical toxicity (including certain medications)
What is chronic hepatitis?	A persistent inflammation of the liver
What are causes of chronic hepatitis?	Infection, immune (autoimmune) and metabolic disorders
Which hepatitis viruses are associated with chronic hepatitis?	Usually the parenteral viruses—B, C, and D
How do chronic active hepatitis and chronic persistent hepatitis differ?	Histologically, chronic active hepatitis involves the limiting plate of the portal triad, whereas chronic persistent hepatitis does not.
Which has a better prognosis?	Chronic persistent hepatitis
What is the most common cause of unconjugated hyperbilirubinemia in children?	**Viral hepatitis**
What viruses cause hepatitis?	Hepatitis viruses A, B, C, D, and E; herpes simplex virus; varicella-zoster virus; cytomegalovirus; Epstein-Barr virus; adenovirus; enterovirus; rubella virus; parvovirus; influenza viruses
How does viral hepatitis present?	**Variable**. May range from subclinical ("anicteric") to overwhelming liver necrosis and failure.

What is the typical clinical presentation of symptomatic viral hepatitis?	**Preicteric phase:** fever, malaise, loss of appetite, abdominal pain, RUQ tenderness **Icteric phase:** jaundice, light (clay-colored) stools, dark urine (secondary to bilirubinuria), increased serum levels of hepatic transaminases

HEPATITIS A

How is it spread?	Usually via the fecal-oral route
What are sources of infection?	Contaminated water, foods (including raw shellfish), person-to-person contact (particularly among younger children)
What is the common name for hepatitis A?	**Infectious hepatitis**
What is the chance of an infected child passing the disease to another household member?	About 10%–20%
What is the incubation period?	About 4 weeks, although it can range from 10–50 days
How is a child's presentation different from an adult's?	Children are more likely to have anicteric hepatitis, with subclinical disease.
What is the laboratory diagnosis?	Demonstration of **IgM anti-hepatitis A antibodies** in serum
Is demonstration of IgG anti-hepatitis A antibodies useful?	Somewhat. These titers rise later than IgM and may persist, so the positive IgG antibody does not necessarily represent acute infection.
How can hepatitis A infection be prevented?	Good hygiene and public health measures; immune globulin injections within 2 weeks of exposure can prevent infection or reduce disease
Is there a vaccine for hepatitis A?	Yes

Does hepatitis A lead to chronic hepatitis?	Usually not
Treatment of hepatitis A?	Usually supportive

HEPATITIS B

What is another name for hepatitis B?	**Serum hepatitis**
How is it spread?	Usually via **parenteral** routes, including blood and blood products, sexual transmission, and maternal-child transmission
What is hepatitis Be antigen?	A secreted soluble antigen that is highly associated with infectivity
What is hepatitis B surface antigen (HBsAg)?	The major envelope protein of the virus
What is hepatitis core (HBc) antigen?	The major protein in the viral capsid
Which antigen correlates best with infectivity?	Hepatitis Be antigen
What is the risk to the infant of a known hepatitis B–infected mother?	Depends on her hepatitis Be antigen status; if positive, the risk of transplacental infection is 65%–85%; if negative, the risk is 10%–20%
When does mother-to-infant transmission usually occur?	During delivery
What is meant by "chronic carrier state"?	Patients infected with hepatitis B who have a persistent viral infection
Who are most likely to become chronic carriers?	Infected infants
What are the risks to chronic carriers?	Persistent infectivity; chronic liver disease

How is hepatitis B infection diagnosed?	Usually via serologic testing, looking at serum antibodies against HBsAg and HBc and for the presence of the HBsAg
What is the first serum marker of hepatitis B infection?	Presence of HBsAg
Which antibody usually appears first after an acute hepatitis B infection?	Anti-HBc (at around 15 weeks)
How can hepatitis B infection be prevented?	Universal precautions for health care workers Decreased exposure by high-risk individuals **Hepatitis B vaccine** is available and effective **Hepatitis B immune globulin** for passive immunization
How do you treat an infant born to an infected mother?	Hepatitis B immune globulin and hepatitis B vaccine within 12 hours
Is hepatitis B vaccine recommended for all infants?	Yes

HEPATITIS C

How is it spread?	Usually via parenteral routes; also possibly sexual transmission and mother-to-infant transmission
How is it diagnosed?	Usually by serology (ELISA) or PCR
When does the ELISA test become positive?	It may be up to 8–12 weeks after infection before the ELISA is positive, although it may be positive earlier.
Treatment?	α- and β-Interferon have shown encouraging results.
What is the risk for chronic liver disease?	May be as high as 70% of infected patients

HEPATITIS D

What is another name for the hepatitis D virus?	Delta virus
How is it transmitted?	Usually via blood products
What is its relationship to hepatitis B infection?	Infection with hepatitis B virus (either previous or concurrent) is required
How is it diagnosed?	Demonstration of anti-hepatitis D virus antibodies

HEPATITIS E

How is it spread?	Fecal-oral route
What is the incubation period?	2–9 weeks
How is it diagnosed?	Diagnosis is usually based on epidemiology and exclusion of other viruses.

BILIARY ATRESIA

What is it?	Abnormality of the intrahepatic and/or extrahepatic bile ducts, in which the ducts are either fibrous cords or completely absent
What is the incidence?	1 in 15,000
What are associated defects?	Congenital heart disease Absent inferior vena cava Preduodenal portal vein Intestinal malrotation Polysplenia
What is the etiology?	It is unknown at this time. Biliary atresia appears to be a condition acquired after birth and may be due to a reovirus infection. It appears to be an inflammatory process.

What is so-called correctable biliary atresia?

Biliary atresia in which the intrahepatic and proximal extrahepatic ducts are patent.

What is the natural history of biliary atresia?

Biliary duct obstruction with progressive cirrhosis, portal hypertension, hepatomegaly, and jaundice
Infants with uncorrected biliary atresia are likely to die before 2 years of age.

What are presenting signs and symptoms?

Jaundice and hepatomegaly are usually the initial signs. Acholic stools and dark urine are present. Direct bilirubin and alkaline phosphatase levels are elevated.

How is it diagnosed?

The diagnosis is suggested by obstruction of biliary flow on a nuclear imaging scan. However, final diagnosis is made at laparotomy when it is established that the biliary tree is fibrous.

Treatment?

Surgical correction is the first-line treatment. It involves resection of the atretic gallbladder and biliary ducts up to the point of the liver that lies within the branches of the portal vein (the periportal plate). Roux-en-Y hepaticojejunostomy is performed with the jejunum anastomosed directly to the periportal plate.

What are the outcomes?

Approximately 33% of infants have a successful outcome with no need for liver transplant; 66% of infants ultimately require liver transplant for survival.

When is surgical correction of biliary atresia most likely to be successful?

Before the infant is 8 weeks of age and when bile flow is established after the operation

What is the surgical procedure typically called?

The Kasai portoenterostomy

CHOLEDOCHAL CYSTS

What are they?

These are abnormal dilatations of the extrahepatic biliary system and/or the intrahepatic biliary system. The cysts usually have thick walls of dense connective tissue with strands of smooth muscle. There is little or no muscle lining.

What is the etiology?

Unknown. However there is usually an abnormal entrance of the pancreatic duct into the common bile duct above the sphincter of Oddi. It is postulated that reflux of pancreatic enzymes may cause the formation of choledochal cysts.

What are the five types of choledochal cysts?

Type I: cystic dilatation of the common bile duct

Type II: diverticular malformation of the common bile duct

Type III: a choledochocele at the level of the sphincter of Oddi

Type IV: cystic dilatation of the extrahepatic and intrahepatic common bile ducts

Type V: single or multiple intrahepatic dilatations of the bile ducts

Who are most prone to getting choledochal cysts?

Females and individuals of Asian descent

How do choledochal cysts present in infants?

Jaundice is usually the first presenting sign.

In older children?

A classic triad of **abdominal pain, jaundice,** and a **palpable mass** has been described. However, usually the abdominal pain and jaundice are the two most common presenting signs. Older children with choledochal cysts may also present with onset of **pancreatitis.**

What are typical laboratory findings?

Elevated bilirubin and alkaline phosphatase, suggesting bile duct obstruction; also, the serum amylase is often elevated

What is the most useful diagnostic study?

Ultrasound; occasionally a biliary nuclear scan and/or ERCP may be needed to confirm the diagnosis

Treatment?	**Surgical excision** when possible. This usually entails resecting the dilated portion of the common bile duct and performing a Roux-en-Y choledochojejunostomy. The gallbladder is removed at the same time. In some cases, the cyst cannot be removed in its entirety and, therefore, the inner lining of the cyst should be shelled out from the outer wall of the cyst. This approach works for types I, II, and IV. A type III cyst is usually simply unroofed within the duodenum. Type V cysts represent the most difficult surgical challenge. These are usually drained into a Roux-en-Y jejunal limb.
What is the risk of leaving choledochal cyst tissue behind?	There is a significant incidence of degeneration of the cyst epithelium into **adenosquamous carcinoma.** Unfortunately, type V cysts are probably the greatest threat for this, because they can not be entirely removed and the inner linings are not easily removed either.
What are the outcomes?	Generally the result of surgery for types I, II, III, and IV cysts are quite good. However patients with type V cysts have an increased risk of developing carcinoma and also tend to present with recurring bouts of cholangitis.

PORTAL HYPERTENSION

What are the three types of obstruction that may cause portal hypertension in children?	1. Extrahepatic obstruction (portal vein thrombosis) 2. Intrahepatic venous obstruction 3. Suprahepatic venous obstruction (Budd-Chiari syndrome)
What is the most common type of portal hypertension in children?	Extrahepatic (portal vein thrombosis)
What are the common causes of extrahepatic portal hypertension in children?	Neonatal omphalitis Intra-abdominal infections Dehydration Umbilical vein catheterization Enterocolitis Congenital abnormalities of portal area

What are causes of intrahepatic portal hypertension?

It is usually caused by cirrhosis, which in turn is secondary to the following conditions:
Biliary atresia
Congenital hepatic fibrosis
Cystic fibrosis
α-I-antitrypsin deficiency
Radiation or chemotherapy changes
Hepatitis
Sclerosing cholangitis
Histiocytosis X
Galactosemia
Congenital biliary cirrhosis
Hepatic hemangioma
Glycogen storage disease

What are the common causes of suprahepatic portal obstruction (Budd-Chiari syndrome)?

In most cases the cause cannot be identified. Occasionally (and usually outside of the United States) granulomatous disease may cause this condition. In other cases, oral contraceptive use may cause this condition.

What are the four most common symptoms of portal hypertension?

1. Esophageal variceal hemorrhage
2. Splenomegaly with possible subsequent hypersplenism
3. Ascites
4. Ultimately, liver failure

TREATMENT

How is portal hypertension caused by portal vein thrombosis treated?

Esophageal variceal bleeding is usually the most troublesome complication but rarely requires emergent operative intervention. Usually, the patient is hospitalized and given **IV fluids, vitamin K, H₂ blockers,** and **blood transfusion,** if necessary, to provide adequate support until the bleeding stops. In some cases, direct visualization of the varices with **injection of a sclerosing agent** is required. If a portosystemic shunt is required, a **distal splenorenal** or **mesocaval shunt** are the two most common operations employed.

How is portal hypertension due to liver cirrhosis treated?

Variceal bleeding is treated with sclerosing agents. However, the ultimate course of treatment depends on the prognosis of the hepatic disease. Worsening hypertension may require a **distal splenorenal** or a **mesocaval shunt**. In some cases, **liver transplantation** is required.

How is portal hypertension due to suprahepatic obstruction treated?

Shunts from the portal system to the right atrium have occasionally been successful. In most cases, **liver transplantation** is currently the treatment of choice.

CONGENITAL HEPATIC FIBROSIS

What is it?

A disease characterized by diffuse periportal and perilobular fibrosis. These may form duct-like structures but do not communicate themselves with the biliary system.

What are some associated conditions?

Renal tubular ectasia
Autosomal recessive polycystic renal
    disease
Nephronophthisis

What are the signs and symptoms?

This condition usually becomes evident in early childhood. Hepatosplenomegaly and esophageal variceal bleeding secondary to portal hypertension are characteristic conditions.

What is the treatment?

Usually the hepatocellular function is normal. Therefore, treatment focuses on control of esophageal bleeding. Usually bleeding episodes can be controlled by supportive care or sclerotherapy using endoscopy. In some cases, a portosystemic shunt may be required.

What are the outcomes?

Even if a portosystemic shunt is required, the prognosis from a hepatic standpoint is usually good. However, associated renal conditions may limit long-term survival.

21

Renal Diseases

ACUTE RENAL FAILURE

What is it?	A sudden decrease in glomerular filtration rate to a level that is insufficient to maintain fluid and electrolyte homeostasis
What is oliguria?	Decreased urine output
What are the three classifications of oliguria?	Prerenal: volume depletion or poor cardiac output Renal (or intrinsic): glomerular or tubular injury Postrenal (or obstructive): congenital or acquired urinary tract obstruction (must be bilateral)
What are the most common causes of acute renal failure?	
In infants?	Sepsis, asphyxia/hypotension, congenital heart disease, congenital urinary tract anomalies, renal arterial thrombi
In older children?	Hemolytic–uremic syndrome (HUS), acute glomerulonephritis (usually poststreptococcal), trauma, sepsis
How can you differentiate prerenal oliguria from intrinsic renal failure in infants?	In prerenal oliguria, the kidney responds to hypoperfusion by increasing sodium and water reabsorption. The urine is concentrated (specific gravity > 1.010) and the fractional excretion of sodium (FE_{Na}) is low (< 1%). When glomerular and/or tubular damage has occurred, these functions cannot take place. The urine will be isosthenuric (specific gravity = 1.010) and FE_{Na} will be high (> 2%).

What are the cardiac manifestations of hyperkalemia?

Peaked T waves are seen first, followed by prolonged PR intervals, flattened P waves, widened QRS complexes, and terminally, ventricular tachycardia and fibrillation.

What is the treatment of hyperkalemia?

1. Membrane stabilization: calcium gluconate (100 mg/kg IV) or calcium chloride (10 mg/kg IV)
2. Redistribution: $NaHCO_3$ (1–2 mEq/kg IV) drives K^+ into cells in exchange for H^+ extruded to buffer the bicarbonate. β-agonists (10 mg of albuterol as nebulizer) as well as insulin (0.1 u/kg IV) plus glucose (0.5 g/kg IV) stimulate cellular uptake of K^+.
3. Removal: Kayexalate (Na^+–K^+ exchange resin) used po or per rectum binds K^+ for later excretion; dialysis is the most effective method of removing K^+.

Why are patients with acute renal failure commonly hypertensive?

Fluid overload is the most common cause of hypertension, although acute glomerular diseases (AGN, HUS) are also associated with **high renin** output.

How is hypertension best treated in renal failure?

1. Appropriate **fluid management** is mandatory; diuresis if possible, and dialysis if necessary
2. Vasodilators (e.g., calcium channel blockers, sodium nitroprusside, diazoxide)
3. ACE inhibitors

What is the proper fluid replacement prescription for a child in acute renal failure?

Combine insensible losses, urine output, extrarenal fluid losses (e.g., nasogastric drainage, stool losses), and estimated losses of Na^+ and other electrolytes

What is CAVH, and how is it used in acute renal failure?

Continuous arteriovenous hemofiltration—CAVH utilizes the patient's cardiac output to drive fluid transfer across an extracorporeal membrane. It is most useful for patients with extreme fluid overload.

CHRONIC RENAL FAILURE

What is creatinine clearance (Ccr)?

An estimate of glomerular filtration rate: $Ccr = UV/P \times 1.73/SA = ml/min/1.73\ M^2$, where

  SA = body surface area (M^2)
  U (mg/ml) = urinary creatinine concentration
  V (ml/min) = total urine volume (ml) divided by time (min)
  P (mg/ml) = serum creatinine

A correction factor of 1.73 is used to normalize adult and child creatinine clearance values since a normal adult body surface area is 1.73 M^2.

What is a normal Ccr for an infant?

A normal newborn's Ccr is ≈ 20 ml/min/ 1.73 M^2

At what age is adult level reached?

Normal adult values (80–120 ml/min/ 1.73 M^2) are reached by 2 years of age.

What level of Ccr denotes end-stage renal disease?

$Ccr \leq 10\ ml/min/1.73\ M^2$

What are the most common causes of chronic renal insufficiency/renal failure in the pediatric population?

In infants and preschool children?

Congenital structural anomalies
Obstruction
Hypoplasia/dysplasia

In older children and adolescents?

Acquired glomerular diseases, including glomerulonephritis, HUS, reflux nephropathy, and lupus
Inherited disorders, including Alport syndrome and polycystic kidney disease

How well do children with chronic renal failure grow?

Poorly, both in weight gain and linear growth

Why?

Potential causes include steroid treatment, protein losses (in nephrotic syndrome), sodium wasting, chronic acidosis, renal osteodystrophy, recurrent illness, and malnutrition.

What is the treatment of growth failure?

Aggressive nutritional support, medical management of electrolyte abnormalities, dialysis, and recombinant growth hormone all help. **Early renal transplant may be recommended.**

What is renal osteodystrophy?

Bone demineralization caused by decreased renal function, leading to decreased production of vitamin D and elevated parathyroid hormone levels; demineralization is often severe enough to impair growth and increase the risks of fracture

Why are patients with renal failure anemic?

Because failing kidneys stop producing erythropoietin

How is it treated?

Subcutaneous or IV-recombinant erythropoietin administration reduces the need for transfusions.

What are the hallmark electrolyte abnormalities in chronic renal failure?

Hyperkalemia, uremia (increased BUN), hyperphosphatemia, hypocalcemia, and acidosis

What are the treatment options for children with end-stage renal disease?

1. **Peritoneal dialysis** (the favored modality for children) utilizes the peritoneal membrane for exchange with dialysate and may be done in an automated fashion by the parents at home.
2. **Hemodialysis** is harsher, requires in-hospital treatments, and utilizes needles.
3. **Renal transplantation** (either from living relatives or cadaveric donors) provides long-term and more physiologic renal replacement; there may be problems with rejection or recurrent disease.

NEPHROTIC SYNDROME

What four features characterize it?

1. Edema
2. Proteinuria (> 4 mg/kg/hr)
3. Hypoalbuminemia (< 2.0–2.5 g/dl)
4. Hypercholesterolemia

What are the causes?

Approximately 85% of children with nephrotic syndrome have "minimal change disease." The remaining causes include focal segmental glomerular sclerosis, membranoproliferative glomerulonephritis, membranous nephropathy, systemic lupus erythematosus, and Henoch-Schönlein purpura.

What is minimal change disease?

It is a form of nephrotic syndrome in which light microscopy is normal; immunofluorescence is normal; and electron microscopy shows only fusion of the podocyte foot processes.

What is the source of the edema in nephrotic syndrome?

Although not completely understood, the edema is most likely due to a decreased plasma oncotic pressure secondary to protein loss into the urine. The fluid leakage into the extravascular space also causes decreased perfusion pressure, which results in increased sodium and water reabsorption by the kidney.

How is nephrotic syndrome treated?

>Ninety-five percent of children with minimal change disease go into remission with corticosteroid therapy (typically 2 mg/kg/day of prednisone) within 4 weeks. Two thirds will have relapses, some frequently. Steroid toxicity and/or dependence may lead to treatment with cytotoxic agents, such as cyclophosphamide or chlorambucil. When nephrotic syndrome is a secondary process, treatment or resolution of the primary process usually allows resolution of the nephrotic syndrome.

What is the prognosis of minimal change disease?

The disease usually resolves spontaneously after puberty without renal dysfunction.

What are the complications of nephrotic syndrome?

Infection—pneumococcal and gram-negative infections are the most common; increased susceptibility is due to poor nutrition, loss of immunoglobulins, and immunosuppressive therapy

GLOMERULONEPHRITIS

What is the difference between nephritis and nephrosis?	**Nephrosis** (or nephrotic syndrome): proteinuria, hypoalbuminemia, and edema
	Nephritis: hematuria, decreased creatinine clearance, and hypertension; many chronic glomerular diseases present a picture of nephritis with or without nephrosis
What is the typical presentation of acute poststreptococcal glomerulonephritis (PSGN)?	Gross hematuria, hypertension, mild edema, and decreased renal function 7–14 days following a skin or throat infection with **group A streptococcus**
What is the lab profile of poststreptococcal glomerulonephritis?	**Decreased C3** and **elevated strep titers** (ASO, Streptozyme, or anti-DNase B)
What is the clinical course?	Varying degrees of renal insufficiency and hypertension with resolution of clinical signs after 1 month
How long can urinary abnormalities last?	For up to 2 years
How many children completely recover?	95%; children with severe involvement have all the risks of acute renal failure
Does penicillin help?	May prevent further spreading of nephritogenic strains, but unlike rheumatic fever, treatment of strep infections does not significantly decrease the risk of PSGN
What chronic forms of glomerulonephritis most commonly affect children?	IgA nephropathy, lupus nephritis, membranoproliferative glomerulonephritis, membranous nephropathy, Henoch-Schönlein purpura, focal segmental glomerulosclerosis, and Alport syndrome

VESICOURETERAL REFLUX (VUR)

What is it?

It is "backwash" of urine from the bladder into the ureter and/or kidney and is caused by incompetence of the ureterovesical junction

How does it cause damage?

By exposing the kidney to high pressure during voiding and by increasing the risk of pyelonephritis in the presence of a lower urinary tract infection; these exposures can lead to dilatation and scarring of the collecting system and renal parenchyma

What is the etiology?

It may be primary and isolated (congenital incompetence) or **associated with other urinary tract abnormalities**. Secondary reflux may be caused by increased bladder pressure, inflammation, obstructing lesions (e.g., posterior urethral valves) or previous surgical procedures.

How is it recognized?

Usually during an evaluation for a urinary tract infection, renal insufficiency, hypertension, or voiding problems

How is it diagnosed?

Voiding cystourethrogram (**VCUG**), in which radio-opaque dye is instilled into the bladder until full, and the dye is observed during voiding

What is the grading system?

Grade I: reflux into a nondilated distal ureter
Grade II: reflux into the upper collecting system without dilatation
Grade III: reflux into a dilated collecting system without blunting of calyces
Grade IV: reflux into a dilated system with blunting of calyces
Grade V: massive reflux with gross dilatation and distortion of the ureter and collecting system

What are the complications of VUR?	Renal scarring, leading to **end-stage renal disease** (15%–20% of children on dialysis had VUR) and **hypertension**
What is the natural history?	Risk of renal scarring increases with the degree of reflux. Eighty percent of children with primary grades I and II reflux undergo spontaneous correction with maturation. Higher degrees of reflux are less likely to resolve. Secondary reflux has a less favorable outcome across all grades.
What is the treatment?	1. Prevent infection with antibiotic prophylaxis (commonly, trimethoprim/sulfamethoxazole). If expectant management is undertaken, uroprophylaxis continues as long as the reflux persists. 2. Follow-up VCUGs should be performed every 1-to-2 years to evaluate the progression or regression of the reflux. 3. Children with severe degrees of reflux, breakthrough infections while on uroprophylaxis, or evidence of renal scarring are candidates for surgical correction via **ureteral reimplantation.**

RENAL TUBULAR ACIDOSIS (RTA)

What is it?	Systemic hyperchloremic (i.e., normal anion gap) acidosis resulting from abnormal urinary acidification processes
How does it usually present?	Growth failure in the first year of life
What is type 1 (distal) RTA?	The distal tubule has a deficient H^+ excretion capability, which leads to excess body H^+.
What is type 2 (proximal) RTA?	An inability of the proximal tubule to reabsorb filtered bicarbonate, leading to loss of buffering capacity and acidosis.

What is type 4 RTA?

Distal tubular damage, which is commonly caused by obstructive uropathy, leads to decreased responsiveness to aldosterone; inability to excrete H^+ and K^+ leads to hyperkalemic acidosis

How can you differentiate among these types?

Types 1 and 2 usually cause hypokalemia, whereas type 4 tends to cause hyperkalemia. Types 1 and 2 can be differentiated in an acidotic patient by urine pH: Type 2 patients acidify urine to pH < 5.5 when serum HCO_3^- is less than 16 mEq/L (their distal acidifying mechanisms still work). Type 1 patients cannot acidify the urine because of distal abnormalities, even in the presence of significant systemic acidosis.

How can you differentiate types 1 and 2?

By the replacement of bicarbonate: Type 1 patients typically require only 1–2 mEq/kg/day of $NaHCO_3$ to maintain acid–base balance, because only the small amount of base needed to buffer endogenously formed H^+ is necessary. Type 2 patients are unable to reabsorb bicarbonate, and doses of 10 mEq/kg/day may be needed for acid–base balance.

FANCONI SYNDROME

What is it?

Generalized aminoaciduria, glycosuria, and phosphaturia and is often accompanied by bicarbonate wasting, proteinuria, and hyperkaluria, all of which are due to proximal tubule transport defects

What are common clinical manifestations?

Clinical signs are growth failure and vitamin D–resistant rickets.

What causes it?

It is usually idiopathic; however, it is a common feature of certain inborn errors of metabolism (e.g., cystinosis, galactosemia, Lowe syndrome) or toxic events (e.g., heavy metal poisoning).

What are lab findings?	Normal anion gap hyperchloremic metabolic acidosis, hypokalemia, hypophosphatemia, elevated fractional excretion of phosphate (> 15%), glycosuria in the presence of euglycemia
Treatment?	Evaluation for underlying abnormalities, high doses of vitamin D, phosphate and bicarbonate supplementation

DIABETES INSIPIDUS (DI)

What is central DI?	Loss of antidiuretic hormone (ADH) secretion, resulting in the inability to concentrate urine appropriately despite normal renal function
What are the consequences?	Increased urine output, **hyper**natremia, and dehydration
What is the etiology?	Idiopathic, posttraumatic/postsurgical, congenital malformation, intracranial tumors, CNS infections, histiocytosis, granulomatous disease, familial
What are the signs and symptoms?	**Polyuria, polydipsia, weight loss,** and **growth failure;** patients generally prefer water to other fluids
What signs may indicate that DI is secondary to a tumor?	Neurologic or visual complaints may be present.
What are the diagnostic lab results?	Morning urine specific gravity < 1.010 Low urine osmolarity Normal-to-high serum sodium concentration
What is the water deprivation test?	The test is begun in the morning after a water load of 500 ml/m². Measurements are taken of: 1. Hourly weights and urine output 2. Urine specific gravity and osmolarity on each sample 3. Serum sodium and osmolarity every 4 hours

What constitutes a positive test?	Persistence of dilute urine with osmolarity less than that of plasma, a rise in serum sodium to > 145 mEq/L, a rise of serum osmolarity to > 290 mOsm/kg, and a weight loss of 3%–5% suggest DI. Desmopressin (dDAVP), a long-acting analog of ADH, is given at the end of the test to document responsiveness to ADH.
What radiographic tests should be ordered?	1. Skull radiograph investigating for calcification, enlargement of the sella turcica, erosion of the clinoid processes, or increased width of the suture lines 2. An MRI is ordered to differentiate the posterior from the anterior pituitary. A bright spot is present in the posterior pituitary in normal patients but is absent in patients with lesions of the hypothalamic-neurohypophyseal tract.
What is the treatment?	dDAVP is given intranasally once or twice daily.
What is the differential Dx?	Nephrogenic diabetes insipidus, psychogenic water drinking, impaired thirst mechanism

NEPHROGENIC DIABETES INSIPIDUS

What are the differences between nephrogenic and central DI?	Patients with nephrogenic DI synthesize and secrete adequate ADH, whereas patients with central DI do not.
What is the primary defect in nephrogenic DI?	The defect in nephrogenic DI is the lack of distal tubular response to ADH, leading to inability to concentrate the urine.
What is the etiology of primary nephrogenic DI?	Primary nephrogenic DI is a rare X-linked recessive disorder with profound effects in males, although females may be mildly affected. In some families, the defect is caused by a mutation in the vasopressin receptor. Autosomal dominant and recessive DI have also been described.

What is the etiology of secondary nephrogenic DI?

Secondary nephrogenic DI is more common and often less severe; causes include obstructive uropathy, chronic renal failure, sickle cell anemia, and drug toxicity.

How does it present?

In the more severe forms, nephrogenic DI presents within the first weeks of life, usually as polyuria, polydipsia, failure to thrive, and chronic dehydration. The degree of dehydration is commonly underappreciated because the child continues to urinate. Fever, irritability, and poor feeding are also common.

What are lab findings?

Hypernatremia, hyperchloremia, urine osmolarity < 200 mOsm/kg in the presence of serum osmolarity > 300 mOsm/kg. ADH levels are normal, and there is no response to exogenously administered vasopressin.

What is the treatment?

Insurance of adequate fluid intake is the most important treatment modality. Although somewhat counterintuitive, thiazide diuretics decrease urine output by causing mild sodium depletion, thereby encouraging proximal tubular sodium and water reabsorption. Prostaglandin synthesis inhibitors are also useful for decreasing urine output, although the mechanism of action is unclear.

RENAL STONES

What are the signs and symptoms?

Hematuria (microscopic or gross), abdominal or flank pain, or urinary tract infection

What is the most common chemical composition of a stone?

Calcium oxalate

  Other chemical compositions?

Calcium phosphate, struvite (magnesium ammonium phosphate), uric acid, and cystine

What are predisposing conditions?

Urinary tract anomalies, recurrent UTIs, hypercalciuria, renal tubular acidosis (especially distal), immobilization, hyperoxaluria, cystinuria, hyperparathyroidism, hypocitraturia (citrate is an inhibitor of stone formation)

What are radiographic findings?

Plain abdominal radiograph shows calcium-containing stones, whereas intravenous pyelogram and/or ultrasound documents location of radiopaque and radiolucent stones as well as the degree of obstruction. Ultrasound and voiding cystourethrogram help evaluate urinary tract abnormalities.

What are useful lab studies?

Serum: electrolytes (especially HCO_3^-), calcium, phosphorus, uric acid, creatinine, parathyroid hormone
Urine: urinalysis and culture, urine pH, 24-hour collection for calcium, creatinine, phosphorus, oxalate, uric acid, cystine, and citrate

What is normal calcium excretion?

< 4 mg/kg/day or urinary calcium–creatinine ratio < 0.2

What is the treatment of hypercalciuria?

Limit calcium intake to the RDA, increase fluid intake, and limit sodium intake (sodium restriction increases calcium reabsorption); if stones persist, thiazide diuretics may help

What is the treatment of stones?

1. Hydration and pain management until stone passes
2. Treatment of predisposing conditions may prevent future stones
3. If stones persist, lithotripsy can pulverize some stones without the need for surgery
4. Endoscopic, percutaneous, and open surgery may be needed

HYPERTENSION

What is hypertension in the pediatric population?

Blood pressure increases with age:
Significant hypertension is defined as blood pressures greater than the 95th percentile for age and sex.

Severe hypertension is blood pressure greater than the 99th percentile.

What is the appropriate size for a child's blood pressure cuff?

The cuff bladder width should be large enough to encircle two thirds of the upper arm. Bladder length should be long enough to surround the entire arm circumference.

What happens to readings if the cuff is too large or small?

Cuffs that are too small give erroneously high readings, whereas cuffs that are too large may give erroneously low readings.

What are the most common causes of acute hypertension in infants?

Renal artery occlusion, medications

In children and adolescents?

Acute glomerulonephritis, HUS, medications (including illicit drugs)

What are the most common causes of chronic hypertension in infants?

Renal arterial thrombi (umbilical catheter complication), aortic coarctation, obstructive uropathy, medications

In young children?

Obstructive uropathy, reflux nephropathy, glomerular disease, renal artery stenosis

In adolescents?

Essential hypertension, glomerular disease, reflux nephropathy, renal artery stenosis

How is the diagnosis of essential hypertension made?

By exclusion of secondary causes

What should evaluation include?

1. Studies of renal function and anatomy, and urinary sediment
2. Studies for rare but correctable causes, such as pheochromocytoma, Cushing disease, and aortic coarctation
3. Nuclear scans and/or arteriography for diagnosis of renal artery stenosis may be needed

What medications are used to treat chronic hypertension in children?

Essentially all forms of antihypertensives may be used if monitored appropriately.

When are diuretics used?

For patients with underlying renal disease and fluid overload; often used in conjunction with other medications

22

Genitourinary Disorders

HYPOSPADIAS

What is it?	Malformation of the penis with abnormal ventral placement of the urethral meatus
Where may the meatus be located?	The ventral side of the penis, the scrotum, or on the perineum
What is the etiology?	Incomplete virilization of the penis, possibly associated with androgen insensitivity
What is the incidence?	About 1 per 300 male births; it is the most common penile malformation
What are associated malformations?	1. Chordee (curvature) of the penis is common. 2. Hernias and cryptorchidism are common, but renal and bladder malformations are not. 3. Chromosome abnormalities are uncommon in patients with isolated hypospadias, but should be considered in patients with complex malformations.
Treatment?	Surgical repair, sometimes in stages for severe hypospadias
What are common complications?	Chordee, fistulas, and strictures

CRYPTORCHIDISM

What is it?	Lack of normal descent of the testicle
What is the incidence?	About 1 in 100 male infants

Do undescended testicles usually present unilaterally or bilaterally?

Unilaterally in 75% of cases

At what age is a boy's testicle considered truly undescended?

After 1 year of age

Why?

Because testicles that are undescended at birth usually descend into the scrotum within the first year

What are the consequences of an undescended testicle?

1. After the second year, testicular degeneration occurs, resulting in low spermatogonia counts and degeneration of germinal epithelium. Seminiferous tubules become fibrous. This overall degeneration can cause the formation of sperm antibodies, which can adversely affect fertility even if there is a normal descended testicle on the opposite side.
2. There is an **increased incidence of cancer**, particularly **seminoma**, in an undescended testicle.

Treatment?

Although hormone therapy has been used to induce descent of the testicle, it is almost always unsuccessful. The major treatment of undescended testicle is **orchiopexy**, which is usually performed through an inguinal incision. Occasionally, the spermatic vessels may need to be divided high in the retroperitoneum to allow the testicle to be brought down into the scrotum. The blood supply is then dependent on collateral vessels along the vas deferens.

When should orchiopexy be performed?

No later than 2 years of age. Current recommendations suggest that orchiopexy should be performed between 6 and 12 months of age.

EPIDIDYMITIS

What is it?

Inflammation of the epididymis

What are the two most common causes?	1. Reflux of infected urine 2. STDs caused by gonococci and chlamydia
How does it present?	Unilateral pain in the scrotum
What are physical findings?	A large, tender, and firm epididymis with a normal testicle
Treatment?	Antibiotics appropriate for the identified pathogen; if epididymitis is severe, intravenous antibiotics may be required for 48–72 hours
What should be suspected if epididymitis occurs in a nonsexually active child or a prepubertal child?	These patients may have a urinary tract abnormality. They should be evaluated with a renal ultrasound and a VCUG.

TESTICULAR TORSION

What is it?	The testicle twists upon its blood supply and the vas deferens. The testicle then becomes ischemic and necrotic.
What are the two types of testicular torsion?	1. Extravaginal, which occurs when the torsion of the vessels and the vas deferens is outside of the tunic vaginalis 2. Intravaginal, which occurs when the torsion of the vessels and the vas deferens is within the tunic vaginalis
In which age groups do extravaginal and intravaginal torsion occur?	Extravaginal: predominantly in the neonatal period Intravaginal torsion (also known as the **Bell-Clapper** anomaly): predominantly in older children
How does torsion present?	It usually presents as an acute scrotum with severe scrotal pain and significant scrotal swelling unilaterally.
Differential Dx?	Epididymitis Torsion of the appendix epididymitis Orchitis Acute hydrocele Torsion of the appendix testes

What is the evaluation for testicular torsion?

If testicular torsion is highly suspected, the patient should be brought directly to the operating room. If length of symptomatology is approaching or exceeding 6 hours, it is likely that the testicle is necrotic. If the time course from onset of the symptomatology is shorter and there is a suspicion that an alternative diagnosis is possible, Doppler ultrasound or testicular radioisotope imaging may confirm viability of the testicle and rule out torsion.

Treatment?

A surgical exploration of the scrotum is performed through a midline incision in the scrotum. The affected testicle is unrotated if viability is still thought to be present. If the testicle is necrotic, it is removed. If it is viable, it is fixed in four points in the scrotum. The opposite testicle is routinely fixed in the opposite scrotum at four points as well.

TESTICULAR TUMORS

What are the common types of testicular tumors which affect boys?

1. Germ cell tumor
2. Teratoma
3. Seminoma
4. Gonadal stromal tumors
5. Gonadoblastoma
6. Leukemic and lymphomatous infiltrates
7. Rhabdomyosarcoma

Which of these is the most common type?

Germ cell tumor

Which is the most common germ cell tumor?

The yolk-sac (endodermal sinus) tumor

What are symptoms and signs of the yolk-sac tumor?

Presence of a testicular mass; sometimes a hydrocele may be caused by the tumor and may delay diagnosis

What are common chemical markers?

The most common is alpha-fetoprotein (αFP); however, beta-HCG may also be secreted

What is the surgical workup and treatment?

Biopsy should be performed through an inguinal incision. If a biopsy is done through the scrotum, hemiscrotectomy is also needed in the surgical resection if the biopsy is positive. Orchiectomy is performed through an inguinal incision. If the tumor is isolated to the testicle, surgical resection (orchiectomy) is all that is required. Retroperitoneal lymph node dissection is required if there is evidence of clinically suspicious nodes on CT scan. Extensive tumor will require chemotherapy.

In which patients do gonadoblastomas arise?

Male pseudohermaphrodites and patients with mixed gonadal dysgenesis; these patients are usually not phenotypic males

Treatment?

Usually only orchiectomy, because these tumors are encapsulated and slow-growing

In which patients do seminomas most commonly arise?

Males with cryptorchid testes

What is the treatment of seminoma?

Surgical resection with radiation therapy; these tumors are particularly sensitive to radiation therapy

How are leukemic and lymphomatous infiltrates treated?

After a transscrotal biopsy, these lesions are treated systemically according to the type of disease found.

Which tumors cause precocious puberty?

These are usually the gonadal stromal and sex cord tumors, such as the Sertoli cell and Leydig cell neoplasms; Leydig cells in particular secrete excessive testosterone

Treatment?

Surgical resection (orchiectomy)

How is testicular rhabdomyosarcoma evaluated and treated?

Similar to yolk-sac tumor; bone scan and bone marrow aspirates are needed as well; radiation therapy may be adjunctive, but is rarely needed

What are the outcomes for rhabdomyosarcoma?	Favorable, about 95% 5-year survival
Treatment for teratoma?	Simple orchiectomy

OVARIAN TUMORS

What the four major categories of ovarian tumors in children?	1. Germ cell tumors, including teratoma, dysgerminoma, endodermal sinus tumor, embryonal carcinoma, and choriocarcinoma 2. Gonadoblastoma 3. Sex cord stromal tumors, including granulosa-theca tumor and Sertoli-Leydig tumor 4. Epithelial ovarian tumor, including mucinous, serous, clear cell, endometrioid, mixed, and undifferentiated
Which is the most common ovarian tumor in children?	Teratoma
Are most of these benign or malignant?	Benign
How do they present?	Presence of an abdominal mass and/or pain
What may be a pertinent radiographic finding?	The presence of calcification in 50% of cases
Treatment?	If the tumor is within the capsule of the ovary, unilateral salpingo-oophorectomy is all that is needed. However, if the tumor is grade II or greater, there is an increased chance of malignancy and chemotherapy will be required.
What are dysgerminomas?	They are malignant tumors derived from primordial germ cells.
In what age group do they commonly present?	Prepubertal and adolescent girls.
Are these tumors biologically active?	Minimally

Treatment?	Surgical resection with radiation and chemotherapy
What is an endodermal sinus tumor?	It is an aggressive malignant germ cell tumor that grows rapidly and metastasizes early.
In what age group do they commonly present?	Teenage girls and young adult women
Is there a tumor marker?	Yes, αFP
Treatment?	Surgical resection with chemotherapy
What is the outcome?	There is approximately a 60%–70% four-year survival
What is an embryonal carcinoma?	This is another malignant germ cell tumor that is quite biologically active.
What are the tumor markers?	αFP and beta-HCG
What is the characteristic presentation?	A patient may present with abnormal vaginal bleeding, hirsutism, and precocious puberty due to elevated beta-HCG.
Treatment?	Surgical resection and chemotherapy
What is a choriocarcinoma?	An aggressive germ cell tumor that generally is hormonally active
What is the tumor marker?	Beta-HCG
What are presenting symptoms?	Precocious puberty or menstrual irregularity
Treatment?	Surgical resection with chemotherapy
What is a gonadoblastoma?	These are tumors that arise in dysgenetic gonads.
Treatment?	Surgical resection of the gonadoblastoma as well as the opposite ovary, because it is also at risk for malignant degeneration

What is a granulosa-theca cell tumor?

It is a tumor that has its origin in sex cord or stromal tissue.

What is the presentation?

An abdominal mass and precocious puberty

What is the tumor marker?

Inhibin

Treatment?

Surgical resection

What is a Sertoli-Leydig cell tumor?

Another ovarian tumor of sex cord or stromal origin; these tumors were formerly called arrhenoblastomas

What is the characteristic presentation?

An abdominal or pelvic mass with masculinization because of testosterone production.

Treatment?

Surgical resection

What are epithelial ovarian tumors?

These are tumors of typical ovarian tissue. They are relatively infrequent in children.

What are the tumor markers?

Calcium 125 and carcino-embryonic antigen (CEA)

What is the most typical presentation in children?

Presence of an abdominal mass

How is surgical staging undertaken?

Surgical staging includes:
1. Peritoneal washings for cytology
2. Examination of all peritoneal surfaces and liver
3. Biopsies of the diaphragm and peritoneum
4. Omentectomy
5. Sampling of para-aortic and pelvic lymph nodes

Treatment?

Surgical excision of the tumor with the staging procedures as outlined; adjuvant chemotherapy is needed in all stages above stage I as well as in some stage I cases

What are poor prognostic indicators?	Advanced stage Aneuploidy C-fms oncogene

VAGINAL ATRESIA

What is complete vaginal atresia?	A condition in which the mullerian ducts fail to reach the urogenital sinus, which results in a lack of an opening at the vaginal introitus
In complete vaginal atresia, what is the status of the other reproductive organs?	The ovaries and fallopian tubes are normal. The uterus is bicornuate and rudimentary.
What is proximal vaginal atresia?	It is a failure of the mullerian duct to form the mullerian tubercle.
What is the status of the reproductive organs?	The fallopian tubes and ovaries are normal. The uterus and cervix are hypoplastic or absent.
What is distal vaginal atresia?	Failure of formation of the vaginal plate
What is the status of the reproductive organs?	The cervix, uterus, and fallopian tubes are normal.
What is hydrocolpos?	Filling of the vagina with mucus
What is hydrometrocolpos?	Filling of the vagina and uterus with mucus
What is hematocolpos?	Filling of the vagina with menstrual blood discharge
What is hematometrocolpos?	Filling of the vagina and uterus with menstrual blood discharge
What are common presenting symptoms in distal vaginal atresia?	Colicky abdominal pain once menarche begins due to collection of menstrual blood (i.e., hematocolpos or hematometrocolpos)
How is this treated?	Perineal vaginoplasty

How does proximal vaginal atresia present?	It is more likely to present as lack of menstrual periods, because of the hypoplasia or agenesis of the uterus.
Can abdominal pain occur with proximal vaginal atresia?	Yes, in cases in which the uterus is well formed enough to produce menstrual blood
How is this treated?	Laparotomy to drain the uterus and approximate it to the distal vagina

VAGINAL TUMORS

What are the two most typical vaginal tumors of childhood?	1. Rhabdomyosarcoma 2. Endodermal sinus tumor
How do these tumors present?	Usually the tumor presents as a mass or swelling of the vagina, with possible associated vaginal bleeding
What should the workup of an endodermal sinus tumor include?	Serum for αFP and beta-HCG; CT scan of the vagina, pelvis, and abdomen; chest radiograph
What is the treatment?	Usually, biopsy of the tumor is performed with subsequent chemotherapy and completion resection. Resection may include removal of the uterus if the tumor extends that far.
What is included in the workup of rhabdomyosarcoma?	Chest radiograph CT scan of the pelvis and abdomen Bone marrow aspirate Bone scan Cystoscopy
How is this tumor treated?	Usually biopsy is followed by chemotherapy and then completion resection. Hysterectomy or pelvic exenteration is rarely required.
What is the five-year survival for rhabdomyosarcoma of the vagina?	Approximately 85%

IMPERFORATE HYMEN

What is the most common cause of vaginal obstruction?	Imperforate hymen
What is imperforate hymen?	Persistence of an epithelial membrane at the opening of the vagina
How does it usually present?	Often imperforate hymen does not present until adolescence. The adolescent girl experiences episodes of lower abdominal pain but no menstruation. After a time, a lower abdominal mass may be present, representing hydrometrocolpos or metrocolpos.
How is this treated?	The hymen is incised with a cruciate incision. The raw edges of the hymen ring are then sutured with absorbable sutures to promote epithelialization of the edges of the new open hymen ring.

23

Endocrine Disorders

DIABETES

DIABETES INSIPIDUS (SEE CHAPTER 21)

DIABETES MELLITUS

What is it?
Absent or diminished insulin secretion or action resulting in **hyperglycemia** and abnormal energy metabolism

What are the two types?
Type I: insulin-dependent diabetes mellitus (IDDM); there is a loss of pancreatic-cell function, resulting in a loss of insulin secretion; it is the **most common type seen in childhood**
Type II: non–insulin-dependent diabetes mellitus (NIDDM); there is continuous insulin production but at a decreased rate or there is an insulin receptor defect; more common in adults

What is the etiology?
Exact etiology is unknown, but is probably associated with a combination of genetic and environmental factors; autoimmune processes important in most cases

How does IDDM present?
Most commonly **polyuria, polydipsia, and weight loss;** symptoms often occur insidiously over weeks to months; presents less often with diabetic ketoacidosis (DKA)

How is IDDM diagnosed?
Random blood sugar > 200 mg/dl or fasting blood sugar > 140 mg/dl and elevated glycosylated hemoglobin level; Islet cell antibodies may be present

Why is glycosylated hemoglobin important?
It provides an estimate of the average blood glucose level for the preceding 2–3 months

What are the goals of IDDM management?

Normal growth and development and prevention of early and late complications; specific goals for blood sugar ranges and glycosylated hemoglobin vary by age

What are the four main components of management of IDDM?

1. **Insulin**: given as a combination of short-acting (regular) and long-acting (NPH, lente, or ultralente) 2–3 times daily before meals; recombinant human insulin is less immunogenic and thus generally preferred over beef or pork insulin
2. **Diet:** avoidance of simple sugars; attention to fat intake, appropriate distribution, and total number of calories; consistency in meal/snack times
3. **Exercise:** aerobic exercise lowers blood sugar without additional insulin and aids general overall fitness; patients should exercise after a meal/snack to avoid hypoglycemia.
4. **Glucose monitoring:** 3–4 times daily before meals/snacks

What are the acute complications of IDDM?

Hypoglycemia can occur with overinsulinization or vigorous exercise, or if the patient skips meals. DKA may be caused by poor patient compliance with insulin therapy or severe illness.

What are signs and symptoms of hypoglycemia?

Hunger, diaphoresis, and tremulousness due to sympathetic discharge
Deprivation of glucose to the CNS can lead to lethargy, bizarre behavior, slurred speech, loss of consciousness, and seizures

What is the treatment of hypoglycemia?

If awake and alert, oral glucose-containing fluids and foods or glucose tabs/gel; if unconscious, intramuscular glucagon

What are late complications of IDDM?

Retinopathy, nephropathy, neuropathy, and large vessel atherosclerosis

Can these be prevented?

Good glucose control can decrease the frequency of these complications by up to 75% and potentially prevent them.

What is DKA?

A potentially life-threatening condition occurring in IDDM that is characterized by severe hyperglycemia, with resulting electrolyte disturbances and metabolic acidosis

What are signs and symptoms of DKA?

Polyuria, polydipsia, fatigue, dehydration with tachycardia and hypotension, abdominal pain, nausea, and vomiting; Kussmaul respirations, obtundation, and coma may occur

What are causes of DKA?

DKA may be the initial presentation of IDDM. In known diabetics, DKA may be triggered by illnesses or noncompliance with insulin therapy.

What are the metabolic derangements in DKA?

Severe hyperglycemia

↓ serum CO_2 (with respiratory compensation)

↑ BUN and Hct (dehydration with hemoconcentration)

Normal or low Na (pseudohyponatremia is artifact due to lipemic serum or hyperglycemia)

Normal or increased **serum K^+** due to cellular shifts from acidosis; **however, total body K^+ depletion is present and potentially life-threatening**

Positive serum and urine ketones

How is DKA treated?

IV fluids and correction of electrolytes (especially K^+); fluids alone lower the glucose level and correct acidosis

$NaHCO_3$ is reserved for severe acidosis ($CO_2 < 12$)

IV insulin: 0.1 U/kg bolus then infusion at 0.1 U/kg/hr

Dextrose (5%–10%) is added to IV fluids when the glucose level reaches 250–300 mg/dl and insulin infusion is decreased to 0.05 U/kg/hr

What are cautions in DKA treatment?	SLOW correction of hyperglycemia and dehydration; too much fluid too quickly or rapid shifts in osmolarity may cause cerebral edema and herniation; insulin dosage should be tapered to avoid hypoglycemia during the latter phase of DKA treatment
What is the treatment of NIDDM?	Diet and exercise are first-line treatments. If unsuccessful, treatment includes oral hypoglycemic agents and then insulin.
What is the team approach?	A diabetes management system that incorporates the physician, nurse educator, nutritionist, social worker, psychologist, and the patient to achieve goals.

PARATHYROID HORMONE (PTH) DISORDERS

HYPERPARATHYROIDISM

What is it?	Elevated levels of PTH, causing hypercalcemia and hypophosphatemia
What does PTH do?	PTH mobilizes calcium from bone and causes decreased renal tubular reabsorption of phosphorus
What are the signs and symptoms?	Those related to hypercalcemia include nausea, vomiting, constipation, lethargy, weakness, and confusion. Hypertension and renal colic occur secondary to kidney stones. Fractures also occur.
What are diagnostic lab findings?	Elevated serum calcium (total and ionized), low phosphorus, and elevated PTH (relative to elevated serum calcium)
What might radiographs show?	Subperiosteal bone resorption
What is the etiology?	Genetic (familial) hyperfunction of all the parathyroid glands (hyperplasia) or a solitary adenoma in nonfamilial cases

Is this condition common in children?	No
What is the treatment?	1. Hyperplasia: subtotal parathyroidectomy (usually 3½ glands), or total parathyroidectomy with reimplantation of pieces of half gland in sternocleidomastoid or brachialis muscle 2. Adenoma: removal of adenomatous gland
What are associated syndromes?	Multiple endocrine neoplasia (**MEN**): **Type I:** tumors of the parathyroids, anterior pituitary, and pancreatic islet cells **Type IIa:** hyperparathyroidism, pheochromocytoma, and medullary thyroid carcinoma
What causes secondary hyperparathyroidism?	Chronic renal or hepatic disease and vitamin D deficiency

HYPOPARATHYROIDISM

What is it?	Low levels of PTH
What are the metabolic results?	Hypocalcemia and hyperphosphatemia
What are the signs and symptoms?	Those related to hypocalcemia, including tetany, seizures, abdominal pain, numbness of the face or extremities, and carpopedal spasm
What is Chvostek's sign?	Twitching of the muscles innervated by the facial nerve, which is elicited by tapping 1-2 cm anterior to the earlobe just below the zygomatic process
What is Trousseau's sign?	Carpal spasm that occurs after inflating a blood pressure cuff on the upper arm to above systolic pressure for up to 3 minutes
What is the treatment?	Vitamin D and calcium supplements

What is the etiology in children?	Sporadic, autoimmune, or DiGeorge syndrome
What is DiGeorge syndrome?	Dysgenesis of the third and fourth pharyngeal pouches, resulting in hypoplasia of the thymus and parathyroid glands and anomalies of the great vessels; frequently associated with a submicroscopic deletion of chromosome 22
What is transient neonatal hypoparathyroidism?	Decreased parathyroid responsiveness due to prematurity, hypomagnesemia (infants of diabetic mothers, malabsorption), or maternal hyperparathyroidism
Differential Dx of transient neonatal hypoparathyroidism?	Early hypocalcemia (first 3 days of life): secondary to asphyxia Late hypocalcemia (at or after the end of the first week): due to a high phosphate load (cow's milk or swallowed maternal blood), intestinal calcium malabsorption, or presentation of idiopathic hypoparathyroidism

PRECOCIOUS PUBERTY

What is it?	Onset of puberty before 8 (females) or 9 (males) years of age
What is usually the first sign of puberty in males?	Enlargement of the testes
What is the first sign of puberty in females?	Breast enlargement
Is precocious puberty more common in boys or girls?	Girls
What is the most common cause of precocious puberty in girls?	Idiopathic precocious puberty
What is meant by central precocious puberty?	Precocious puberty secondary to increased release of releasing factors and gonadotropins

Name some causes of central precocious puberty.

1. Idiopathic true precocious puberty
2. CNS trauma, tumor, hamartoma, or malformation
3. Postinfectious or postinflammatory
4. Chronic exposure to sex steroids

What is pseudoprecocious (incomplete, or peripheral) puberty?

Puberty caused by release of hormones by mechanisms other than the usual hypothalamic-pituitary-gonadal axis

What are some causes of pseudoprecocious puberty?

Exogenous hormones
Hormone-producing tumors (e.g., adrenal, ovarian, testicular)
Congenital adrenal hyperplasia

What is premature adrenarche?

Premature appearance of secondary sexual hair

How does premature adrenarche differ from precocious puberty?

Premature adrenarche has no other features of puberty, such as physical changes in genitalia or breasts or linear growth

How do you evaluate premature adrenarche?

Most patients require no laboratory testing. Careful clinical follow-up is key to excluding precocious puberty.

What is premature thelarche?

Premature breast development

How does premature thelarche differ from precocious puberty?

In premature thelarche, there are no other signs of pubertal development.

How should you evaluate premature thelarche?

Careful and frequent clinical follow-up; most patients require no additional testing unless there are other changes suggestive of puberty

What is the initial evaluation of precocious puberty?

Detailed history (including evaluation of growth data) and physical examination

What comprises the lab evaluation?

Guided by history and physical, it may include serum follicle-stimulating hormone (FSH), luteinizing hormone (LH), estradiol, testosterone, cortisol, bone age

What other radiographic studies are indicated?

Depending on clinical and screening lab test findings, an MRI of the head and ultrasound of the pelvis (ovaries) or abdomen (adrenal glands, other masses) may be indicated.

GYNECOMASTIA

What is it?

Breast tissue enlargement in the male

What are the four types of isolated gynecomastia?

1. Benign adolescent hypertrophy, which is characterized by a small (approximately 3 cm) subareolar mass that ultimately resolves spontaneously
2. Physiologically induced gynecomastia, which may be due to sporadic elevation in estrogen or other causes (e.g., hormone ingestion)
3. Gynecomastia stimulated by obesity
4. "Apparent gynecomastia," which is due to pectoral muscle hypertrophy

Gynecomastia may be associated with other symptoms in various endocrine and genetic conditions.

What are treatments of the various isolated types?

Excision of breast tissue through a submammary incision may be used for physiologically induced gynecomastia and, in some cases, benign adolescent hypertrophy when it is too bothersome for the adolescent. Obesity-induced gynecomastia should be evaluated after the patient has adhered to a diet and exercise regimen to lose weight. If gynecomastia persists, resection of breast tissue may be necessary. No treatment is needed for pectoral muscle hypertrophy.

DELAYED PUBERTY

What is it?

Delay in the onset of development of secondary sexual characteristics

After what age is puberty considered delayed?

If there has been no development of secondary sexual characteristics by **13 (females)** or **14 (males) years of age**

What is hypergonadotropic hypogonadism?
Delayed puberty associated with increased levels of FSH and LH

What is its pathophysiology?
The pituitary is functioning, but there is lack of peripheral (end-organ) response

What is hypogonadotropic hypogonadism?
Delayed puberty associated with decreased levels of FSH and LH

What is its pathophysiology?
Implies a central problem in gonadotropin production or release; this may include a structural abnormality, tumor, hypopituitarism, or nutritional problem

What is the most common cause of delayed puberty in boys?
Constitutional delay of puberty

Other causes in males?
Gonadal failure or dysgenesis, Klinefelter syndrome, hypopituitarism, CNS tumors, certain malformation syndromes, nutritional disturbances

What are causes of pubertal delay in girls?
Turner syndrome, gonadal dysgenesis from other causes, gonadotropin deficiency, CNS abnormality, inadequate nutrition (including that resulting from anorexia nervosa)

How is delayed puberty evaluated?
Careful history and physical examination
Hand and wrist radiograph to determine bone age (if there is short stature)
Thyroid tests
Serum gonadotropins

In the evaluation of delayed puberty in boys, what findings indicate the need for chromosome studies?
Evidence of poor testicular development
Dysmorphic features
Unexplained mental retardation or developmental delay

In girls?
Short stature
Features of Turner syndrome
Unexplained mental retardation or developmental delay
Dysmorphic features

What is the treatment of delayed puberty in boys?

Ideally, treat the underlying cause. If this is not possible, consider a brief course of testosterone by injection. A longer course may be indicated if there is no spontaneous puberty within 12 months.

What is the treatment of delayed puberty in girls?

Ideally, treat the underlying cause. If this is not possible, consider a low-dose conjugated estrogen, increasing the dosage gradually over about 1 year to mimic natural pubertal levels. Menarche can be achieved later by adding a progestational agent in a cycling regimen: usually 16 days of estrogen only, then 10 days of both estrogen and progesterone, then 5 days off of both agents.

GROWTH HORMONE (GH) DEFICIENCY

What is GH?

It is anterior pituitary hormone that causes growth of all tissues, especially bone and cartilage. It promotes mineralization of bones and has a role in carbohydrate and lipid metabolism.

What are common causes of GH deficiency?

Idiopathic
Congenital
Secondary to CNS trauma or infection
Effect of surgery, chemotherapy, or
    irradiation for CNS tumors
Histiocytosis
Sarcoidosis

How does it present?

Symptomatic hypoglycemia; microphallus in males; growth velocity decreases after 6–12 months

Are newborns with GH deficiency usually of normal size?

Yes, because GH is not necessary for fetal growth

How does it present in childhood?

Short stature with growth velocity < 5 cm/yr; mild truncal obesity; frontal bossing; flat nasal bridge; high-pitch voice; delayed dental development; sometimes hypoglycemia

What are diagnostic findings?	Delayed skeletal development (bone-age radiograph), low serum IGF-1 and IGF-BP3, and abnormal response to GH stimulation tests (random GH levels are not helpful because of pulsatile secretion)
What are associated conditions?	Panhypopituitarism; septo-optic dysplasia (blindness and absence of septum pellucidum)
What is the differential Dx?	Genetic short stature, constitutional delay of growth and adolescence (CDGA), Turner syndrome, chronic diseases, psychosocial dwarfism, nutritional dwarfism, chronic glucocorticoid therapy, skeletal dysplasias
What is the treatment for GH deficiency?	Recombinant GH via daily subcutaneous injection

PANHYPOPITUITARISM

Which hormones are affected in panhypopituitarism?	Anterior pituitary hormones, including adrenocorticotropic hormone (ACTH), GH, thyroid-stimulating hormone (TSH), LH, FSH, and prolactin
What are the causes?	Idiopathic, effects from treatment of CNS tumors, trauma, congenital midline defects, familial; hypothalamic disease can produce symptoms identical to primary pituitary disorders
What is septo-optic dysplasia?	Panhypopituitarism associated with optic nerve hypoplasia (blindness) and absence of the septum pellucidum; posterior pituitary hormones may also be deficient
What are the complications?	Hypoglycemia, prolonged jaundice, apnea, and hypotonia; microphallus in males
How is panhypopituitarism diagnosed?	1. Low GH concentration (< 7 ng/dl) in response to hypoglycemia or GH stimulation tests, low TSH and T_4, and a low morning cortisol level with abnormal response to ACTH stimulation

2. In newborns, low TSH, LH, and
FSH levels (LH and FSH normally is
low in children after the newborn
period until puberty; not helpful prior
to adolescence)

What is the treatment?

Replacement hormones:
Hydrocortisone
GH
L-thyroxine (T_4)
Estrogen or testosterone at puberty
    easier than achieving pulsatile patterns
    of LH and FSH that are needed for
    gonadal steroid synthesis

THYROID DISORDERS

HYPERTHYROIDISM

**What are common causes
of hyperthyroidism?**

Graves disease, autonomous thyroid
nodules, subacute thyroiditis, pituitary
adenomas, McCune-Albright syndrome;
in infants, neonatal thyrotoxicosis due to
maternal Graves disease

What is Graves disease?

Hyperthyroidism secondary to diffuse
thyroid hyperplasia ("diffuse toxic goiter")

**What causes Graves
disease?**

Autoimmune etiology—circulating
thyroid-stimulating immunoglobulins
(IgG) bind to TSH receptors

**What are findings on
thyroid function tests?**

Elevated T_4 levels; TSH is very low or
undetectable due to feedback
suppression by high T_4 levels

**Which sex is affected
more?**

Females, approximately 4:1

**At what age are children
affected?**

Two thirds of childhood cases occur
between 10–15 years of age.

**What are signs and
symptoms of Graves
disease?**

Increased appetite; heat intolerance;
diaphoresis; weight loss; frequent loose
stools; difficulty sleeping; weakness and
inability to participate in sports; emotional
lability; deterioration of school
performance; nervousness; proptosis/
exophthalmos; tachycardia; warm, moist,

smooth skin; tremor; thyroid gland is diffusely enlarged, smooth, nontender and firm

How is Graves disease diagnosed?

Elevated T_4, T_3, and T_3 resin uptake; low or suppressed TSH

What is Graves ophthalmopathy?

Lymphocytic infiltration of the conjunctiva, extraocular muscles, and retrobulbar tissues; may cause redness and edema of the conjunctiva, decreased mobility of the eye, and proptosis; severity not necessarily associated with disease course

What is a thyroid storm?

A rare, life-threatening complication of Graves disease; uncontrolled exaggerated hyperthyroidism leads to marked hyperthermia, tachycardia, vomiting, diarrhea, and CNS symptoms (apathy, confusion, coma); cardiac failure may occur

What can cause a thyroid storm?

Infection, surgery, trauma, or noncompliance with antithyroid medications

What is the natural history of Graves disease?

Waxing and waning hyperthyroidism of variable duration; eventual *hypo*thyroidism results from autoimmune destruction of thyroid tissue

What is the treatment of Graves disease?

Antithyroid medications to block thyroid hormone production:
Propylthiouracil (PTU), which also blocks peripheral conversion of T_4 to T_3
Methimazole
Propranolol for relief of adrenergic symptoms

What treatment should be considered for failure of medical therapy, patient noncompliance, or recurrent hyperthyroidism?

Radioactive iodine (^{131}I) or subtotal thyroidectomy

Differential Dx of Graves disease?	Hyperthyroidism due to: 1. Subacute or Hashimoto thyroiditis (early phases) 2. Autonomous thyroid nodule(s) 3. Factitious hyperthyroidism (excessive ingestion of thyroid hormone preparations) 4. Excessive TSH production (pituitary adenoma or pituitary resistance to thyroid hormone)
What is neonatal Graves disease?	Neonatal hyperthyroidism due to transplacental passage of thyroid-stimulating immunoglobulins (IgG)
How does neonatal Graves disease present?	Jitteriness, hyperactivity, stare, increased appetite, poor weight gain, tachycardia, and thyroid enlargement in an infant born to a woman with Graves disease
What is the treatment of neonatal Graves disease?	PTU, iodide solution (Lugol solution), and propranolol
What is the natural course of neonatal Graves disease?	Resolves over the first few months of life as maternal immunoglobulins are cleared from the infant's circulation

HYPOTHYROIDISM

What are two categories of hypothyroidism in children?	**Congenital hypothyroidism** due to thyroid gland agenesis, dysgenesis, or enzymatic defects **Juvenile hypothyroidism,** which is acquired and usually occurs after the first year of life
Which is more serious?	Congenital hypothyroidism
Why?	Thyroid hormone is needed during at least the first 2 years of life for normal brain growth and development
What may occur if diagnosis is delayed?	Delay in diagnosis past 6 weeks of age can lead to mental retardation

How does congenital hypothyroidism present?

At birth, infants most often appear normal but may have prolonged jaundice. If untreated, symptoms develop over 1–2 months and include:
Poor feeding
Lethargy
Hypotonia
Constipation
Coarse facial features
Large protruding tongue
Large open fontanelles
Hoarse cry
Umbilical hernia
Cool, dry, mottled skin
Developmental delay

What constitutes newborn screening for congenital hypothyroidism?

A battery of screening labs (which differ slightly by state) that are obtained by heelstick blood specimen and sent to state labs as a dried blood specimen on special filter paper. These labs are taken before a newborn is discharged from the hospital but repeated later if discharge occurs before 48 hours of age since there are hormonal fluctuations around the time of birth. Thyroid hormone (T_4) is screened for in every state. If low, a serum thyroid panel is obtained to document hypothyroidism (i.e., low T_4, low T_3 resin uptake, elevated TSH).

What is the incidence of congenital hypothyroidism?

1:4000 births

What is the role of the thyroid scan?

Before starting treatment, a technetium 99-m scan should be obtained:
1. Absent uptake–thyroid agenesis
2. Abnormal location of uptake–ectopic gland
3. Increased uptake–enzymatic defect
All conditions require lifelong treatment.

What is the treatment for congenital hypothyroidism in a newborn?

L-thyroxine ASAP!

What is the differential Dx?

1. Transient hypothyroidism due to maternal blocking antibodies (low T_4, elevated TSH)

2. Thyroxine-binding globulin (TBG) deficiency (i.e., low total T_4, normal free T_4, nl TSH)
3. Sick euthyroid syndrome, characterized by sick preterm infants (low T_4, nl TSH)

What is the treatment strategy?

Due to the risk of developing CNS abnormalities, treat until 2–3 years of age, then stop and recheck T_4 and TSH in 3–4 weeks. If abnormal, treat for life. If normal, repeat again for 4–6 weeks. If again normal, therapy can be discontinued, but ensure follow-up labs in 2–3 months.

What are signs and symptoms of juvenile hypothyroidism?

Slow growth; cold intolerance; decreased appetite; constipation; coarse puffy face; flattened nasal bridge; stocky habitus; dull, dry, thin hair; rough, dry, sallow skin; delayed relaxation phase of deep tendon reflexes; school performance is usually *not* impaired

What is the etiology?

Most commonly autoimmune destruction secondary to chronic lymphocytic thyroiditis **(Hashimoto thyroiditis)**. Other conditions include:
1. Surgical or radioactive iodine ablation for treatment of hyperthyroidism
2. Goitrogens (iodides in cough syrups, antithyroid drugs)
3. Ectopic thyroid dysgenesis

What are the diagnostic findings?

Low T_4, low T_3 resin uptake, elevated TSH
Thyroid antimicrosomal and antithyroglobulin antibodies often positive in Hashimoto thyroiditis
Delayed bone age, which can indicate duration of hypothyroidis

What is the treatment for juvenile hypothyroidism?

Oral L-thyroxine

SIADH

What is it?

Syndromes of **I**nappropriate **A**nti**d**iuretic **H**ormone: excess ADH results in

	expansion of vascular volume and hyponatremia
What are common causes?	It is associated with pulmonary and CNS diseases (e.g., pneumonia, pulmonary TB, bacterial meningitis, intracranial tumors/trauma) and some chemotherapeutic agents. In preterm infants in intensive care nurseries, SIADH occurs in association with positive-pressure ventilation and bronchopulmonary dysplasia.
What are signs and symptoms?	Water retention and weight gain; symptoms may progress to lethargy, confusion, and seizures secondary to hyponatremia
What is the treatment?	Fluid restriction; symptomatic hyponatremia may require careful infusion of hypertonic (3%) saline

ADRENOCORTICAL INSUFFICIENCY

What is it?	Adrenal insufficiency, resulting in decreased cortisol and aldosterone production
What is Addison disease?	Primary adrenocortical insufficiency usually due to an autoimmune process
What are other common causes of adrenocortical insufficiency?	Congenital adrenal *hypo*plasia, bilateral adrenal hemorrhage (Waterhouse-Friderichsen syndrome), trauma, thrombosis, infection (TB), tumors, drugs, adrenoleukodystrophy (a CNS demyelinating disorder)
What are the signs and symptoms?	Weakness, fatigue, anorexia, abdominal pain, nausea, vomiting, weight loss, salt-craving, hypoglycemia, postural hypotension, and increased pigmentation (especially at pressure points, lips, nipples, buccal mucosa, and scarred areas of skin)

What are diagnostic findings?	Elevated ACTH and a low morning serum cortisol level that fails to rise with ACTH stimulation
	There may be fasting hypoglycemia, hyponatremia, hyperkalemia, and elevated plasma renin activity
What is the treatment?	Glucocorticoid and mineralocorticoid replacement
When must glucocorticoid be increased above normal replacement levels?	It must be increased 2–3 fold during illnesses and up to 5 fold for trauma and surgery.
What is an adrenal crisis?	A life-threatening episode that is often triggered by an illness or injury; it is characterized by fever, weakness, abdominal pain, vomiting, hypotension, dehydration, and shock.
How is it treated?	Rehydration; correction of hyponatremia, hyperkalemia, and metabolic acidosis; and intravenous glucocorticoids in stress doses

CUSHING DISEASE AND SYNDROME

What is Cushing disease?	Bilateral adrenal hyperplasia *secondary* to increased ACTH production caused by pituitary adenoma, resulting in increased cortisol production
What is Cushing syndrome?	Increased cortisol production due to adrenal tumors (including carcinomas), ectopic ACTH production by nonpituitary tumors, or exogenous glucocorticoids
What characterizes these conditions?	A constellation of signs and symptoms, which are due to excess cortisol production or exogenous glucocorticoids and include:
	Rounded face ("moon facies")
	Obesity
	Stretch marks
	A hump on the upper back ("buffalo hump")
	Masculinization
	Impaired growth
	Hypertension

What are two laboratory findings in these conditions?	1. Elevated serum cortisol levels with loss of diurnal rhythm 2. Elevated 24-hour urinary-free cortisol
What is the dexamethasone suppression test?	Dexamethasone (1 mg) is given at 11 pm, and cortisol is measured at 8 AM the next day. Failure to suppress cortisol to < 5 ug/dl suggests Cushing disease or syndrome. If result is positive, low- and high-dose dexamethasone suppression tests are performed to differentiate between central and non-central or adrenal causes.

PHEOCHROMOCYTOMA

What is it?	A rare tumor of chromaffin cells, which are derived from neural crest tissue
Location of the tumor?	Most commonly in the adrenal medulla; most of the remainder occur along the abdominal sympathetic chain, including the organ of Zuckerkandl and renal hilus; extra-adrenal tumors may be referred to as paragangliomas
What are the signs and symptoms?	Hypertension (sustained or paroxysmal), headache, vomiting, pallor, sweating, visual disturbances, weight loss, and sometimes tachycardia and tremor; hypertensive encephalopathy can be life-threatening
What are the laboratory findings?	Abnormally high serum levels of catecholamines (e.g., epinephrine and norepinephrine) and high urine levels of their metabolites (e.g., metanephrine, normetanephrine, and VMA)
What is the treatment?	Surgical excision **(preoperative control of hypertension with α-blockers is mandatory)**
What are associated conditions?	MEN: **Type IIA:** Pheochromocytoma, medullary thyroid carcinoma, hyperparathyroidism **Type IIB:** Pheochromocytoma, medullary thyroid carcinoma, multiple neuromas

AMBIGUOUS GENITALIA

What does ambiguous genitalia (intersex anomaly) refer to?

A constellation of conditions with a variety of causes in which the genitalia are not phenotypically normal for either sex

What are the four major classifications?

1. Female pseudohermaphroditism
2. True hermaphroditism
3. Male pseudohermaphroditism
4. Mixed gonadal dysgenesis

What are the typical karyotypes, gonads, and urinary steroid findings for each classification?

1. Female pseudohermaphroditism:
   Barr body smear: positive
   Karyotype: 46 XX
   Urinary steroids: positive
   Gonads: normal ovaries
2. True hermaphroditism:
   Barr body smear: positive
   Karyotype: 46 XX
   Urinary steroids: negative
   Gonads: testes, ovary, or ova testis
3. Male pseudohermaphroditism:
   Barr body smear: negative
   Karyotype: 46 XY
   Urinary steroids: negative
   Gonads: testes
4. Mixed gonadal dysgenesis:
   Barr body: negative
   Karyotype: 45 X or 46 XY
   Urinary steroids: negative
   Gonads: dysgenetic and streak ovaries

What is the cause of female pseudohermaphroditism?

This condition, also know as adrenogenital syndrome, is usually due to an enzyme deficiency (most commonly, 21-hydroxylase, 11-hydroxylase, 3-beta-hydroxysteroid dehydrogenase). The deficiency causes an excess formation of intermediate steroids, which cause masculinization of external genitalia.

What other conditions are associated with adrenogenital syndrome?

The enzyme deficiencies cause deficiency of mineralocorticoids and glucocorticoids, which can result in **salt wasting** and **hypertension**.

What is male pseudohermaphroditism (testicular feminization syndrome)?

The genotypic male develops as a phenotypic female because of one of the following:
1. Inadequate testosterone production
2. Inadequate conversion of testosterone to dihydrotestosterone caused by 5-alpha reductase deficiency
3. Deficiencies in androgen receptors

How is this condition discovered?

A female may present with virilization of external genitalia; testes may be discovered during inguinal hernia repair in a female; or a female may present with lack of menses at puberty

What are these patients at risk for?

The testes are at risk for degeneration into **seminoma** or **gonadoblastoma** if left in place. Therefore, both testicles should be removed after appropriate discussion with the family and the patient.

What is mixed gonadal dysgenesis?

It is a condition associated with a mixed karyotype pattern of 45 X or 46 XY.

What are these patients at risk for?

The gonads are prone to developing gonadoblastoma, seminoma, or dysgerminoma.

What is the recommended treatment?

Removal of gonads; hormone replacement at puberty

What is the cause of true hermaphroditism?

It is thought to be the result of a translocation of the short arm of the Y chromosome to an autosome where **testes-determining factor** maintains its ability to develop a primordial gonad into a testis.

How should the gonads be treated?

Any intact testis or testicular tissue of a mixed gonad should be removed.

What is the general diagnostic approach for any patient with an intersex abnormality?

1. Obtain a history for any maternal drug ingestion that may suggest the presence of progestational agents.
2. Obtain a history of any genital abnormalities in relatives or unexplained deaths in infants (which may have been due to electrolyte abnormalities caused by salt wasting).

3. Perform physical exam to assess gonadal symmetry, phallus size and shape, and evaluation of vaginal size.
4. Buccal smear for Barr bodies
5. Urinary steroids
6. Karyotype
7. Serum electrolytes
8. Retrograde genitogram

In general, what does the genitalia in patients with intersex anomalies look like?

Usually the genitalia reflect a phallus that is suggestive of a hypertrophic clitoris with a small vagina. When the phallus is large enough to be a penis, it often has a chordee and hypospadias.

What gender should a child with an intersex anomaly be reared as?

If there is any question about the ability to provide an adequate phallus, then the patient should be reared as a female. If the anomaly is present at birth, it is imperative to assign a gender as soon as possible, so that the appropriate operative procedure and social development can occur.

What are appropriate phallus sizes for a male infant?

At term: 3.5 ± 0.4 cm
At 34 weeks gestation: 3.0 ± 0.4 cm
At 30 weeks gestation: 2.5 ± 0.4 cm (as measured along the dorsum from the base to the tip of the stretched glans)

What is the surgical approach to perineal reconstruction?
　For infants who will be raised as females?

Cystoscopy is used to assess the urethral and vaginal openings because, in many of these patients, these two orifices join to form a common opening at the perineum. If the vaginal opening is distal to the urethral opening, reconstruction is performed at about 6 months of age. For more proximal openings, reconstruction is performed in a staged fashion with clitoral recession and labial-scrotal reduction at approximately 6 months of age and vaginal repair at 2–3 years of age.

For infants who will be raised as males?

Reconstruction is performed in a staged manner. The first stage involves a release of the chordee; subsequent operations repair the hypospadias.

In which intersex anomaly can patients still be fertile?

Female pseudohermaphroditism

SEIZURE

What is a seizure?	A paroxysmal event arising from cerebral gray matter that interferes with normal brain function
What is a tonic–clonic seizure?	Rhythmic, generalized, jerking movements and loss of consciousness; incontinence is common; postictal lethargy is characteristic; this type is very common in children
What is an absence seizure?	Brief episode (5–10 seconds) of staring and loss of consciousness, which may occur many times each day; there is no postictal state, the patient is unaware of the seizure, and it is rare
What is a partial complex seizure?	It is characterized by a sensory (smell, taste) hallucination and often an affective experience (e.g., fear, depersonalization) and is followed by loss of consciousness while the patient engages in repetitive, meaningless motor activity (automatism). A postictal state follows.
Are seizures dangerous?	Not necessarily—prolonged seizures may cause hypoxia or hypoglycemia, but the main danger is the underlying cause of the seizure or the accidents that may occur during the seizure
What causes seizures?	Seizures are symptoms. Be careful to check for a CNS infection or metabolic problem, especially hypoglycemia. Seizures may also be triggered by fever. However, in children the underlying cause is frequently never found; this constitutes an **idiopathic seizure disorder**, commonly called **epilepsy**.

Are brain tumors a cause?	Rarely
Are EEGs helpful?	An EEG will help characterize a seizure. However, it neither diagnoses nor rules out idiopathic seizure disorder; this must be done clinically.
Should treatment be started after the first seizure?	Most clinicians do not treat a single seizure.
How are seizures treated?	Acutely—severe seizures may require a benzodiazepine (e.g., Valium); if possible, treat the underlying cause
When should a child diagnosed with seizure disorder be treated with chronic anticonvulsants?	When a second seizure occurs, especially if it occurs soon after the first
What are some drugs used to treat seizure disorder?	Phenytoin, carbamazepine, valproic acid, and phenobarbital
What is the prognosis for seizure disorder?	Most seizure problems resolve spontaneously. If a child is seizure-free for 2 years on therapy, then therapy may be weaned over a 4- to 6-month period.

ARNOLD-CHIARI MALFORMATION

What is it?	Elongation and downward displacement of the medulla and cerebellum into the spinal canal
What are its consequences?	Obstruction of the fourth ventricle, resulting in obstructive hydrocephalus and possibly brain stem compression
What are associated conditions?	Most commonly neural tube defects, especially myelomeningocele
How is it treated?	Shunting, to relieve hydrocephalus; posterior fossa decompression if necessary

CEREBRAL PALSY (CP)

What is it?	A nonprogressive movement and posture disorder due to brain injury or malformation that occurs early in development; it is not an etiologic diagnosis but a clinical syndrome (a manifestation of static encephalopathy) that refers only to motor disability
What are the etiologies?	1. **Prenatal (55%)**: genetic factors, toxins, placental factors, and infection 2. **Perinatal (35%)**: prematurity and sequelae; asphyxia 3. **Postnatal (10%)**: infection, trauma, and asphyxia
What is the incidence?	Approximately 2 per 1,000 children
What are the signs and symptoms?	Delay in motor development with abnormalities in muscle tone, movement patterns, and reflexes
How is it diagnosed?	Diagnosis is based on clinical history and physical examination. Laboratory tests are often needed to confirm suspected brain injury (e.g,. porencephalic cyst), rule out a progressive or degenerative neurologic process (e.g., astrocytoma, metachromatic leukodystrophy), or to define etiology (e.g., chromosome analysis).
How is CP classified?	1. **Spastic,** which is subclassified topographically by the distribution of spasticity: diplegic, hemiplegic, triplegic, or quadriplegic 2. **Extrapyramidal,** which is subclassified by the quality of muscle tone or movement disorder: hypotonic, choreoathetoid, dystonic, or ataxic 3. **Mixed** includes both spastic and extrapyramidal components
What are associated disabilities?	Mental retardation (60%) Seizures (20%–30%) Hearing and/or visual impairments Learning disabilities

Attention deficits
Dysphagia
Malnutrition
Poor growth
Constipation
Gastroesophageal reflux
Joint contractures and scoliosis, which
frequently require surgery

Does CP range in severity?

Yes. A broad range of severity exists, from minimal, with little or no functional disability, to severe, with total dependence for mobility, self-care, and feeding.

What is the treatment?

Treatment is geared toward maximizing functional abilities, managing concurrent medical problems, and preventing secondary disabilities. Treatment often requires the expertise of many disciplines, such as pediatrics, neurology, orthopedics, speech pathology, physical and occupational therapy, special education, psychology, audiology, and orthotics.

INTRACRANIAL HEMORRHAGE (ICH)

What are causes of ICH in the newborn?

Trauma, asphyxia, primary hemorrhagic condition, congenital vascular anomaly, and prematurity

What commonly causes subdural hemorrhages in the infant?

A large-for-gestational-age term infant with cephalopelvic disproportion

What may be the cause of a subarachnoid hemorrhage in an otherwise healthy neonate?

Seizure or trauma

What is intraventricular hemorrhage?

Hemorrhage into the ventricles from the subependymal germinal matrix; this matrix is gelatinous with immature fragile blood vessels

What are predisposing factors for intraventricular hemorrhage in infants?

It is mostly a condition of the premature neonate. Other risk factors include respiratory distress syndrome, hypoxia or hypotension, reperfusion of ischemic tissue, pneumothorax, and hypertension.

When do most cases of intraventricular hemorrhage occur?

80%–90% of cases occur between birth and day 3 of life.

What are clinical manifestations?

Physical signs may include a bulging fontanel, decreased muscle tone, lethargy, apnea, somnolence, and seizures. There may be hemodynamic changes, including hypotension and bradycardia. In some cases, there may be no clinical manifestations.

How is diagnosis made?

Most commonly by head ultrasonography

What are the four grades of intraventricular hemorrhage?

Grade I: bleeding confined to the germinal matrix subependymal region with ≤ 10% of the ventricle involved
Grade II: intraventricular bleeding with 10%–15% filling of the ventricle
Grade III: greater than 50% involvement with dilation of the ventricle
Grade IV: grade III hemorrhage with associated intraparenchymal lesions

What is the prognosis for intraventricular hemorrhage?

The likelihood of neurologic sequelae increases significantly with increased grade.

What are long-term sequelae?

1. Hydrocephalus requiring ventriculoperitoneal shunt
2. Long-term seizure disorder
3. Significant development delay

What is the mortality rate with grade IV hemorrhage?

50%

GUILLAIN-BARRÉ SYNDROME

What is it?   It is an acute demyelination of peripheral nerves. It is an autoimmune syndrome and often follows a trivial viral infection.

What are the signs and symptoms?
Extremity weakness usually beginning distally and extending promixally, progressing over several days
Painful sensory complaints
Areflexia
Autonomic involvement (e.g., hypotension, arrhythmias) may occur and is dangerous.

What laboratory studies are used?
CSF protein is usually very elevated within a few days of onset. EMG and nerve conduction velocity studies are helpful. Pulmonary function tests help predict respiratory failure.

Differential Dx?
Diphtheria-associated polyneuropathy
Tick paralysis
Be very careful about misdiagnosing early Guillain-Barré as conversion reaction

What is the treatment?
General supportive care
Plasma exchange if symptoms are severe or rapidly progressing
Rarely, a patient may require mechanical ventilation.

What is the prognosis?   Most patients make a complete recovery.

MYASTHENIA GRAVIS

What is it?   An autoimmune disorder with neuromuscular junction dysfunction that leads to weakness

What are the symptoms?   **Rapidly fatigable weakness;** double vision is common; upper airway weakness may be present and is very dangerous

How is it diagnosed?	Largely on a clinical basis—history of fluctuating weakness and physical findings of rapidly fatigable weakness
What does EMG show?	Rapid loss of activity following repetitive stimulation of the same muscles
What is Tensilon (edrophonium)?	A very short-acting acetylcholinesterase inhibitor; administered intravenously
How is Tensilon used in assessing myasthenia gravis?	In myasthenia, Tensilon usually produces a rapid, dramatic increase in strength. A positive test is consistent with (but does not diagnose) myasthenia gravis.
What is the treatment?	Acetylcholinesterase inhibitors (e.g., pyridostigmine, Mestinon) Immunosuppressive drugs (e.g., steroids) Thymectomy

CREUTZFELDT-JAKOB DISEASE

What is it?	It is one of a collection of subacute spongiform encephalopathies that result in spongy degeneration of the cerebral cortical grey matter. Other diseases in this classification include kuru in humans and "mad cow" disease.
What is the etiology?	The infecting agent was once believed to be a virus. However, its characteristics suggest that it may be an infectious protein (prion).
How is the disease transmitted?	In humans, it usually occurs by iatrogenic means. It may be transmitted by contaminated neurosurgical instruments, transplantation of contaminated cornea, contaminated cortical electrodes, injections of contaminated pituitary-derived growth hormone or gonadotropins, grafts of contaminated dura matter, and drugs or grafts derived from pools of contaminated donors.

What are associated symptoms?	Patients usually first experience sensory disturbances, confusion, or inappropriate behavior. Symptoms progress over weeks or months to dementia and coma.
How is the diagnosis made?	Usually clinically, although brain biopsy can provide definitive diagnosis and is usually performed only if another treatable condition is considered in the differential diagnosis
Is there any treatment for Creutzfeldt-Jakob disease?	No
What is the prognosis?	Death usually occurs within one year of onset of symptoms.

NEURAL TUBE DEFECTS

What are they?	Defects secondary to abnormal closure of the neural tube, including: 1. Myelomeningocele 2. Meningocele 3. Encephalocele 4. Anencephaly 5. Rachischisis (spina bifida)
What causes neural tube defects?	Usually not known; most cases are isolated (sporadic), but there is an increased recurrence risk in families, suggesting multifactorial inheritance
What is the incidence of neural tube defects?	Varies with geography, ethnicity, and other factors; possibly 1 to 4 of every 1000 births
What is anencephaly?	Failure of the cranial portion of the neural tube to close, with associated cranial and brain malformations
What is the prognosis for anencephaly?	Most infants are stillborn or die shortly after birth; survival beyond several days is uncommon.
What is encephalocele?	A defect in the posterior cranium with herniation of membranes (and sometimes brain tissue) through the opening

What is the prognosis?	Varies, depending on the amount of brain tissue involved in the process and the possibility of underlying brain abnormalities
How is it evaluated?	Imaging studies (e.g., ultrasound, MRI, CT scan) are indicated to help assess the brain and plans for surgery, if indicated.
What is a meningocele?	A neural tube defect involving vertebral arch malformation with protrusion of the meninges
Is the spinal cord usually normal?	Yes
How is a meningocele evaluated?	CT scan and MRI to rule out neural tissue involvement; a head CT should also be performed to rule out hydrocephalus
What is myelomeningocele?	A neural tube defect usually involving malformation of the vertebral arches with involvement of the spinal cord
What are complications of myelomeningocele?	Generally, complications depend on the location of the defect and the degree of spinal cord and nerve involvement. Common complications include Arnold-Chiari malformation and hydrocephalus, neurogenic bladder, loss of motor function below the "neurologic level" of lesion, lack of sphincter control, and club foot or contractures.
What is rachischisis (spina bifida)?	An abnormality in which the vertebral column is separated in the midline
What may be associated with spina bifida occulta?	1. Syringomyelia 2. Diastematomyelia 3. Tethered cord 4. Dermoid cyst

How can neural tube defects be prevented?	It has been shown that infants born to women who take folic acid prenatally and during early pregnancy have a lower incidence of neural tube defects.

MACROCEPHALY AND HYDROCEPHALUS

What is macrocephaly?	Large head size (i.e., greater than 95th percentile), regardless of the cause
What is hydrocephalus?	Increased CSF within the cranium
What are two types of hydrocephalus?	Communicating and noncommunicating
What is the difference?	Noncommunicating hydrocephalus is caused by obstruction of CSF flow, whereas communicating hydrocephalus is caused by decreased absorption or overproduction of CSF.
What is X-linked hydrocephalus?	A genetic form of hydrocephalus, usually affecting **males**, in which there is **stenosis of the aqueduct of Sylvius**. The gene is located on the X-chromosome.
What is the most common genetic cause of hydrocephalus?	Neural tube defects

MISCELLANEOUS NEUROLOGIC CONDITIONS

What is spinal muscular atrophy (SMA)?	Disease of anterior horn cells, frequently progressive. Most are inherited as autosomal recessive traits.
What is Werdnig-Hoffmann disease?	Also known as spinal muscular atrophy type I, it is an early-onset progressive disorder. The age of onset is usually before 6 months of age, with survival beyond 3 years uncommon. A late infantile and more slowly progressing disease is called SMA type II.

**What is Kugelberg-
Welander disease?**

A juvenile onset form of spinal muscular
dystrophy; age of onset usually in first
decade, but may be later; also known as
SMA type III

What is Reye syndrome?

Metabolic encephalopathy, frequently
associated with liver dysfunction and
fatty changes in the liver

What is the cause?

Unknown—seen following certain viral
infections (varicella, influenza), and
epidemiologically related to the use of
aspirin in some patients

**How is the diagnosis
made?**

Elevated hepatocellular enzymes in
serum, hyperammonemia, exclusion of
other diagnoses (such as medium-chain
acyl-CoA dehydrogenase deficiency)

25

Neoplastic Diseases

NEUROBLASTOMA

What is it?

An embryonal tumor of neural crest cell origin

What is the incidence?

There are 8.5 cases per 1 million children, with about 500 new cases yearly in the United States. It is the **second most common solid tumor of infancy and childhood** (brain tumors being the most common).

Where does neuroblastoma originate?

In the sympathetic nervous system:
Adrenal medulla: 50%
Para-aortic sympathetic ganglia: 24%
Mediastinum: 20%
Neck: 3%
Pelvis: 3%

Which children may be at increased risk for neuroblastoma?

Those with **other neural crest–related conditions** (neurocristopathies), such as Hirschsprung disease, Klippel-Feil syndrome, Waardenburg syndrome, and Ondine curse; also at increased risk are children with Beckwith-Wiedemann syndrome, adrenal hyperplasia, fetal alcohol syndrome, or those whose mothers took Dilantin during pregnancy

What are presenting symptoms?

These depend on the site of origin. The most common presenting symptom is an abdominal mass, which is found in more than 50% of patients. Other symptoms include respiratory distress, Horner syndrome, proptosis, bilateral orbital ecchymosis ("panda eyes"), paraplegia or cauda equina, bladder or vascular compression, opsoclonus and nystagmus (dancing-eye syndrome).

What diagnostic studies are used?

CT scan or MRI is generally used. Metastatic workup includes bone scan and long bone radiographs. Bone marrow aspirates are also performed. Metaiodobenzylguanidine (MIBG) scanning may be helpful in identifying primary tumor and metastases if the origin is unknown; however, a biopsy of the primary tumor is usually needed for definitive diagnosis.

What are useful tumor markers?

1. **Urine vanillylmandelic acid, homovanillic acid, and metanephrine levels,** which are collected in a 24-hour sample.
2. Other tumor markers include serum **neuron-specific enolase (NSE)** and serum **ferritin**
3. Markers from the tumor itself will include the **n-*myc* oncogene and the *trk* proto-oncogene**
4. Flow cytometry is used to determine DNA ploidy
5. Integrity of chromosome 1p

What are the stages?

The International Neuroblastoma Staging System:

Stage I: localized tumor that is completely excised

Stage IIa: unilateral tumor with incomplete excision, microscopic residual, and negative lymph nodes

Stage IIb: unilateral tumor with complete or incomplete excision, with positive local lymph nodes

Stage III: tumor infiltrating across the midline or unilateral tumor with contralateral lymph node involvement

Stage IV: dissemination of tumor to distant lymph nodes, bone, bone marrow, liver, or other organs

Stage IV-S: localized primary tumor as defined for Stage I or II with dissemination limited to liver, skin, and/or bone marrow

[There are a variety of staging systems similar to the International Neuroblastoma Staging System; of these, the more widely used systems include the Pediatric Oncology Group (POG) and the Evans System.]

What is unique about stage IV-S?

Most newborn infants and 30% of infants younger than 1 year of age present with this stage. This stage has an unusually good survival rate despite the dissemination aspect. Usually no treatment is needed other than excision of the primary tumor. Chemotherapy or radiation therapy may be required if an enlarged liver compromises the infant's respiratory or nutritional status.

What are favorable prognostic factors?

1. Younger than 1 year of age
2. Less than 3 n-*myc* copies
3. Normal serum NSE and ferritin levels
4. DNA aneuploidy or hyperploidy
5. High *trk* proto-oncogene expression
6. Intact heterogenous chromosome 1p

What is the treatment?

For stages I and II, primary surgical excision with follow-up chemotherapy. For stages III and IV, preoperative chemotherapy is usually needed to shrink the tumor before resection can be undertaken. Bone marrow transplantation may be used in stage IV tumors.

What is overall survival rate?

Overall survival rate for infants younger than 1 year of age is 72% and older than 1 year of age is 32%; however, survival is about 90% for children with stages I and II in both groups, with significantly worse prognosis for stages III and IV. Stage for stage, children younger than 1 year of age have a better prognosis.

WILMS TUMOR

What is it?

An embryonal tumor of renal origin

What is the incidence?

There are about 500 new cases in the United States each year.
Wilms tumor represents slightly more than 10% of all childhood cancer cases.

What is the age at diagnosis?

Usually between 1–4 years of age

What are associated conditions?

1. Sporadic aniridia
2. Hemihypertrophy
3. Beckwith-Wiedemann syndrome
4. Neurofibromatosis
5. Genitourinary tract anomalies

What are the signs and symptoms?

The tumor usually presents as a large, palpable, painless abdominal mass. Gross hematuria may be noted in 10%–15% of cases. Elevated blood pressure may be noted in 20% of cases.

How is it diagnosed?

The tumor is usually assessed and identified via CT scan. Ultrasound is used to assess for vena caval extension. Chest radiograph or CT scan rules out pulmonary metastases. Ultimate diagnosis and staging are determined during surgical excision.

What are the stages?

Stage I: unilateral tumor without capsular involvement; it is completely resected

Stage II: unilateral tumor with renal capsule involvement; it is completely resected

Stage III: unilateral tumor with regional lymph node involvement, preoperative tumor rupture, or significant intraoperative tumor spill

Stage IV: metastasis to lung, bone, brain, liver, or distant lymph nodes

Stage V: bilateral renal tumors

What is the treatment?

Surgical excision is followed by chemotherapy, depending on the stage. Radiation is needed for advanced stage tumors.

What are the two pathology types?

1. Favorable histology (89%) includes blastema, epithelial, mixed, cystic, and glomerular types.
2. Unfavorable histology includes anaplastic types.

(Clear and rhabdoid histology were considered unfavorable histology, but are now considered individual tumor types separate from Wilms tumor.)

What is the prognosis?

The current overall survival rate for patients is 80%. In patients with favorable histology, overall survival rate is 90%. Survival rate approaches 95%–100% for stages I and II tumors.

What is mesoblastic nephroma?

It is a renal tumor that usually presents in infants younger than 3–4 months of age. Its presentation may be similar to that of Wilms tumor. However, 95% are benign and surgical resection is the only treatment necessary.

What is nephroblastomatosis (nodular renal blastema)?

It is a capsular nest of primitive metanephric epithelial rests around the rim of the kidney. If found, these may progress to Wilms tumor. Patients are treated with chemotherapy when these rests are found.

HODGKIN DISEASE

What is it?

A malignant lymph node disorder of unknown etiology

What is the incidence?

5% of childhood malignancies; 6 cases per 1 million children

At what age is it most common?

The first peak is 15–40 years of age, and the later peak is 45–55 years of age; 15% of patients are younger than 16 years of age.

What is the most frequent presenting finding?

Painless cervical lymphadenopathy

What are other presenting signs and symptoms?

Enlarged axillary or inguinal lymph nodes may be the first presenting sign. Children with mediastinal involvement may have respiratory distress, but this is more common in non-Hodgkin lymphoma. Other symptoms may include fever, night sweats, and weight loss (i.e., the "B" symptoms).

How is the diagnosis made?

Diagnosis must be made by histologic examination.
Reed-Sternberg cells must be found.

What are the four histologic types?

1. Lymphocyte predominance
2. Nodular sclerosing
3. Mixed cellularity
4. Lymphocyte depletion

Which is the most common histologic type in children?

Nodular sclerosing (> 65%)

Which histologic type has the best prognosis?

Lymphocyte predominance

Which histologic type has the worst prognosis?

Lymphocyte depletion

What is the staging classification?

The Ann Arbor Classification:

Stage I: involvement of a single lymph node region or a single extralymphatic organ

Stage II: involvement of two or more lymph node regions on the same side of the diaphragm, or localized involvement of an extralymphatic organ or site and of one or more lymph node regions on the same side of the diaphragm

Stage III: involvement of lymph node regions on both sides of the diaphragm; other lymphatic organs may be involved

Stage IV: diffuse or disseminated disease

(Stages are further classified as "A" or "B," depending on whether or not "B" symptoms are present.)

How is staging accomplished?

Staging involves clinical assessment, chest radiograph, abdominal and chest CT scans, bone marrow biopsy, lymphangiography, and staging laparotomy.

Why is staging laparotomy performed?

Because it will upstage a patient from stage I or II in approximately 25% of cases and downstage a patient from stage III in approximately 25% of cases

What is involved in a staging laparotomy?

1. Splenectomy
2. Core liver biopsies of each lobe
3. Lymph node biopsies from the celiac region, splenic hilum, porta hepatis, para-aortic region, and bilateral iliac regions
4. Oophoropexy in girls (i.e., move the ovaries to the midline so that if radiation is needed, they are not in the field of radiation to the iliac regions)

What are the complications of staging laparotomy?

The most common complication is intestinal obstruction. Other complications include post-splenectomy sepsis, atelectasis, wound infection, pleural effusion, abscess, pancreatitis, and thrombotic episodes.

How is Hodgkin disease treated?

Treatment depends on disease stage. Generally, a combination of chemotherapy and radiation is used. In some older children with stage I or II disease, radiation therapy alone may be sufficient. In lower stages, chemotherapy alone may also be sufficient.

What are the complications of therapy?

1. Most complications are due to the specific agents used and include:
   Myelosuppression and cardiac toxicity (Adriamycin)
   Pulmonary fibrosis (bleomycin)
   Gonadal dysfunction or sterility (alkylating agents)
   Neurologic impairment (vincristine, vinblastine)
2. Other complications include growth impairment due to radiation and development of second neoplasms.

What are the most common second neoplasms?

Acute nonlymphoblastic leukemia
Non-Hodgkin lymphoma
Thyroid carcinoma
Parathyroid adenoma
Soft tissue sarcoma
Osteogenic sarcoma
Breast carcinoma
Basal cell carcinoma

What is the prognosis of Hodgkin disease?	Overall survival of children with Hodgkin disease reaches 98%. The youngest children have the best prognosis. Even children and adolescents with stages III and IV disease can expect to have a 75%–85% 5-year survival rate.

NON-HODGKIN LYMPHOMA

What is it?	It is a heterogenous group of lymphoid tumors.
What is the incidence?	7%–10% of all pediatric malignancies; it is the third most common pediatric malignancy (after leukemia and brain tumors)
What are the three most common types in childhood?	1. Lymphoblastic lymphoma (LBL) 2. Small non-cleaved cell (Burkitt and non-Burkitt lymphoma) 3. Large-cell lymphoma (histiocytic)
What are possible causes of non-Hodgkin lymphoma?	Viral infections and immunodeficiency have been implicated. In particular, Burkitt lymphoma of the endemic type, normally found in Africa, is usually associated with Epstein-Barr virus. However, in the United States, where sporadic Burkitt lymphoma occurs, the Epstein-Barr virus is involved in only 10%–20% of cases.
What are some of the associated immunodeficiency conditions?	HIV Wiskott-Aldrich syndrome Bloom syndrome Ataxia-telangiectasia Severe combined immunodeficiency disease X-linked lymphoproliferative syndrome Patients immunosupressed for organ transplantation
How are non-Hodgkin lymphomas classified?	According to: Morphology Immunophenotype Histochemical staining Cytogenic markers Molecular analysis

What are presenting signs and symptoms:

In LBL?

Usually presents as an anterior mediastinal mass with respiratory symptomatology or superior vena caval syndrome

In non-Burkitt lymphoma or Burkitt lymphoma of the sporadic type?

Usually presents with abdominal symptoms, which represents tumor involvement of the bowel, manifesting as intussusception or obstruction; the endemic type of Burkitt lymphoma presents with involvement of the eye or the jaw

In large-cell lymphomas?

They are usually extranodal and present with widely disseminated disease.

How is the diagnosis made?

By a biopsy of an involved lymph node, bone marrow biopsies, or cytologic evaluation of pleural fluid or ascites

What tests are needed for complete workup?

1. CBC with differential
2. Liver and renal function tests
3. Serum uric acid, calcium, phosphorus, LDH, and electrolytes
4. Chest radiograph
5. Chest and/or abdominal CT scan
6. Bone scan
7. Spinal tap

How is non-Hodgkin lymphoma treated?

It depends on the type of lymphoma. Generally chemotherapy is used. Radiation therapy may be needed to shrink large mediastinal tumors when respiratory distress is present. Bone marrow transplant may ultimately be needed.

What is tumor lysis syndrome?

This can result when tumor is destroyed during treatment. It causes hyperuricemia, which can compromise renal function. This syndrome is particularly characteristic during treatment of lymphoma.

How is tumor lysis treated?

During treatment, hydration is very important. If tumor lysis occurs, allopurinol is administered and $NaHCO_3$ is added to the IV fluid in order to alkalinize the urine and increase the solubility of uric acid to facilitate renal clearance. If hyperphosphatemia occurs, alkalinization must be halted because calcium phosphate may precipitate. Diuretics must be used with caution; they may lower the urine pH, enhancing hyperuricemia.

LEUKEMIA

What is the incidence of leukemia in childhood?	1:2800 before 15 years of age
What are some of the clinical features on presentation?	Fatigue, fever, pallor, petechiae, purpura, lymphadenopathy, hepatosplenomegaly, bone or joint pain, weight loss, anorexia, headache
What are the laboratory findings on presentation?	Thrombocytopenia Anemia Low (or high) total white blood cell count (WBC)
What are predisposing conditions?	Down syndrome, Fanconi anemia, and Bloom syndrome
How are leukemias classified?	According to: Cell morphology Chromosome abnormalities Staining properties Surface antigens Clinical behavior (rapidity of onset)
What is the most common leukemia in childhood?	**Acute lymphoblastic leukemia (ALL)**

ALL

How common is ALL?	It accounts for **85%** of childhood leukemias.
At what age is the peak incidence of ALL?	4 years of age
What are good prognostic features?	Child is 3–7 years of age WBC < 10,000/μl

What are poor prognostic features?	Child < 1 year or > 10 years of age WBC > 50,000/μl
How is it diagnosed?	By examination of a bone marrow aspirate; may also use cell surface marker studies and karyotype
What are the types of ALL?	Pre pre-B-cell T-cell Pre-B-cell B-cell
What is induction?	Initial treatment phase
What medications are used for induction in ALL?	Usual medications include a corticosteroid, vincristine, and L-asparaginase.
How successful is induction in ALL?	98% of patients achieve remission.
What is consolidation (intensification)?	Treatment regimens in some protocols that lead to further reduction in malignant cells
What is remission?	Absence of leukemia cells in bone marrow, with normalization of peripheral blood counts and marrow precursors
What is maintenance therapy?	Treatment designed to further reduce the chance of recurrence of the leukemia
What are commonly used maintenance drugs?	Methotrexate 6-Mercaptopurine Prednisone L-asparaginase
What is CNS prophylaxis?	Treatment to prevent leukemia relapse in the CNS
Why is this necessary?	The CNS is a relative sanctuary for leukemia cells, and typical systemic medications may not adequately penetrate the CNS.

What are the methods of CNS prophylaxis?	Intrathecal medications (e.g., methotrexate, hydrocortisone, ARA-C) and radiation

ACUTE MYELOCYTIC LEUKEMIA (AML)

What is the incidence of AML?	1 in 15,000 children each year; it accounts for 15%–20% of childhood acute leukemia
What are some presenting signs and symptoms?	Fever, anemia, pallor, pain (particularly bone pain), bleeding, bruising, hepatosplenomegaly, DIC, skin nodules
What are poor prognostic features at presentation?	Organomegaly High WBC DIC Certain chromosome abnormalities indicate a poor prognosis.
How many subtypes of AML are there?	At least seven (based on FAB classification system)
What conditions predispose a child to AML?	Fanconi anemia, Down syndrome, Bloom syndrome, Wiskott-Aldrich syndrome
What is the significance of chromosome abnormalities in AML?	Chromosome abnormalities are common in AML, and some may be associated with an improved prognosis. Chromosome 7 abnormalities are associated with a relatively poor prognosis.
What is the treatment for AML?	It is usually more intense than that for ALL. Induction medications may include ARA-C, daunorubicin, and other more experimental drugs. **Bone marrow transplantation** should be considered if there is a suitable donor.
What is the outcome of AML?	Most patients achieve an initial remission, but long-term survival is worse than that for ALL.

RETINOBLASTOMA

What is it?
The most common childhood eye tumor. It arises from primitive cells prior to differentiation.

What is the incidence?
About 1 in 20,000 children

How does it present?
It may present with **strabismus** and/or abnormal red reflex.
The reflex actually appears white (**leukocoria**) because of reflection of light off the tumor surface.

Is retinoblastoma hereditary?
About 40% of cases are familial; the remainder are sporadic.

What causes retinoblastoma?
It is caused by loss of function of both copies of the retinoblastoma gene, a tumor-suppressor gene, on chromosome 13.

For what other tumors are patients with retinoblastoma at risk?
Osteosarcomas, particularly in patients with hereditary retinoblastoma

RHABDOMYOSARCOMA

What is it?
This is a soft tissue tumor of skeletal muscle origin that may occur in a variety of sites.

What is the incidence?
It is the most common soft tissue sarcoma in infants and children, representing 10%–15% of all solid tumors and 6% of all pediatric cancers. It is more common in boys than in girls and in whites than in blacks.

What are associated conditions?
Children with neurofibromatosis and basal cell nevus syndrome have an increased rate of rhabdomyosarcoma.

Are there familial tendencies?
There may be familial occurrences. Also, female relatives of children with rhabdomyosarcoma may have an increased risk of breast cancer.

Are there any specific biologic markers?	No
What are the most common ages of presentation?	There are two peak instances: The first is 2–5 years of age and the second is 12–18 years of age.
What are important prognostic criteria?	1. Site 2. Stage 3. Histology
What are the stages of rhabdomyosarcoma?	Stage I: completely resected localized disease Stage II: grossly resected tumor with residual disease or positive lymph nodes Stage III: gross residual disease Stage IV: metastatic disease
What are the primary sites of rhabdomyosarcoma in children?	Orbit, paratesticular, vagina, uterus, extremity, bladder or prostate, perianal, retroperitoneal, chest wall, head and neck
What are sites where prognosis is relatively favorable?	Orbit, vagina, vulva, and paratesticular
What are favorable histologies?	Embryonal, non-osseous Ewing, botryoid, mixed, undifferentiated, and pleomorphic
Which physiology type has the best prognosis?	Embryonal cell type
What are unfavorable histologies?	Alveolar, anaplastic, and monomorphous round cell
What are the signs and symptoms?	They vary according to the site of tumor.
How is it diagnosed?	Usually by biopsy or at excision of the tumor after primary workup
How is tumor evaluation carried out?	This also depends on the site of the tumor. Usually MRI or CT imaging is required. Chest radiographs and bone scan are also required to rule out distant spread.

What is the treatment?	Generally surgical excision is desired, but this may not be possible if the tumor is involved in vital structures. In these cases, chemotherapy and radiation may be required before tumor resection. When the tumor can be primarily resected, chemotherapy and often radiation therapy are needed as adjuvant treatment. A significant exception is when the primary tumor arises in the orbit. In these cases, chemotherapy and radiation, without surgery, will result in a 90% survival rate.
What is the prognosis?	Overall survival rate during the second intergroup rhabdomyosarcoma sarcoma (IRS) trial was 63% for 5 years.

OSTEOGENIC SARCOMA

What is it?	It is a bone tumor characterized by spindle cells. It may occur in various cytologic forms, including osteoblastic, chondroblastic, fibroblastic, telangiectatic, giant-cell type, and malignant fibrous histiocytoma-like.
How common is osteogenic sarcoma?	There are fewer than 500 new cases yearly, but it is the most common malignant bone tumor in children.
What three sites are most commonly affected?	**Distal femur, proximal tibia,** and **proximal humerus**
Is there a gender difference?	**Males** outnumber females 2 to 1.
Which portions of the bone are most commonly affected?	The **medullary cavity** and the **metaphysis**
How do these tumors present?	Persistent pain after minor trauma is the typical history. A mass may be palpable.
What are the radiographic findings?	Characteristically, there is periosteal elevation with a **"sunburst"** pattern of soft tissue calcifications.

What is the mode of spread for these tumors?	The tumor most commonly spreads to the lung through the blood system.
What is the tumor marker for osteogenic sarcoma?	**Alkaline phosphatase**
What is the treatment?	Although surgical resection was often the initial treatment, currently preoperative chemotherapy and resection using limb salvage techniques comprise the most common treatment strategy.
What is the outcome?	Overall survival rate is 60%–75%.

EWING SARCOMA

What is it?	It is a sarcoma that normally develops in the bone marrow and consists of **small blue round cells.**
What bones are most commonly affected?	The **femur, humerus, ribs,** and **flat bones** (e.g., the scapula). However, any bone may be affected.
What part of the bone is most commonly affected?	The midshaft
In what age-group and gender does Ewing sarcoma most commonly present?	Male adolescents
What are typical presenting symptoms?	**Bone pain** followed by swelling is usually the initial symptom. Bone necrosis can ensue, causing fever, and thus Ewing sarcoma is often misdiagnosed as osteomyelitis.
What are typical radiographic findings?	Disruption of the bony cortex with layers of new periosteal bone formation, resulting in an **"onionskin"** appearance.
What is the treatment?	Usually a combination of chemotherapy and radiation is performed before surgical resection of the involved bony region.

What is the outcome?	Usually limb salvage can be achieved. The overall survival rate is approximately 75%.
Where does the tumor most commonly metastasize?	The **lungs**

MEDULLOBLASTOMA

What is it?	It is a tumor of the **posterior fossa.**
Where does it originate?	From the **roof of the fourth ventricle**
What are typical symptoms?	Signs and symptoms of **increased intracranial pressure,** including headache, vomiting, diplopia, and papilledema; **in infants, a bulging fontanel may be present**
What is the most useful diagnostic study?	MRI
What is the age of onset?	Generally younger than 7 years of age
What is the treatment?	Surgical removal with associated radiation therapy; if there is residual tumor after surgical removal, chemotherapy may also be needed
What is the outcome?	Generally, children younger than 2 years of age have a poorer outcome than older patients. For older patients who do not require chemotherapy, there is a 5-year survival rate of 70%. If chemotherapy is required, the survival rate is about 60%.

ASTROCYTOMA

What is it?	It is a tumor of **glial origin** that tends to be cystic in nature.
Where does it occur?	Either in the **cerebellar** or in the **intracerebral region**

What are the symptoms and signs?	It depends on the location of the tumor: 1. Cerebellar tumors are usually manifested by headache, vomiting, diplopia, papilledema, or hydrocephalus. 2. Tumors of the cerebral tissue may result in epilepsy, upper motor neuron signs, or even growth arrest of the opposite extremity.
What is the most useful diagnostic study?	MRI
What is the treatment?	Surgical removal of the tumor is required. Follow-up radiation therapy may be required for high-grade astrocytoma or tumors that show residual progression postoperatively.
What is the outcome?	Generally, cerebellar tumors have a much better outcome than cerebral tumors. Five-year survival rate for cerebellar tumors is 90%, whereas for cerebral tumors it is about 30%–80%. The worse the grade, the poorer is the prognosis.

HEPATOBLASTOMA

What is it?	A malignant tumor of the liver that may be related to maldevelopment of the liver
What are the four types?	1. Fetal or well-differentiated 2. Embryonal (immature and poorly differentiated) 3. Mixed epithelial and mesenchymal 4. Anaplastic
At what age is hepatoblastoma most commonly seen?	Usually before 4 years of age; two thirds of patients are younger than 2 years of age
What are associated conditions?	Hemihypertrophy Beckwith-Wiedemann syndrome Fanconi anemia Fetal alcohol syndrome Cirrhosis Tyrosinemia TPN-cholestasis Type I glycogen storage disease

What are the signs and symptoms?	A large right upper quadrant mass is usually the presenting sign. Nausea and vomiting may also be present.
What are pertinent laboratory values?	Commonly serum bilirubin, αFP, and HCG are elevated.
What are the components of the diagnostic workup?	Workup should include serum tumor markers, a plain chest and abdominal radiograph, ultrasound examination to rule out involvement of surrounding structures or the vena cava, a CT scan of the abdomen, a bone marrow aspirate, and bone scan.
What is the treatment?	Tumor resection is the primary treatment. The extent of resection should follow anatomic lines in the liver according to the location of the tumor. Chemotherapy may be required as initial treatment for exceptionally large tumors in order to reduce the tumor to a resectable size.
What percent of children with hepatoblastoma have surgically resectable tumors?	Less than 50%
What is the outcome?	Children with Stage 1 disease with a complete resection and chemotherapy may have an 85%–90% survival rate. This survival rate may be slightly higher if histology is pure fetal. Overall survival rate for all cases of hepatoblastoma is 50%.

HEPATOMA

What is it?	Hepatocellular carcinoma—it is an epithelial malignancy similar to that seen in adults
What are risk factors for hepatoma?	Chronic hepatitis from hepatitis B virus Cirrhosis Hemihypertrophy Beckwith-Wiedemann syndrome Fanconi anemia Fetal alcohol syndrome Type I glycogen storage disease Tyrosinemia

In which lobe of the liver is hepatoma commonly found?	The **right** lobe
Where does the tumor commonly spread?	It first spreads intrahepatically via lymphatic and vascular channels. It may then extend along the hepatic veins and vena cava. Hematogenous spread is to the lung, brain, and bone marrow.
What is a favorable variant of hepatoma?	**Fibrolamellar carcinoma**
What are the clinical manifestations of hepatoma?	Right upper quadrant mass, nausea and vomiting, abdominal pain, weight loss, anemia

What are important laboratory values?

1. CBC
2. SGOT and SGPT
3. Alkaline phosphatase
4. Bilirubin, which is almost always normal except in advanced cases
5. Serum αFP, which is elevated in 50% of childhood cases
6. Serum ferritin, which is elevated in virtually all cases

What are important diagnostic tests?

1. Ultrasound determines that the mass is solid.
2. CT scan delineates the extent of the tumor as well as vascular involvement.
3. Bone marrow aspirate and bone scan are needed for evidence of tumor involvement in those regions.
4. A hepatic angiogram may help determine liver and tumor anatomy and vascular variations.

How is hepatoma staged?

Stage I: total resection of the specimen with clean margins

Stage II: total gross resection with microscopic residual disease

Stage III: unresectable tumor or gross residual disease

Stage IV: metastatic disease

What is the preferred treatment?	Complete resection is required for any chance of complete cure. If the tumor is too large for resection initially, chemotherapy may be used in attempt to shrink the tumor. Postoperative chemotherapy is always needed.
What are the most effective chemotherapeutic agents?	Doxorubicin and cisplatin may be the most effective, although actinomycin D, vincristine, cyclophosphamide, etoposide, 5-fluorouracil, and others have been used.
What are three major metabolic concerns following hepatic resection?	1. Hypoalbuminemia 2. Hypoglycemia 3. Hypothrombinemia
What is the overall survival rate for children with hepatoma?	15%

SACROCOCCYGEAL TERATOMA (SCT)

What is it?	A teratoma is a tumor consisting of tissue from some or all of three primitive germ-cell layers (i.e., endoderm, mesoderm, ectoderm); tissue may reveal itself in varying stages of maturity; **sacrococcygeal area is the most common site for teratomas.**
When is an SCT usually noted?	Is usually obvious on prenatal ultrasound or at birth
Where else may teratomas be found?	Ovary, testicle, head and neck, mediastinum, retroperitoneum
What are the signs and symptoms?	In sacrococcygeal area, tumor protrudes from presacral space and pushes the rectum forward. The tumor may weigh as much as the infant! Tumors in other sites may present as physical deformities or as a result of compression of surrounding structures, such as the lung or trachea.

What are characteristic radiologic findings?	**Calcifications** in 50% of cases
What is the malignant potential?	Low in infants, but increases with age
Which serum tumor markers should be checked for?	HCG (choriocarcinoma) and αFP (yolk sac carcinoma); these markers are also monitored in follow-up to detect recurrence
What is the treatment?	Surgical removal
What is the vascular source of an SCT?	Presacral vessels; these must be removed with the coccyx to minimize the potential for recurrence and malignancy
What is the outcome?	If the tumor is benign, outcome is excellent (but it is necessary to monitor for recurrence of malignant tissue). If malignancy is present, outcome is generally poor. If the primary tumor has malignant components, recurrence is common, even if original tumor is thought to be completely excised.

MELANOMA

What is the incidence of melanoma in children?	It accounts for 1%–3% of all pediatric malignancies.
What are risk factors for melanoma?	1. Fair-skinned children are more prone to melanoma than are darker skinned children.
	2. Familial atypical mole melanoma syndrome
	3. Xeroderma pigmentosum
	4. Increased numbers of melanocytic nevi
	5. Acquired nevi, especially in areas of chronic irritation or trauma
	6. Giant congenital nevus
	7. Atypical nevi
	8. Excessive (especially intense and intermittent) sun exposure
	9. Family history
	10. Immunosuppression
	NOTE: In 30%–50% of cases, melanoma will occur at a site without a previous nevus.

What are Clark's levels of tumor invasion?

Level I: tumor cells above basement membrane
Level II: invasion of papillary dermis
Level III: tumor cells at junction of papillary and reticular dermis
Level IV: invasion of reticular dermis
Level V: invasion of subcutaneous fat

What are Breslow's classifications of tumor thickness?

In situ
< 0.76 mm
0.76–1.5 mm
1.5–4 mm
> 4 mm

What is the mortality of melanoma determined by?

Thickness of tumor and level of invasion into the skin

What is the overall mortality rate?

40%

What is the treatment?

If detected early, local excision with an appropriate margin according to location and depth of the melanoma may be all that is needed. However, for more extensive tumors, adjuvant chemotherapy is needed. The role of lymph node dissection is controversial, although resection of the appropriate nodal group may benefit survival in early stage lesions.

What are preventive measures?

Avoidance of intense sun and use of protective clothing and sunscreen

26

Skin, Soft Tissue, Nail, and Hair Disorders

SKIN

LYMPHANGIOMA

What is it?	A benign tumor of the lymphatic system that consists of large or small saccules of lymph fluid
What is "cystic hygroma"?	This term is usually used to describe a large, primarily cystic lymphangioma of the neck
When do lymphangiomas present?	Usually at or soon after birth
Where are they located?	Anywhere in the body, but most commonly the neck, axilla, mediastinum, groin, and lower abdomen
What are the symptoms?	Often asymptomatic; however, lymphangiomas of the neck, tongue, or glottic regions may cause respiratory distress; infection or inflammation may be a presenting symptom, but a lymphangioma usually presents as a painless mass
Do lymphangiomas regress?	No
What is the treatment?	Surgical excision (re-excision may be necessary in 10%–15% of cases) Sclerosing agents have been tried with minimal success

HEMANGIOMA

What is it?	Abnormal proliferation of vascular endothelial cells, resulting in tumors of varying sizes and types composed of abnormal blood vessels
How do they present?	Although most are visible on the skin, hemangiomas may involve any organ. Presentation may relate to the effect on the involved organ. In addition, large hemangiomas (particularly of the liver) may cause heart failure due to arteriovenous shunting or purpura due to consumption of platelets (**Kasabach-Merritt syndrome**).
How are they diagnosed?	Cutaneous lesions are easily diagnosed by physical exam. Ultrasound or CT may be required for intracorporeal lesions.
May hemangiomas be multiple?	**YES!** Discovery of one hemangioma should prompt a search for others. Ask about any evidence of airway obstruction.
What is the typical course of a hemangioma?	Growth over the first 1–1.5 years followed by involution; 80% are gone by 5 years of age.
What is the treatment?	If functional difficulties should arise, oral or injected steroids may be initially used; α-interferon has also been effective.
What are indications for medical therapy?	1. Obstruction of vision 2. Thrombocytopenia 3. Obstruction of luminal organs 4. Uncontrollable hemorrhage or ulceration 5. Repeated infection 6. Cardiac compromise because of arteriovenous shunting

What are indications for surgical resection?	Any previously listed indication that does not respond to medical therapy or if symptoms are too severe to wait for medical results

ATOPIC DERMATITIS (ECZEMA)

What is it?	A common **inflammatory skin disorder** of infancy and childhood in which the acute phase is characterized by an **itch–scratch cycle;** usually noninfectious
How does it present?	Often presents as an erythematous, papulovesicular eruption that can progress to a scaly, lichenified dermatitis over time; it is worse in the winter and is usually seen on the face, neck, and antecubital and popliteal fossae
What is the prevalence?	Approximately **1%** of the general population and **3%–5%** of children younger than 5 years of age. Ninety percent of eczema presents before 5 years of age.
What is the pathogenesis?	Unknown—patients with moderate-to-severe atopic dermatitis frequently have elevated **IgE**, which is caused by disordered control of its synthesis
What are the phases of atopic dermatitis?	The distribution of the rash varies among three distinct phases: 1. In **infancy** it affects the cheeks, scalp, trunk, and extensor surface of the extremities. 2. In the **childhood** phase it affects the flexor surfaces, especially the antecubital and popliteal fossae, wrists and ankles. 3. In the **adult** phase, the lesions are generally on the face, back, feet, and neck.
Individuals with atopic dermatitis are often prone to what types of skin infections?	*Staphylococcus aureus* β-Hemolytic streptococci Herpes simplex Molluscum contagiosum Fungal infections

With what is atopic dermatitis associated?	May be seen in families with a high incidence of allergies and/or asthma
What is the differential diagnosis?	Seborrheic dermatitis Psoriasis Scabies Contact dermatitis Drug reactions Zinc deficiency Severe combined immunodeficiency
What is the prognosis?	80%–90% outgrow it by puberty
What is the treatment?	Therapy is directed at controlling the dryness, inflammation, and pruritus. Environmental control plays an important role. Bath oils, mild nonirritating soap, and moisturizer or emollients help control the dryness. Topical corticosteroids are used to control inflammation. Antihistamines are used to control itching. Antibiotics or antifungals are used to control infections on an as-needed basis.
What types of steroids should be avoided in infants?	Strong fluorinated steroids on the face

IMPETIGO

What is it?	A cutaneous infection of either staphylococcal or streptococcal origin
What are the two types?	Bullous and non-bullous
Which is more common?	**Non-bullous**—accounting for approximately 70% of cases of impetigo
What is the presentation of non-bullous impetigo?	Generally a small vesicle or pustule forms on a predisposing lesion and may spread to a honey-colored, approximately 2-cm, clustered lesion; it is usually more common during warm weather

What are predisposing lesions?	Chickenpox Insect bites Abrasions Lacerations Burns
What is the treatment?	These lesions usually resolve on their own within 2 weeks. Antibiotic therapy is rarely needed.
Who typically gets bullous impetigo?	Infants and young children
What is the most common bacterial cause?	**Staphylococcus** (80%)
What are the characteristics of bullous impetigo?	Transparent, flaccid bullae develop on the affected skin.
What is the treatment?	Either topical or oral antibiotics
What are potential complications of impetigo?	Cellulitis Osteomyelitis Septic arthritis Pneumonia Septicemia
What is a rare renal complication?	Post-streptococcal glomerulonephritis

CELLULITIS

What is it?	Acute inflammation of the dermis and subcutaneous fat, usually caused by bacterial invasion of the skin
What are some etiologic agents?	*Streptococcus pyogenes* (group A) and *S. aureus* are most common. *Streptococcus pneumoniae* and *Haemophilus influenzae* also cause cellulitis.
Which are most common in newborns?	Group B strep, *E. coli*
In infants and young children?	*H. influenzae*

What is the clinical picture?

1. Skin is red, tender, edematous, warm, and may be indurated. Borders are indistinct and not elevated.
2. Enlarged, tender regional **lymph nodes**, lymphangitis
3. Fever, chills, malaise, poor appetite

What are the mechanisms of spread?

Local spread: break in skin (e.g., wound, bite, excoriation, impetigo, folliculitis, carbuncle, varicella)
Hematogenous spread
Direct extension from deeper infection

Is blood culture useful?

Yes, in patients with **systemic illness** (fever, toxicity, leukocytosis) or **facial cellulitis** and in **newborns** and those who are **immunocompromised**; low sensitivity in other patients

Is tissue aspiration useful?

The yield is up to 50% positive. A positive yield is higher in immunocompromised patients. (**Note:** This can be a painful and traumatic procedure. Carefully weigh risk versus benefit.)

What is the treatment?

Antibiotic therapy is aimed at the most likely causative organisms. **Adjunctive therapies** include warm compresses, bed rest, elevation, and pain control.

Who warrants IV antibiotics?

Newborns and immunocompromised patients as well as patients with high fever, systemic toxicity, vomiting, periorbital/orbital cellulitis, or who show no improvement after 2 days of oral therapy almost always warrant IV antibiotics. Outpatient therapy with IM ceftriaxone is an alternative in patients with reliable follow-up.

What is erysipelas?

It is a skin infection usually caused by **group A β-hemolytic streptococcus**; most often occurs in neonates and infants

What are clinical features of erysipelas?

Onset is preceded by malaise, myalgia, systemic illness. Skin lesion is characterized by rapid expansion, and has sharply demarcated erythematous and elevated advancing edge. Lesion may have irregular, fluid-filled blisters. It often involves the umbilical stump in neonates.

What is periorbital cellulitis?

Inflammation of soft tissues of the eye superficial to the orbital septum

What causes it?

Trauma, insect bites, or severe conjunctivitis with spread of infection to surrounding area; may also result from bacteremia, sinusitis, and hematogenous spread

What are causative organisms?

S. aureus: usually when trauma, insect bite, or other skin infection (e.g., impetigo) is present
H. influenzae: with bacteremia
S. pneumoniae: with bacteremia
Group A β-hemolytic streptococci

What is the clinical presentation?

Eyelid, conjunctivae, and surrounding area are swollen, red, warm, and indurated. **Purple hue** to the skin is associated with *H. influenzae*. Fever and systemic toxicity may be present.

What comprises the evaluation of periorbital cellulitis?

CBC, blood culture, and wound/lesion culture (if appropriate)
Must rule out true orbital cellulitis. If unable to do so clinically, obtain ophthalmology evaluation and/or CT scan looking for orbital involvement (e.g., EOM entrapment, proptosis, optic nerve swelling).
Lumbar puncture should be performed if meningitis is not ruled out clinically.

What is the treatment?

Intravenous antibiotics, directed against usual pathogens, are necessary. Ceftriaxone, with or without nafcillin, is a typical choice.

What are three possible complications of true orbital cellulitis?	1. Compression or stretching of the optic nerve and visual loss 2. Cavernous sinus thrombosis 3. Meningitis
What is buccal cellulitis?	Infection of the skin and subcutaneous tissues of the cheek.
What age group is this most common in?	Occurs almost exclusively in children 6 months to 3 years of age
What are common causative organisms?	Usually caused by hematogenous spread of *H. influenzae* or *S. pneumoniae*
What other condition is commonly associated with buccal cellulitis?	Up to 90% incidence of accompanying **meningitis**
What is the treatment?	Often requires IV antibiotics

HYPER- AND HYPOPIGMENTATION

What are hyper- and hypopigmentation?	These terms refer to either an increase or decrease in skin pigmentation, respectively.
What are the causes of pigmentation changes?	Pigmentation changes may be local or generalized and are due to a wide variety of defects, including: 1. Absence of melanocytes 2. Defective melanocytes 3. Overproduction of melanin 4. Pigmentation changes induced by hormones 5. Focal developmental defects 6. Postinflammatory sequelae
What are freckles?	Light or dark brown macules that are usually less than 3 mm in diameter. The edges are poorly defined and they occur in sun-exposed areas.
Who are they common in?	Fair-haired individuals
What determines formation of freckles besides sun exposure?	Predisposition to freckles may be a familial trait.

What is the histology of a freckle?

Increased melanin and pigment in the epidermal base cells

What are they a risk factor for?

Melanoma

What are lentigines?

These are small, round, dark brown macules. They can occur anywhere in the body and are generally less than 3 cm.

Are these related to freckles?

No. They have no relation to sun exposure.

What is their histology?

Lentigines represent increased numbers of melanocytes with dense deposits of melanin in elongated, club-shaped, epidermal rete ridges.

In what conditions are lentigines found?

1. Addison disease
2. Pregnancy
3. Lentiginosis profusa
4. LAMB syndrome—Lentigines, Atrial myxoma, Mucocutaneous myxomas, Blue nevi
5. Leopard syndrome
6. Peutz-Jeghers syndrome

What are café au lait spots?

These are uniformly hyperpigmented macular lesions with sharp demarcation. The hue is determined by the natural skin tone. The deeper the color of the natural skin tone, the deeper is the color of the café au lait spot. They may be quite large in size.

What is the histology?

Increased numbers of melanocytes and melanin in the epidermis

Are café au lait spots found in otherwise healthy children?

Yes—10% of healthy children have café au lait spots. Such a child typically has one to three spots.

With what conditions may café au lait spots be associated?

1. McCune-Albright syndrome
2. Neurofibromatosis (von Recklinghausen disease)
3. Russell-Silver syndrome
4. Multiple lentigines
5. Ataxia telangiectasia

6. Fanconi anemia
7. Tuberous sclerosis
8. Bloom syndrome
9. Epidermal nevus syndrome
10. Gaucher syndrome
11. Chédiak-Higashi syndrome

Incontinentia Pigmenti

What is incontinentia pigmenti (Bloch-Sulzberger syndrome)?

It is an ectodermal disorder comprised of dermatologic, dental, ocular, and CNS abnormalities.

How is this disease transmitted?

By an X-linked dominant gene that is lethal in males

What are the cutaneous manifestations?

These occur in four phases:
First: erythematous linear streaks and plaques of vesicles
Second: blisters on the distal limbs that become dry and hyperketotic, thus forming verrucous plaques that involute within 6 months
Third: this stage develops over weeks to months and involves hyperpigmentation on the trunk; however, this hyperpigmentation may also be present on the limbs, axillae, and groins; the hyperpigmentation may take on the appearance of macular whorls, reticulated patches, flecks, and linear streaks
Fourth: hypopigmented, hairless, anhidrotic patches

What is the treatment?

No treatment is needed for the skin changes because they are benign. Treatment is directed towards the ocular, dental, and CNS abnormalities.

Albinism

What is it?

It is a collection of conditions in which there is failure of melanin production in the skin, hair, and eyes.

How is the specific type of albinism determined?	According to: 1. Clinical manifestations 2. Morphology of the melanosomes 3. Hair bulb incubation test, in which hair bulbs are incubated to test for the presence of tyrosinase (presence or absence of tyrosinase may help determine which type of albinism is present)
What is partial albinism?	Also called piebaldism, it is characterized by sharply demarcated amelanotic patches on the forehead, anterior scalp, ventral trunk, elbows, and knees.
How is this condition transmitted?	Autosomal dominant trait
What is the histology of the depigmented regions in partial albinism?	Absence of melanocytes and melanosomes
How does the defective gene occur?	Mutation in the KIT proto-oncogene

Waardenburg Syndrome

What is it?	This syndrome is characterized by lateral displacement of the medial canthi with dystopia canthorum; broad nasal root; heterochromic irises; congenital deafness; a white forelock; and cutaneous hypopigmentation.
What is the inheritance pattern?	**Autosomal dominant** with variable penetrance and expression

Tuberous Sclerosis

What is it?	This is a multisystem condition, involving the **eye, kidney, heart, skin,** and **CNS** (see Chapter 29).
What is the classic triad?	**Hypopigmented skin lesions** with **epilepsy** and **mental retardation**

What are the hypopigmented skin lesions called?	**Ash-leaf** lesions
Where are they most commonly found?	The trunk
How is this condition inherited?	Autosomal dominant trait
What is the prognosis for tuberous sclerosis?	It varies. Some patients are healthy, whereas others may have severe mental retardation, seizures, or cardiac tumors.

Other Conditions with Deficient Pigmentation

What is Chédiak-Higashi syndrome?	It is a condition characterized by abnormal neutrophil function due to improper fusion of granulocytes. In addition, melanocytes do not function properly, thus failing to dispense pigment. Albinism of hair and skin ensues. There is also abnormal platelet aggregation.
What is hypomelanosis of ito (incontinentia pigmenti achromians)?	This condition results in **hypomelanosis** (i.e., hypopigmented macules shaped in demarcated whorls, streaks, and patches). These lesions are essentially the negative image of those hyperpigmented lesions found in incontinentia pigmenti.
What are associated abnormalities?	Anomalies of the **CNS** as well as the **musculoskeletal** and **ophthalmic** systems

VITILIGO

What is it?	Acquired, sharply circumscribed depigmented macules of varying size and shape
What causes vitiligo?	The cause is unknown, but it may be due to an autoimmune mechanism. It tends to occur in **areas of frequent trauma.**

What are associated conditions?	Hypothyroidism, hyperthyroidism, adrenal insufficiency, pernicious anemia, diabetes
What is the course of vitiligo?	Spontaneous repigmentation occurs in about 10%–20% of patients. However, in most patients, progression of depigmentation occurs.
What is the treatment?	Oral or topical psoralen compounds can be administered together with exposure to sunlight or UV light sources. Repigmentation may be partial and may take many months to occur. Topical steroids are occasionally useful. In general, it is important to protect depigmented areas from excessive sunlight because there is no protection normally provided by melanocytes.

STURGE-WEBER DISEASE

What is it?	It is a condition characterized by a constellation of symptoms. The most obvious symptom is a **facial hemangioma (port wine stain).** Seizures, hemiparesis, intracranial calcifications, and mental retardation may be components of this condition. (**Note:** Not all patients with a facial port wine stain have Sturge-Weber disease.)
What is the etiology?	It is thought to be due to anomalous development of the vascular bed during cerebral vascularization.
What are the clinical manifestations?	The facial hemangioma, which is present at birth, is always noted first. It may extend to the lower face, the trunk, and the mucosa of the month and pharynx. The facial hemangioma frequently occurs in the distribution of the trigeminal nerve. Seizures and mental retardation may ensue. If present, the seizures usually occur within the first year of life and become increasingly refractory to therapy. Ocular manifestations include buphthalmos and glaucoma.

How is the diagnosis made?	The constellation of symptoms plus the presence of **intracranial calcifications** on skull radiograph suggest the diagnosis. CT scan of the head may show **unilateral cortical atrophy** and **ipsilateral dilation of the lateral ventricle.**
What is the treatment?	Generally treatment is focused on the control of seizures. Some advocate hemispherectomy or lobectomy to prevent mental retardation. The facial hemangioma may be treated by laser therapy if desired. Ocular pressures also need to be monitored because of the risk for development of glaucoma.

PROTEUS SYNDROME

What is it?	A disturbance of ectodermal and mesodermal growth
What is the etiology?	Unknown
What are the clinical manifestations?	Asymmetric overgrowth of the extremities, verrucous skin lesions, angiomas, lipomas, bone thickening, macrocephaly, excessive muscle growth
What is characteristic of the muscle anomaly?	Abnormal portions of muscle undergo muscular dysgenesis histologically. Abnormal and normal zones of muscles do not follow anatomic planes.
What is the treatment?	Currently there is no known treatment.

MONGOLIAN SPOTS

What are they?	Bluish areas of increased dermal melanocytosis, frequently found across the lumbosacral and gluteal regions of newborns
In which infants are they commonly found?	The incidence is higher in infants whose natural skin color is dark.

| Are mongolian spots malignant? | No. They are thought to be benign, but may be mistaken for bruises. |

CONGENITAL MELANOCYTIC NEVI

| What are they? | Darkly pigmented nevi present at birth; sizes vary |
| Is there a risk of malignancy? | Yes. Some authors recommend removal in childhood. |

TINEA VERSICOLOR

| What is tinea versicolor? | A superficial fungal disease caused by *Pityrosporum orbiculare* |
| What are characteristic lesions? | Round to oval lesions, sometimes with a fine scale, that may be either hyper- or hypopigmented |

RASHES

What causes diaper rash?	Several possible causes, including irritation from urine and stool, candidal overgrowth, allergic reaction, and bacterial infection
What is seborrheic dermatitis?	Oily, yellow, scaly eruption, usually involving the scalp, but may also involve cheeks, trunk, and diaper area
What is the etiology?	The exact cause is unknown, but outbreaks can be associated with stress, poor hygiene, and excessive perspiration
What are viral causes of a rash?	Measles (rubeola), rubella, roseola, "fifth disease," enterovirus
Describe the rash associated with:	
Measles?	Maculopapular, purplish-red rash that generally starts on the face and spreads to extremities; lasts 7–10 days; **Koplik spots** may be seen in the mouth
With rubella?	Maculopapular rash that spreads from face to extremities; shorter duration than measles rash

With roseola?	Macular rash, often at the end of the febrile illness
With "fifth disease" (erythema infectiosum)?	"Slapped cheek" appearance on face; mottled/reticular rash on trunk and extremities
With enteroviruses?	Variable: may be maculopapular or macular; usually on abdomen, chest, palms, and soles
What are some bacterial causes of rash?	*S. pyogenes* (scarlet fever), *S. aureus* (staphylococcal scalded skin syndrome and toxic shock syndrome)
Describe the rash associated with:	
Scarlet fever?	Usually diffuse and erythematous, with a sandpaper quality; may have darker lines in skinfold areas (Pastia's lines); may desquamate, particularly on the face
With staphylococcal scalded skin syndrome?	Generalized, painful, and beefy red; may show blister and/or bullae formation
With toxic shock syndrome?	Diffuse, but usually not tender; may see erythema of conjunctivae, lips, mucosa, palms, and soles

NAIL

INGROWN TOENAIL

What is it?	Side of nail burrows into adjoining skin, resulting in swelling, granulation tissue, erythema, and sometimes infection
Which toe is usually affected?	Large toe
What is the treatment?	Soak toe in warm, soapy water to clean and provide symptomatic relief. Antibiotics are needed for infection. However, removal of one third to one half of toenail on affected side is ultimately needed.

**What are important
aspects of nail removal?**

This can be done under local anesthesia
with a digital block.
Removal of matrix of nail bed will keep
nail from regrowing.
Excess granulation tissue is removed.

**How is recurrence
prevented?**

Unfortunately, if nail regrows,
recurrence is common.
Ingrowth may be prevented by cutting
nails straight across and by teasing the
skin away from the nail with a cotton
swab as the nail regrows.

HANGNAIL

What is it?

Growth of nail material along the lateral
aspect of the nail where it joins into the
skin; it is commonly deep-seated and
tends to curl away from the normal nail;
discomfort is encountered when this
area is rubbed or caught on clothes or
fabric

How is it treated?

By pulling it out (In some cases,
freezing or providing a local anesthetic
beforehand can help)

NAIL (SUBUNGUAL) HEMATOMA

What is it?

Blood clot collected under nail bed
secondary to trauma. It can be very
painful.

What is the sign?

Bluish collection underneath nail with
swelling

What is the treatment?

Heat the end of a paper clip over a
flame and rest it on nail. This will melt
the nail over the hematoma and drain it.
Immediate relief is usually the rule.

**What condition may exist if
a hematoma-looking lesion
exists without a history of
trauma?**

MELANOMA

PARONYCHIA

What is it?	An area of inflammation or abscess formation involving the folds of tissue at the base (or at the lateral base) of the fingernail
What is the treatment?	Often, warm soaks induce drainage, leading to resolution. Antibiotics may be needed for the surrounding cellulitis. Occasionally, a small incision is needed for drainage.

FELON

What is it?	Infected collection (essentially a small abscess) in pulp of distal finger pad
What are the signs and symptoms?	Swelling with tenseness and sometimes erythema of finger pad. Extremely tender to touch.
What is the treatment?	Surgical drainage with incision in midfinger pad parallel to direction of finger. Antibiotics may be needed for cellulitis. Incisions in lateral aspects of finger are to be avoided despite description of this in older sources; these incisions may damage digital nerves and vessels.

HAIR

TRICHOTILLOMANIA

What is it?	Irregular areas of incomplete hair loss due to compulsive pulling, twisting, or breaking of the hair
What causes this behavior?	In some children, this may be a benign behavior; in others, it may represent an obsessive-compulsive disorder.

What is the treatment?	If a benign habit, treatment of concurrent thumb sucking (which is usually present) may resolve the hair-damaging behavior. In children with obsessive-compulsive disorder, medical therapy with behavioral modification may be necessary.

ALOPECIA

What is it?	Partial or complete hair loss (distinguished from hypotrichosis, which is deficient hair growth)
What are the causes of true alopecia?	1. Inflammatory dermatoses 2. Mechanical trauma 3. Drugs 4. Infection 5. Endocrine disorders 6. Nutritional imbalance 7. Disturbance of the hair
What are some causes of alopecia in children?	Alopecia areata, tinea capitis, and trichotillomania
What is the treatment?	Usually alopecia will resolve when the underlying cause is treated; it is rarely primary or congenital.
What is alopecia areata?	Focal hair loss, believed to be immune-mediated
How is it treated?	Most children require no treatment. Steroids are helpful in some cases, but relapses may occur.

HYPERTRICHOSIS

What is it?	Excessive hair growth in inappropriate areas; it may be localized, generalized, permanent, or transient; the pattern of hair growth is not in a sexual distribution
What is the etiology?	It may have racial and/or familial forms. It is also associated with a variety of conditions, including: Local trauma Malnutrition Anorexia nervosa

Chronic inflammatory dermatoses
Hamartomas or nevi
Endocrine disorders (e.g.,
   hypercortisolism)
Congenital and genetic disorders (e.g.,
   Cornelia de Lange syndrome)
A wide variety of drugs, including
   Dilantin, steroids, cyclosporin,
   minoxidil, and streptomycin

HIRSUTISM

What is it?

Excessive hair growth in appropriate areas (i.e., in a sexual pattern)

What are common causes?

1. Hyperprolactinemia
2. Gonadal tumors
3. Endocrine insensitivity
4. Adrenal conditions (e.g., enzyme deficiencies, neoplasms, Cushing syndrome)
5. Drugs (e.g., minoxidil, Dilantin, cyclosporin, steroids, oral contraceptives, Dyazide diuretics)
6. Congenital anomalies (e.g., trisomy 18, Cornelia de Lange syndrome, Hurler syndrome, juvenile hypothyroidism)

What is the treatment?

Treatment of the underlying cause

TINEA CAPITIS

What is it?

A superficial fungal infection, usually caused by *Trichophyton tonsurans* or *Microsporum canis*

How is tinea capitis diagnosed?

Broken-off hair shafts may give a "black-dot" appearance (*T. tonsurans*) or may show yellow-green fluorescence with a Wood's lamp. Both may show hyphae and spores under microscopic exam using KOH.

How is it treated?

Topical antifungal agents may be used, but systemic treatment with griseofulvin may be required.

27

Infectious Diseases

MENINGITIS

What is it?	Inflammation of the meninges
What are common clinical findings?	Fever, headache, stiff neck, mental status changes, CSF leukocytosis
What are the two classes of meningitis?	**Septic** (usually bacterial) **Aseptic** (usually viral)

BACTERIAL MENINGITIS

How does bacterial meningitis present?	Highly variable and age dependent
In neonates and infants?	Nonspecific signs of serious illness, including **tachypnea, lethargy, irritability, poor feeding, jaundice, hypoglycemia, and vomiting**; child may be febrile, afebrile, or hypothermic; later signs include **bulging fontanelle, seizures,** and **poor muscle tone**
In older children?	May have more classic meningeal signs, including **Kernig's** and/or **Brudzinski's signs, headache, photophobia, vomiting, mental status changes** (e.g., lethargy, disorientation); **petechiae/purpura** are signs of a poor prognosis
What are the most common causative organisms from birth to 1 month of age?	Group B streptococcus, *Escherichia coli, Listeria monocytogenes*
1–3 months of age?	*Haemophilus influenzae,* group B streptococcus, *Streptococcus pneumoniae*
3 months to 3 years of age?	*H. influenzae, S. pneumoniae, Neisseria meningitidis*

Older than 3 years of age?	*N. meningitidis, S. pneumoniae, H. influenzae* (less common by age 7–8 years of age) (**Note:** Immunization against *H. influenzae* has decreased meningitis due to this bacteria.)
How is diagnosis made?	**Lumbar puncture** is required for diagnosis.
For what should CSF be sent?	For culture, cell count, glucose, and total protein
What CSF findings suggest meningitis?	CSF leukocytosis (usually > 1000) with **predominance of PMNs, elevated protein,** and **relative hypoglycemia** (< 60%–70% of serum glucose) are suggestive. **Gram stain** may show bacteria; culture will reveal specific organisms.
What problems occur when interpreting CSF?	"Bloody" spinal taps are common in pediatrics. This may confound both protein and WBC levels. Previous treatment with antibiotics (e.g., amoxicillin for otitis) renders culture results inaccurate and may decrease WBC. Viral meningitis can have CSF profile similar to bacterial meningitis early in its course. Repeat lumbar puncture may be necessary.
What other findings are suggestive of meningitis?	**High peripheral WBC** with left shift (caution: WBC may be low) **Thrombocytopenia** with **decrease in hematocrit** is suggestive of DIC. **Blood cultures** may be positive in 80%–90% of cases.
What should precede lumbar puncture if high intracranial pressure (ICP) is suspected?	If elevated ICP is suspected (papilledema, focal neurologic signs), CT scan should precede lumbar puncture. **Do not delay treatment in a seriously ill patient.**
What is the treatment? **Birth to 4 weeks of age?**	Ampicillin and gentamicin are commonly used.

1–3 months of age?	Ampicillin and third-generation cephalosporin
3 months of age?	Third-generation cephalosporin (**Note:** Determination of antibiotic sensitivities is essential. Treatment before culture should cover likely organisms in the patient's age group and clinical setting.)
What is the duration of treatment?	It depends on the patient's age, the causative organism, and the patient's response to treatment. General guidelines: *H. influenzae* and *S. pneumoniae*: 10–14 days *N. meningitidis*: 14 days Group B streptococcus: 14–21 days *E. coli*: 21 days Repeat lumbar puncture to ensure sterilization of CSF is often recommended.
What are other components in the management of meningitis?	**Fluid restriction** to two-third maintenance (when intravascular volume is restored) may help prevent cerebral edema. Follow **head circumference** in infants. Close monitoring of glucose, acid–base and volume status, and tissue oxygenation are essential.
Are steroids indicated?	Steroids have been shown to have some benefit in decreasing hearing loss in *H. influenzae* meningitis. Use varies with institutions.
What are complications of meningitis?	SIADH, cerebral edema, toxic encephalopathy, brain-stem herniation, cranial nerve palsies, deafness, seizures, subdural effusion, cerebral infarct, cortical vein thrombosis, DIC, paresis, mental retardation, hydrocephalus, visual impairment, mental and motor delays
Who suffers most from complications?	Complications are most common in newborns with gram-negative infection and in patients with pneumococcal disease (up to 50%). Sensorineural

hearing loss is the most common complication (up to 20% in *H. influenzae* meningitis). Mortality is higher in *S. pneumoniae* and *N. meningitidis*.

VIRAL MENINGITIS

How does aseptic meningitis present?

It presents in a manner similar to septic meningitis–headache, vomiting, stiff neck, and/or photophobia. Other indicators of viral-type infection, such as **fever, malaise, myalgia, GI symptoms,** and/or **rash**, are present. The clinical course is usually more indolent; classic meningeal signs may be absent. Mental status is usually unaffected, unless associated encephalitis or increased ICP have developed. It is **prudent to treat as if bacterial until culture results are available.** Some viruses (e.g., herpesvirus, rabies, arbovirus) also cause encephalitis and its accompanying complications.

What does the lumbar puncture show?

CSF pleocytosis is the hallmark, but usually less than in bacterial meningitis (i.e., ≤ 500). Differential shows **CSF lymphocytosis** (may show higher percentage of neutrophils early in course). Glucose and protein levels are normal or elevated.
Other specific findings vary with etiology.

What are viral causes?

Enteroviruses (e.g., coxsackievirus, echovirus) are the most common, especially in summer and early fall. Others include **Epstein-Barr, mumps, influenza, herpesvirus,** and **adenoviruses.** Rarely, **rabies** and **arboviruses** are causes. **Poliovirus** is a possible cause in endemic areas or unimmunized populations.

How is it diagnosed?

Many viruses can be cultured from CSF. Enteroviruses can be cultured from stool. Influenza, mumps, and adenovirus may be cultured from the nasopharynx. Serum titers (acute and convalescent) may be helpful. Herpesvirus can be difficult to verify; CT, MRI, and EEG may be useful.

How is viral meningitis treated?

Treatment is primarily supportive. Dehydration and pain sometimes necessitate hospitalization. Acyclovir is used for herpes.

What is the clinical course?

Symptoms usually last 1–3 weeks. Headache may be severe.

What are nonviral causes of aseptic meningitis?

Mycobacteria: *Mycobacterium tuberculosis*

Fungal: *Cryptococcus neoformans* and *Coccidioides immitis* are most common (should be considered in immunocompromised patients)

Rickettsia: Rocky Mountain spotted fever (RMSF), Q fever, typhus, and *Ehrlichia* (should be considered when tick bite or farm animal exposure is in child's history)

Spirochetes: leptospirosis, Lyme disease, syphilis

Others (very uncommon): *Naegleria fowleri* and acanthamoeba (amebic meningitis); *Toxoplasma gondii*, cysticercosis, and trichinosis (all parasites)

CONJUNCTIVITIS

What is it?

Inflammation of the conjunctiva

How does infectious conjunctivitis present?

Erythema (injection) of sclera and/or inner surface of eyelids, often accompanied by increased tearing and/or discharge; eyelids may stick together; pain is uncommon, although patients may complain of roughness or itching

What causes conjunctivitis?

Infection (e.g., bacteria, viruses), allergy, and chemicals

Do viruses or bacteria more commonly cause conjunctivitis?

Bacteria

Which bacteria are the most common causative agents in young children?

H. influenzae and *S. pneumoniae* are most often isolated.
Moraxella catarrhalis, Staphylococcus aureus, and α-hemolytic streptococcus are possible pathogens, but are also found in uninfected eyes.

Which infectious agents in newborns need to be particularly ruled out?

Chlamydia trachomatis and Neisseria gonorrhea

Which is the most common virus isolated?

Adenovirus; herpesvirus and enteroviruses uncommonly cause conjunctivitis

What other condition is often associated with conjunctivitis?

Approximately 25%–33% of patients with conjunctivitis also have **otitis media;** 75% of these infections are bacterial.

How is it diagnosed?

Based on culture; in the newborn period, a rapid test is available for *N. gonorrhea* and *C. trachomatis*

How is it treated?

It will usually resolve without treatment in 7–10 days. Topical antibiotics include trimethoprim-sulfa-polymyxin B, erythromycin, bacitracin, gentamicin, and Sulamyd. *S. pneumoniae* and *H. influenzae* are often resistant to aminoglycosides.

When are systemic antibiotics indicated?

Systemic antibiotics are indicated when otitis media is simultaneously present and if the patient cannot tolerate topical therapy.

What is EKC?

Epidemic keratoconjunctivitis

What causes EKC?

Adenovirus type 8

What are the symptoms?

Very contagious—it is associated with a preauricular node, and presents with eye pain and photophobia

How does allergic conjunctivitis present?	Itching, redness, tearing, and photophobia; usually bilateral; seasonal exacerbations and recurrent disease are common
What is a characteristic physical finding?	Hallmark on physical exam is papillary hyperplasia with edema, leading to "cobblestoning" of conjunctiva.
What are associated features?	History and/or presence of other atopic disease; may have angioedema of eyelids
What is vernal conjunctivitis?	A **chronic** form of conjunctivitis characterized by severe itching, photophobia, blurry vision, and lacrimation
What are characteristic physical findings?	Exam reveals **large papillae** on the upper eyelids.

OTITIS MEDIA

What are the three types of otitis media?	1. Acute otitis media (AOM) 2. Otitis media with effusion (OME) 3. Chronic otitis media (COM)

AOM

What is it?	Infection of fluid in middle ear space
Why is otitis media more common in infants?	**Anatomy:** The eustachian tube is designed to drain fluid from the middle ear space to the nasopharynx, and to protect against reflux of nasopharyngeal pathogens. Infants have a relatively horizontal angle to the eustachian tube, which becomes more vertical and widens as they grow. **Infections:** Babies have frequent colds, which cause eustachian tube obstruction. Viruses also damage the ciliated epithelium of the tube. Both of these factors inhibit fluid drainage from the middle ear and allow colonization of pathogens that migrate up the tube from the nasopharynx.

What are the clinical signs of otitis media?

Prior or current URI, fever, fussiness, sleeplessness, "pulling at ears" or ear pain, decreased hearing, vomiting, poor appetite

What are the physical findings?

URI evidence on exam
Eardrum is swollen, opaque, and discolored (red, yellow, or gray)
Normal landmarks are obscured
Mobility is decreased or absent on pneumatic otoscopy
Fluid may or may not be visible through tympanic membrane (TM)

Which is the most diagnostic finding?

Lack of TM mobility on pneumatic otoscopy or by tympanogram

What are the most common bacterial pathogens?

S. pneumoniae is the most common (30%–40%) followed by *H. influenzae, M. catarrhalis,* and *Streptococcus pyogenes,* in that order. *S. aureus* is an uncommon cause. Gram-negative enterics cause up to 15% of cases in infants < 6 weeks of age.

Viral pathogens?

Believed to cause up to 30% of AOM cases, viral pathogens include respiratory syncytial virus (RSV), influenza, adenovirus, and coxsackievirus.

Why treat otitis media?

Treatment is thought to prevent conductive hearing loss as well as rare complications, such as mastoiditis, meningitis, and cholesteatoma.

What are the considerations in choosing antibiotics?

1. Many infections are minor or viral and will resolve without therapy. In some countries, AOM is only rarely treated with antibiotics.
2. Nearly 100% of *M. catarrhalis*, 20% of *H. influenzae*, and 25% of pneumococcus cases are β-lactamase producing and thus resistant to penicillins.
3. **Compliance:** It is not easy to give medicine to a baby. TID or more frequent dosing requires medication to be given at day care or school.

4. **Cost:** New cephalosporins are effective but expensive.
5. **Resistance:** Third-generation cephalosporins have an unnecessarily wide spectrum and could contribute to emerging drug resistance in the community.

What are the usual choices of antibiotics?

Many practitioners prescribe amoxicillin initially; other antibiotics include erythromycin-sulfisoxazole (Pediazole) and trimethoprim-sulfamethoxazole (Bactrim).

What are some reasons to change antibiotics?

Treatment failure—no improvement in 2–3 days on initial antibiotic with good compliance
Recurrence—another episode of AOM within 6 weeks
Side effects—diarrhea, GI upset, allergic reactions

What are some second-choice antibiotics?

Amoxicillin/clavulanic acid (Augmentin), cefuroxime, cefixime, and cefpodoxime

What are the pros and cons of these antibiotics?

Augmentin produces diarrhea, but is less expensive and is effective against β-lactamase-producing *H. influenzae*. With cephalosporin, there is less frequent dosing and it causes diarrhea less frequently, but these are more expensive and could contribute to the emergence of resistant bacteria.

What is recurrent otitis media?

Three or more episodes of AOM in 6 months, or 4 or more episodes in 12 months, with documented clinical resolution in between episodes

How can it be prevented?

Prophylactic antibiotic therapy with amoxicillin, sulfisoxazole, or trimethoprim-sulfamethoxazole can be effective in preventing otitis, and thus decrease need for tympanostomy tubes.

OME

What is it?	Fluid (effusion) in the middle ear space without infection; it occurs alone, secondary to URI, or as a sequela of AOM
What are the symptoms?	Often asymptomatic but can manifest as hearing loss, "plugged ears," vertigo, or clumsiness
What are the signs?	Fluid seen behind TM; decreased mobility on pneumatic otoscopy and tympanogram
What is the clinical course?	Spontaneous resolution in majority (> 50% by 3 months and 75% by 6 months); more rapid resolution following AOM (90% by 3 months)
What are the complications?	1. Hearing impairment may cause abnormal language development and contributes to behavioral problems. 2. School performance may be decreased. 3. Predisposes to AOM and subsequent COM.
What is the treatment? **Duration < 3 months?**	Observation only; obtain hearing assessment in > 3 months
Duration up to 6 months without hearing loss?	Antibiotics may cause more rapid resolution, but are not necessary because there is a high spontaneous resolution rate.
Duration of 3 months with bilateral hearing loss?	Antibiotics should be given with close follow up for resolution of effusion and restoration of hearing.
Duration > 3 months with bilateral hearing loss?	Myringotomy with tympanostomy tube placement is indicated.

Are steroids beneficial?	The benefits of steroid use in OME have not yet been conclusively shown, and they may have adverse effects. They are not currently recommended.
Do decongestants help?	Decongestants and antihistamines are not usually effective.
Is tonsillectomy or adenoidectomy helpful?	No

COM

What is it?	Inflammation of the middle ear and/or mastoid with otorrhea through the TM for > 3 months
What are the complications?	Mastoiditis, labyrinthitis, cholesteatoma
What is a tympanocentesis?	Also called **myringotomy with aspiration**, it involves puncturing through the TM to collect and drain fluid from the middle ear space.
What are the indications?	It is indicated for critically ill or immunocompromised patients, neonates, and for patients in which AOM is unresponsive to two or more full courses of antibiotics (assuming good compliance).
What are tympanostomy tubes?	Also called **PE tubes**, these small plastic or metal tubes are surgically placed in TM to drain and ventilate middle ear space.
What are the indications?	1. Recurrent AOM unresponsive to prophylactic antibiotics 2. OME with bilateral hearing impairment 3. Severe retraction or atelectasis of TM 4. Chronic suppurative complications
What are the complications?	Tympanosclerosis or atrophy, dislocation into middle ear, cholesteatoma, extrusion, prolonged otorrhea, and general anesthesia

What are risk factors for otitis media?	Passive smoke, day care attendance, horizontal bottle feeding, anatomic defects of oral pharynx; first episode of otitis at less than 2 months of age

THRUSH

What is it?	Overgrowth of *Candida albicans* in oral cavity
Who gets it?	Infants, children on antibiotics, immunosuppressed children, and those with chronic systemic disorders
What are the clinical features?	Soft, creamy white plaques on buccal mucosa, tongue, palate, and lip commissures; these lesions do not scrape off easily and leave an ulcerated red base when removed
What is the treatment?	For infants, nystatin suspension is a good first choice. If it fails, gentian violet may be effective. For older children not at risk for aspiration, Mycelex Troches are effective.
What are prevention and control measures?	For formula-fed infants, sterilize nipples and pacifiers by boiling them for 5 minutes or placing them in a sterilizer; this prevents reinfection. In breast fed infants, mother's nipples can be a source of infection. Ask mom about sore, red, cracked nipples; she may need treatment as well.

PHARYNGITIS/STREPTOCOCCAL PHARYNGITIS

What is pharyngitis?	Sore throat
What is the most common cause?	90% are viral
What is streptococcal pharyngitis?	Pharyngitis caused by group A β-hemolytic streptococci
What are complications of streptococcal pharyngitis?	Acute rheumatic fever; also local complications (e.g., peritonsillar abscess)

How is the diagnosis made?	Throat culture is the standard, although the rapid antigen tests are also useful.
Can streptococcal pharyngitis be diagnosed purely on clinical grounds?	Not with consistency; the clinical features overlap with the more common viral causes
How is streptococcal pharyngitis treated?	The treatment of choice is penicillin, in a form and dosage of adequate coverage for 10 days; it may be an oral penicillin or a long-acting injectable penicillin. Patients allergic to penicillin can be treated with erythromycin.

GINGIVOSTOMATITIS

What is it?	Inflammation of the gingiva and oral mucosa
What is the usual cause?	It is usually caused by primary infection with herpes simplex virus (HSV) type 1. HSV type 2 can also cause infections.
At what age is it commonly seen?	6 months–3 years of age
What are the symptoms?	There is a prodrome of headache, fever, malaise, and local lymphadenopathy followed by erythema, swelling, and pain of gingiva and palatal mucosa. Grouped vesicles and ulcerations occur on oral mucosa. Bleeding and crusting may occur. It most frequently involves anterior gingiva and palate. Dehydration can follow when pain prevents adequate fluid intake.
How is the diagnosis made?	It is usually made clinically. A Tzanck prep of the base of oral lesions will show multinucleated giant cells and intranuclear inclusions. Culture fluid from vesicles to confirm HSV. Assess hydration status.

How can HSV gingivostomatitis be differentiated from hand-foot-mouth disease or aphthous stomatitis?	1. Hand-foot-mouth disease (coxsackievirus) lesions typically involve the posterior palate and pharynx. 2. Aphthous stomatitis lesions are found on buccal, lingual, and inner lip mucosa.
What is the clinical course?	Lesions heal spontaneously in 1–2 weeks without scarring.
What are common complications?	Complications include pain, secondary infection, and dehydration.
Can it recur?	Reactivation of HSV, leading to recurrent infections, is common. These tend to be less severe with fewer and more localized lesions.
What three treatments are helpful?	1. Pain control: Systemic therapy with acetaminophen and/or ibuprofen is usually sufficient, but occasionally codeine is required. Some physicians give Benadryl-Maalox suspension (1:1 mix) for local pain relief; viscous lidocaine can be added for children > 6 years of age. 2. Oral hygiene: Rinsing with chlorhexidine or glycerine-peroxide mix (younger children) should replace brushing, which may be too painful. 3. Hydration: Cold liquids are best tolerated. Gelatin, popsicles, and ice cream are useful. Citrus and carbonated beverages are painful to drink. Occasionally, IV fluids are needed.
When is antiviral therapy indicated?	Systemic therapy with acyclovir is indicated only in immunocompromised patients.

LYMPHADENITIS

What is lymphadenitis (also called adenitis)?	Swelling and inflammation of lymph nodes.

| What are the most common causes of lymphadenitis in children? | 1. Reaction of a lymph node to other local infection
2. Involvement of staphylococcal infection
3. Atypical mycobacterium
4. Cat-scratch disease
5. Mononucleosis
6. Lymphoma
7. Toxoplasmosis
8. Brucellosis
9. Tularemia
Management of lymphadenitis will involve management of the primary disease process. |

MASTITIS

What is it?	It is an infection of the breast tissue. It may manifest as simply a cellulitis or may reflect development of an abscess.
What is the most common scenario for development of mastitis?	Lactation and breast feeding
What are other possible causes in nonlactating women?	Human bites or diabetes mellitus
What is the most common causative bacteria?	*S. aureus*
What is the treatment?	Warm compresses with an antibiotic that includes coverage of *S. aureus* is usually sufficient. Rarely, if an abscess is present, incision and drainage are needed. If a woman is breast feeding, continuation of breast feeding can also help alleviate symptoms by keeping the breast from overengorging.

GASTROENTERITIS

| What are the signs and symptoms of acute gastroenteritis? | Variable, but may include:
Nausea
Vomiting
Diarrhea
Abdominal pain
Flatulence |

What is the cause of most cases of acute gastroenteritis?	Most cases of acute gastroenteritis in the United States are **viral** in origin.

VIRAL GASTROENTERITIS

Which viruses are most common in children?	Rotavirus, adenovirus, "Norwalk" agent
How are the viruses spread?	Usually via the fecal-oral route, but they may also be spread by respiratory route; good hygiene and hand washing help reduce the risk of infection
How is viral gastroenteritis diagnosed?	1. Detection of viral antigens in stool 2. Viral culture (may not be available in some hospitals) 3. Exclusion of bacterial causes by culture
How is viral gastroenteritis treated?	Usually supportive; prevent dehydration by IV or oral fluid and electrolyte management, depending on severity of condition
Do most children with acute viral gastroenteritis need IV fluids?	No
Can viral gastroenteritis be easily distinguished from bacterial gastroenteritis?	Although there is overlap in symptoms, bacterial causes are more likely associated with bloody diarrhea, stool leukocytes, and tenesmus. Children with viral gastroenteritis may have non-GI symptoms such as cough, nasal discharge, and myalgia.

BACTERIAL GASTROENTERITIS

Name some bacteria that cause acute gastroenteritis.	*Salmonella* *Shigella* *Campylobacter jejuni* *E. coli* *Yersinia enterocolitica* *Clostridium difficile* Food poisoning: *Clostridium perfringens* and *S. aureus* (toxin)

How is acute bacterial gastroenteritis diagnosed?

1. Stool culture (*Salmonella, Shigella, Campylobacter, E. coli, Yersinia, C. difficile, C. perfringens*)
2. Serologic testing (*Yersinia*)
3. Toxin assay (*C. difficile*)
4. Toxin assay in food (*S. aureus*)

How is it treated?

Supportive treatment (IV or orally) for fluid and electrolyte loss. Antibiotic therapy may not be indicated for all patients, because illnesses may be self-limited. Extraintestinal infections (including sepsis) are indications for antibiotic treatment; infants may be given antibiotics more readily than older children.

What are common antibiotics for treatment of uncomplicated bacterial gastrointestinal infections?

For *Salmonella*?

Ampicillin; amoxicillin; ampicillin plus trimethoprim-sulfamethoxazole

For *Shigella*?

Trimethoprim-sulfamethoxazole

For *Campylobacter*?

Erythromycin

For *E. coli*?

Trimethoprim-sulfamethoxazole; ampicillin; gentamicin

For *C. difficile*?

Vancomycin; metronidazole

Why not treat *Salmonella* infection?

Treatment may prolong the "carrier state" and may not significantly alter the clinical course.

When should *Salmonella* infection be treated?

When patient is a young infant (< 3 years of age) or when patient has an immune deficiency, a systemic disease (e.g., sepsis, osteomyelitis), or typhoid fever

What oral rehydration regimen is recommended for gastroenteritis?

The **WHO** oral rehydration solution, which includes:
Glucose: 90 mmol/L
Sodium: 80 mmol/L
Potassium: 20 mmol/L
Chloride: 80 mmol/L
Base (citrate): 30 mmol/L
Final total osmolality = 300 mosm/L

What commercially available oral fluids are useful?	Several, including Pedialyte, Ricelyte, and Infalyte
What are indications for IV fluid?	Inability to drink liquids, severe vomiting, shock or impending shock, coma
Which IV fluid should be used?	It depends on the situation. Ringer's lactate or normal saline for volume expansion is used in severely dehydrated patients, followed by calculated replacement and maintenance fluids, depending on the severity of the dehydration.
Should you feed a child with acute gastroenteritis?	In general, yes, but judiciously. In most children, it may promote healing and help prevent malnutrition.

URINARY TRACT INFECTION (UTI)

What does the term UTI refer to?	Usually infection of the urethra and bladder; the term grossly encompasses ascending infections up to the kidney as well
Who are the patients most at risk?	In the infant stage, infections generally affect males and females equally. However, uncircumcised male infants may have a slightly higher risk. In older children, females are affected more frequently than males.
What are the most common etiologic agents?	*E. coli* accounts for 70%–90% of infections. This is followed by *Klebsiella* and *Proteus* infections. However, staphylococcal and viral species are also found in UTIs.
What is the pathophysiology in infants and children?	Infection usually results from either bacteremia or migration from the urethra. In older children, UTIs more commonly occur because of ascending bacteria from the lower urinary tract.

What is acute bacterial cystitis?

It is infection of the bladder itself. It is characterized by hyperactivity of the detrusor muscle and a decreased functional capacity of the bladder.

What are symptoms of a UTI?

In infants?

Symptoms may include fever, weight loss, failure to thrive, nausea, vomiting, diarrhea, and jaundice.

In older children?

The older child may experience fever, urinary frequency, pain during urination, incontinence, bed wetting, and abdominal pain. The child may also have foul-smelling urine, and hematuria may be present.

How is urine obtained for analysis and culture?

In infants and small children?

A sterile collection bag may be used, but specificity of cultures from this method is not as good. Occasionally, a catheterized specimen or a specimen from a suprapubic puncture may be needed.

In older children?

A good midstream urine specimen for culture can usually be obtained.

What findings suggest infection?

Pyuria suggests infection; however, infection can occur in the absence of pyuria. Conversely, pyuria can be present without infection. Microscopic hematuria may be present. An alkaline pH may suggest *Proteus* infection. A culture of the specimen should be sent. Usually a result of 100,000 colony-forming units per ml are diagnostic of infection. Occasionally, infection may be present with a slightly lower colony-forming unit count.

How are UTIs treated?

Generally trimethoprim-sulfametho-xazole, nitrofurantoin, and amoxicillin are the antibiotic agents of choice. If symptoms are not severe, it is preferable to wait for culture results before starting antibiotics. However, if symptoms are bothersome, antibiotic therapy should be started after the cultures are sent.

If UTI is diagnosed, what further workup is required?

Children with UTIs should have a follow-up voiding cystourethrogram to assess for any reflux. The presence of reflux may predispose to ascending infection and pyelonephritis. A follow-up urine culture should be obtained after treatment to confirm that the UTI is cleared. Further follow-up cultures should be done at 3-month intervals for 1–2 years after the infection. If vesicourethral reflux is present, prophylaxis may be needed for as long as the reflux persists.

PYELONEPHRITIS

What is it?

It is an infection of the renal parenchyma that is usually caused by ascending infection from the lower urinary tract.

What conditions predispose a child to pyelonephritis?

Recurrent UTI and vesicourethral reflux (VUR)

What are the clinical manifestations?
In infants?

Infants may show signs typical of systemic infection, including fever, weight loss, failure to thrive, and irritability.

In older children?

In older children, fever, chills, and flank or abdominal pain are typical symptoms.

What are important laboratory values?

A WBC, ESR, and C-reactive protein should be evaluated; however, these may not differentiate from lower UTIs. As with UTIs, urinary specimens should also be sent for culture. A urinalysis may reveal **white blood cell casts,** heightening the suspicion for pyelonephritis.

What are appropriate imaging studies?	If pyelonephritis is suspected, renal ultrasound may show hydronephrosis, a perirenal abscess, or pyonephrosis. The latter condition may require prompt drainage. In addition, renal scanning may confirm the presence of acute pyelonephritis by revealing filling defects in the renal parenchyma.
What is the treatment?	Intravenous antibiotics to cover the suspected or cultured organisms
What are complications of pyelonephritis?	These may include arterial hypertension and renal insufficiency secondary to chronic renal damage. However, the overall prognosis for appropriately treated pyelonephritis is quite good.
How are renal or perirenal abscesses or infections associated with obstructed urinary tract treated?	Antibiotic therapy with surgical drainage of the infected and obstructed areas

DACTYLITIS

What is it?	This is an infection of the volar fat pad of the distal portion of the finger or thumb. It is usually blistering in nature.
What is the etiology?	Usually this condition occurs spontaneously. In rare cases, dactylitis may be the first manifestation of **sickle cell disease** in an infant.
What are the most common bacteria?	Group A β-hemolytic streptococcus Group B β-hemolytic streptococcus S. aureus
What is the treatment?	Incision and drainage of the blistering lesion as well as penicillin or erythromycin therapy

SEXUALLY TRANSMITTED DISEASES (STDs)

Which age group has the highest rate of STDs?	Adolescents

What are some common STDs?	1. Gonorrhea 2. Syphilis 3. Chlamydia 4. Chancroid 5. Herpes 6. Human papilloma virus (HPV) 7. Trichomonas 8. Gardnerella (*Haemophilus vaginalis*)
If organisms that are usually sexually transmitted are found in younger children, what should be suspected?	Child sexual abuse

GONORRHEA

What is the offending organism in gonorrhea?	*N. gonorrhea*
What are typical symptoms? **In men?**	A purulent discharge that causes burning on urination (dysuria)
In women?	There may be a purulent vaginal discharge with vulvar vaginitis. Dysuria may occur.
What is the most common complication?	Pelvic inflammatory disease (PID)
How is the diagnosis made?	By bacterial culture
What is the treatment?	Ceftriaxone
What is the duration of treatment?	Duration of treatment may depend on whether the disease is local or whether complications, such as PID or disseminated disease, have occurred.

SYPHILIS

What is the offending agent in syphilis?	*Treponema pallidum*

What are the symptoms of syphilis?

Primary syphilis?

A painless chancre appears at the site of inoculation approximately 2–6 weeks after infection. There may be associated adenitis. The chancre heals spontaneously within 4 to 6 weeks.

Secondary syphilis?

Two to ten weeks after the chancre heals, a nonpruritic maculopapular rash occurs. Pustules may develop. Condylomata may occur around the anus and vagina. There may be an associated flu like illness with lymphadenopathy. Thirty percent of people infected with secondary syphilis develop meningitis. After 1–2 months, the infection becomes latent but may recur up to the first year.

Tertiary syphilis?

This late-stage manifests with neurologic, cardiovascular, and granulomatous lesions. The VDRL and RPR detect antibodies against a cardiolipin-cholesterol-lecithin complex. This test is not specific for syphilis. The FTA-ABS and MHA-TP tests, which are more specific diagnostic tests, detect antibodies to *T. pallidum*.

How is syphilis treated?

A single dose of penicillin is adequate for primary, secondary, and latent secondary disease. Treatment must be adjusted for tertiary disease, neurosyphilis, and congenital syphilis.

What is the transmission rate of syphilis from an infected mother to an infant?

Virtually 100%

What is the fetal or perinatal death rate of infected infants?

40%

When should infants be treated for syphilis?

When there is evidence of the infection in the mother or if adequacy of treatment in the mother is in question

CHLAMYDIA

Which of the chlamydia species is most commonly involved in sexually transmitted infection?	*C. trachomatis*
What is another common term for chlamydia infection?	Nongonococcal urethritis (NGU)
What are clinical manifestations?	These can be very similar to gonorrhea and include burning during urination as well as a urethral discharge. Perihepatitis, conjunctivitis, sterility, and PID are symptoms of chlamydia that has spread beyond its local site.
How is the diagnosis made?	Isolation of the organism in tissue culture from the urethra in men and from the endocervix in women; chlamydia may also be detected by fluorescent antibody tests, ELISA, DNA probe, and PCR assay.
What is the treatment?	Doxycycline, cefoxitin, erythromycin, and azithromycin may be adequate medications. In pregnant women, erythromycin or amoxicillin is recommended.
What symptoms may occur in infants of infected mothers?	Conjunctivitis, pneumonia, and infection of the rectum and vagina

CHANCROID

What is chancroid?	This is a lesion characterized by a painful, purulent, sharply delineated ulcer. There is no induration and this helps to distinguish it from a syphilis chancre. Lymphadenopathy may be associated with this condition.
What is the treatment?	Ceftriaxone

GENITAL HERPES

What is the offending agent in genital herpes?	HSV type 2; however, 10%–25% of cases may be caused by HSV type 1
What are clinical manifestations?	
In women?	The vulva and vagina may be involved with vesicles and ulcers. However, the cervix is the primary site of infection. The disease is often subclinical; however, virus may still be shed thus infecting a partner.
In men?	Vesicles or ulcers occur on the penis. The scrotum is less frequently involved. Characteristically, there may be associated pain along affected nerve roots in the perineal region in both genders.
What is the treatment?	There is no cure. Symptomatic and shedding phases may be shortened by the use of acyclovir.
For what other disease are women with HSV at risk?	**Cancer of the cervix;** these women should obtain yearly Pap smears

HUMAN PAPILLOMA VIRUS (HPV)

What is it?	This term encompasses at least 75 different types of virus that contain DNA.
What are the manifestations of sexually transmitted HPV?	Genital warts (also called condylomata acuminata)
How is the diagnosis made?	Usually by physical examination; however, application of 3% acetic acid to a lesion may show a characteristic whitening
What is the treatment?	Topical treatments include trichloroacetic acid, liquid nitrogen, and podophyllin. Other treatments include bleomycin, interferon, and topical 5-fluorouracil. Laser therapy is often required for those lesions that do not respond to medical therapy.

What are two complications of infection with HPV?	1. Cervical dysplasia and cervical cancer 2. Development of respiratory papillomas, which may become malignant

TRICHOMONAS INFECTION

What is the offending agent in *Trichomonas* infections?	*Trichomonas vaginalis*
What are the clinical manifestations of *Trichomonas* infection? **In women?**	There is a frothy, malodorous vaginal discharge, which may be accompanied by vulvar or vaginal irritation, dysuria, and dyspareunia.
In men?	Men are usually asymptomatic, but approximately 10% may experience NGU.
How is the diagnosis made?	**Wet mount** examination of vaginal or urethral secretions will show the trichomonas. This test is successful in about 70% of cases. Cultures may be needed to obtain a definitive diagnosis.
What is the treatment?	**Metronidazole**—however, **it should not be used in pregnant women.** Clotrimazole should be used in the first trimester of pregnancy if infection is suspected.

GARDNERELLA

What are the manifestations of *Gardnerella* infection?	It is usually associated with a foul-smelling vaginal discharge.
How is it diagnosed?	**10% potassium hydroxide** is added to a wet preparation. This results in the emission of a fishy odor. Clue cells, which are epithelial cells ringed with the rod-shaped organism, are also evident on the wet prep.

What is the treatment?	Metronidazole

PID

What is it?	It is a condition that may be caused by a variety of sexually transmitted organisms that have ascended through the vaginal tract into the cervix and uterus. Subsequent migration may occur toward the tubes.
What are the clinical manifestations?	Lower abdominal pain, which can be severe; there may be associated fever
What are physical findings?	Extreme tenderness on motion of the uterus and adnexa (**chandelier sign**). There may also be a purulent discharge from the cervical region.
How is the diagnosis made?	Usually a combination of history, physical exam, and culture of secretions will lead to the diagnosis. However, treatment is usually initiated on the basis of history and physical exam before an absolute organism is identified.
What is the differential diagnosis?	Appendicitis, ovarian cyst, ovarian tumor, ectopic pregnancy, UTI, inflammatory bowel disease
How is PID treated?	Intravenous antibiotics are usually necessary. The antibiotic chosen should include coverage for gonorrhea and *Chlamydia* species.
What are complications of PID?	1. Sterility 2. Increased risk of ectopic pregnancy 3. Chronic pain 4. Dyspareunia 5. Increased risk of recurring PID

COMMON VIRAL SYNDROMES

MEASLES

What is another name for measles?	Rubeola

What are the signs and symptoms of measles?	Fever, cough, coryza, conjunctivitis, maculopapular rash, Koplik spots (enanthem)
How is measles spread?	Usually by direct contact with infectious secretions, but sometimes via airborne route
What is the incubation period?	8–12 days from exposure to onset of symptoms, and 14 days from exposure to appearance of rash
What are complications of measles?	Pneumonia, croup, diarrhea, encephalitis, SSPE
What is SSPE?	Subacute sclerosing panencephalitis
When can SSPE occur?	Long after the illness; average incubation period is 10.8 years
What is the treatment for measles?	Supportive; vitamin A is useful in some studies
Is isolation of the patient necessary?	Respiratory isolation for 4 days after onset of rash; longer for immunocompromised patients

MUMPS

What is it?	It is a systemic viral disease, most notable for swelling of the salivary glands. The mumps virus is a member of the paramyxovirus group, which include measles, parainfluenza, and Newcastle disease virus.
How is mumps spread?	Direct contact via respiratory exposure
What is the incubation period?	12–25 days, although it is usually 16–18 days
What are complications?	**Orchitis**, arthritis, pancreatitis, hearing loss, mastitis, renal involvement
Is isolation of the patient necessary?	Respiratory isolation for 9 days after onset of parotid swelling

What is the treatment?	Supportive

RUBELLA

What is another name for rubella?	German measles
What are the clinical features?	Generalized lymphadenopathy (usually suboccipital, postauricular, cervical nodes), maculopapular erythematous rash
How is rubella spread?	Direct or droplet contact from nasopharyngeal secretions
What is the incubation period?	14–21 days, but it is usually 16–18
Is isolation of patient necessary?	Contact isolation for 7 days after the onset of rash (postnatal infections)
What is the treatment?	Supportive
What are the complications?	Polyarthralgia/arthritis, thrombocytopenia, encephalitis; **major concern is congenital rubella**
What is congenital rubella?	Rubella infection in a fetus, acquired as a consequence of maternal infection during pregnancy
What are complications of congenital rubella?	**Ophthalmologic:** cataracts, microphthalmia, glaucoma, chorioretinitis **Cardiac:** PDA, peripheral pulmonic stenosis, ASD, VSD Sensorineural deafness Microcephaly Mental retardation Growth retardation Thrombocytopenia Ecchymoses/purpura ("blueberry muffin" baby)
Is isolation of a child with congenital rubella necessary?	Contact isolation until 1 year of age or until nasopharyngeal and urine viral cultures are consistently negative for rubella

FIFTH DISEASE

What is another name for fifth disease?	Erythema infectiosum
What is its cause?	Parvovirus B19
What are the clinical features?	Fever, systemic illness (usually mild), and a "slapped cheek" rash on the face
What are the complications?	Arthralgia, arthritis, bone marrow suppression; **may cause hydrops fetalis to the fetus of a woman infected in the first half of pregnancy**
How is it spread?	Respiratory secretions and blood
What is the incubation period?	4–20 days
What is the treatment?	Supportive; immunoglobulin may be helpful in chronic infections in compromised patients

ROSEOLA

What is it?	A systemic viral infection, characterized primarily by high fever for 3–7 days, followed by a maculopapular rash; may have respiratory or GI signs
What are the complications?	Child may have febrile seizures; encephalitis is rare.
What causes roseola?	Human herpesvirus type 6
Other names for roseola?	Exanthem subitum; sixth disease
How is it spread?	Respiratory secretions
What is the incubation period?	Thought to be 9 days
Is isolation of an infected child necessary?	No
What is the treatment?	Supportive

VARICELLA

What is another name for varicella?	Chicken pox
What are the clinical features?	Systemic febrile illness with fever, generalized vesicular rash
What is the cause?	Varicella-zoster virus
What are the complications?	Bacterial infection of skin lesions, thrombocytopenia, arthritis, pneumonia
How is varicella virus spread?	Direct contact, airborne spread, contact with zoster lesions
What is the incubation period?	10–21 days, but it is usually 14–16 days
When is a child infectious?	1–4 days before lesions erupt, and 7–10 days afterward
What is the treatment?	Supportive and symptomatic; **salicylates should be avoided;** antiviral agents (acyclovir) can modify course of disease if administered early
How can chicken pox be prevented?	VZIG (given after exposure) can modify the course or prevent disease; it is used mainly in immunocompromised patients; a varicella vaccine has been developed and approved
What is zoster?	A painful vesicular eruption in a dermatomal distribution
What causes zoster?	Latent varicella virus (after primary systemic infection)

HIV AND AIDS IN PEDIATRICS

What is the most common mode of transmission of HIV in pediatric patients?	Most pediatric HIV is acquired prenatally or perinatally from HIV-positive mothers

What are other modes of transmission?

Contaminated blood products
Sexual transmission, including sexual abuse
Shared needles
Accidental exposure
Breast-feeding from infected mother

Has screening of blood products affected the risk of HIV from this source?

Yes—the risk of HIV from blood products has been significantly reduced but has not been eliminated

What is the risk of perinatal transmission of HIV?

About 20%–30% of infants born to untreated infected women will be infected.

How is congenital HIV infection diagnosed?

Antibody screen in child
Viral culture
PCR for viral DNA

Does a positive antibody screen in a child indicate congenital infection?

No. Transplacentally acquired antibody from an antibody-positive mother can persist for months (perhaps up to 18 months) in the child. More direct identification of the virus is indicated.

What can be done to reduce the risk of perinatal HIV?

Treatment of an infected mother during pregnancy can reduce the risk of infection in her child.

Are newborns infected with HIV clinically ill?

Not necessarily; most may be well at birth

What are early clinical features of HIV infection?

May be nonspecific:
Fever
Lymphadenopathy
Hepatosplenomegaly
Poor weight gain or poor linear growth
Diarrhea
Parotid gland swelling or inflammation
Candidiasis
Persistent or recurrent pneumonia

What is the clinical course of perinatally acquired HIV?

Variable—20%–30% will develop early immune compromise and AIDS

What is the survival in pediatric HIV infection?

Median survival is about **8 years.**

Is the CD4 count useful in monitoring pediatric HIV infection?

Yes, but values must be interpreted in the context of age-adjusted normal values.

How is pediatric HIV infection treated?

Careful surveillance of immune status
Nutritional support
Intravenous immunoglobulin therapy
Antiretroviral therapy
Prophylaxis for common complicating infections

What are complications of pediatric HIV infection?

Pneumocystis carinii pneumonia
Recurrent bacterial disease
Lymphoid interstitial pneumonitis
Encephalopathy
Mycobacterium avium infections
Nephropathy
Cardiomyopathy
Wasting syndrome

What is LIP?

Lymphoid interstitial pneumonitis

What is the cause of LIP?

Not established; it may be viral, perhaps the Epstein-Barr virus

What are the symptoms of LIP?

Cough, usually dry, and respiratory distress; it is a chronic course with exacerbations

How is LIP diagnosed?

Definitive diagnosis is by lung biopsy. It is suspected in patients with suggestive clinical course unresponsive to antibiotics.

What are radiographic findings?

Chest radiograph may show interstitial nodular/reticular infiltrates.

What is the treatment for LIP?

Supportive—steroids and bronchodilators have been used with some improvement in some patients

What is PCP?

P. carinii pneumonia

What is the significance of PCP?

PCP is the most common opportunistic infection in pediatric HIV patients.

What are the symptoms of PCP?	Tachypnea and fever; may have relatively few auscultatory chest findings
How is PCP diagnosed?	PCP may be suspected on clinical grounds. Chest radiograph may show perihilar or interstitial infiltrates. Definitive diagnosis usually requires demonstration of the organism by bronchoscopy, biopsy, and lavage.
What is the prophylaxis for PCP?	**Trimethoprim/sulfamethoxazole** can be used prophylactically.
How is PCP treated?	**Trimethoprim/sulfamethoxazole** or **pentamidine**

TUBERCULOSIS

What are three infecting agents for tuberculosis?	1. *Mycobacterium tuberculosis* 2. *Mycobacterium bovis* 3. *Mycobacterium africanum*
Which infecting agent is the most prevalent?	*M. tuberculosis*
What percent of the world's population is infected with *M. tuberculosis?*	33%
How many people in the United States are infected with *M. tuberculosis?*	10–20,000,000
Which age group has the lowest rate of tuberculosis?	5–14 years of age
How is tuberculosis transmitted?	Transmission is by mucous droplets that become airborne, and is therefore person-to-person.
Is it common for young children to infect others?	No, because often children do not have cough symptoms with tuberculosis and if they do, the cough is not forceful enough to suspend infectious particles.

What is the primary portal of entry of tuberculosis?

The lung

What percent of patients who are infected with tuberculosis develop clinical disease?

Approximately 5%–10%; however, 40% of infected infants develop disease

Which children are at highest risk for developing tuberculosis?

1. Children born in countries with high instances of the disease
2. Poor and indigent children
3. Homeless children
4. Abusers of injected drugs
5. Children exposed to high-risk adults

Which conditions predispose children to become symptomatic with tuberculosis once they are infected?

1. Infection with HIV
2. Immunocompromising diseases, especially malignancy
3. Immunosuppressive drug treatments
4. Infants and children 3 years of age or less

What is the "primary complex" of tuberculosis?

Local infection at the portal of entry, usually the lung, and subsequent infection of regional lymph nodes in that area

What is the Mantoux tuberculin skin test?

This is an intradermal injection containing purified protein derivative. Usually 0.1 ml of 5 tuberculin units is used for initial testing.

What comprises a positive test?

1. In children with high risk of infection, a reactive area ≥ 5 mm
2. For other high-risk adults and children less than 3 years of age, a reactive area ≥ 10 mm is positive
3. For low-risk persons, a reactive area ≥ 15 mm is positive

What factors can cause a false-negative result on the tuberculin test?

1. Young age
2. Malnutrition
3. Immunosuppression
4. Viral diseases (measles, mumps, varicella, influenza)
5. BCG vaccine
6. Overwhelming tuberculosis

What are the clinical manifestations of tuberculosis?

Initially, there is a lung parenchymal focus with involvement of regional lymph nodes. This may result in bronchial obstruction in small children and infants. The clinical manifestations are fairly mild, however. Infants are the most prone to showing signs and symptoms and these are usually nonproductive cough and mild dyspnea. Other generalized systemic symptoms such as fever, night sweats, anorexia, or decreased activity may occur.

What are radiographic findings in children with pulmonary tuberculosis?

Often there will be collapse or consolidation of a lung segment due to bronchial obstruction. There may also be signs of bacterial pneumonia.

What are other possible manifestations of pulmonary disease?

1. Pleural effusion
2. Extension to the pericardium causing pericarditis
3. Upper respiratory tract disease

What other organs may tuberculosis affect?

Essentially any

What are characteristics of CNS involvement?

Meningitis with subsequent **caseous lesion** development. These lesions tend to affect the brain stem most commonly. Early symptomatology may be consistent with typical meningitis but may progress to coma, decerebrate posturing, and eventually death.

What is typical of bone involvement?

Bone involvement is usually centered in the **lower vertebrae.** The resulting spondylitis is called **Pott disease,** which results in kyphosis. Other skeletal structures are rarely affected.

What are manifestations of abdominal disease?

Abdominal lymph nodes may become infected, causing localized peritonitis or even generalized peritonitis if caseous lymph nodes rupture. In the intestine, ulcers may form, which result in pain, diarrhea, or constipation.

What are characteristics of genitourinary disease?

Early symptoms may be virtually silent. However, late symptoms may include dysuria, flank or abdominal pain, and gross hematuria. Subsequent superinfection may occur. Ultimately, hydronephrosis and urethral strictures may develop. In males, epididymitis or orchitis may occur as well.

What are symptoms of perinatal disease?

These usually occur after 2 or 3 weeks of life and include respiratory distress, fever, enlargement of the spleen or liver, poor feeding, lethargy or irritability, lymphadenopathy, abdominal distention, failure to thrive, ear drainage, and skin lesions. Chest radiograph may reveal a miliary pattern. Overall, the symptoms may mimic those seen in the TORCH virus.

How is tuberculosis diagnosed?

By isolation of the bacteria; it is typically seen as an **acid-fast bacteria** on staining with arylmethane; however, it may take 1–6 weeks to confirm growth in culture.

How is tuberculosis treated?

Once tuberculosis is recognized, the most common treatment is **isoniazid (INH)** and **rifampin.** Double drug coverage is necessary because there is always a small portion of bacteria that is resistant to a single drug.

What are the side effects of isoniazid?

Peripheral neuritis and **hepatotoxicity**

What is the side effect of rifampin?

Hepatotoxicity

What is the typical treatment strategy for tuberculosis?

Usually a 9-month course of isoniazid and rifampin will cure 98% of tuberculosis cases. The medications are given daily for the first two months and then twice weekly for the duration of the treatment. If pyrazinamide (PZA) is added, the overall duration of treatment may be shortened to 6 months. However, overall treatment must be tailored to the degree of disease (e.g., a longer course is needed for meningitis). Treatment must also be adjusted if there are possible risks for drug resistance for those medicines chosen.

When should children who do not exhibit tuberculous disease be treated?

Those children with a positive PPD test should be treated with INH for 9 months. INH therapy should also be used for children less than 6 years of age who have been exposed to infected adults and to infants born to mothers who have tuberculosis. If exposed children are negative 3 months after treatment, treatment may be discontinued.

What is the BCG vaccination?

It is a vaccine for bacille Calmette-Guérin

What is its use?

It is probably best used in infants and children to reduce the risk of life-threatening forms of tuberculosis. This is especially true for infants who are at high risk of exposure due to the people they are around or the region in which they live.

Has this vaccine resulted in overall decrease of tuberculosis?

No

PERTUSSIS

What is another name for pertussis?

Whooping cough

What causes pertussis?

Bordetella pertussis

How is it transmitted?

Airborn via respiratory secretions

What is the incubation period?

7–14 days

What are the three stages?

1. Catarrhal
2. Paroxysmal
3. Convalescent

What are characteristics of the cough?

The cough is most obvious in the catarrhal phase. A quick "staccato" cough, such that the patient may not be able to catch his/her breath until the end; the deep breath is the "whoop."

What are complications of pertussis?

Numerous complications are related to infection and to the consequences of violent coughing and pressure. Pneumonia as well as CNS and GI complications are seen.

How is it diagnosed?

Clinical suspicion
Lymphocytosis
Positive culture for *B. pertussis*
Demonstration of organism using
    fluorescent antibody test of
    nasopharyngeal secretions

What is the treatment?

Hospitalization during severe coughing paroxysms; may need suction, supplemental oxygen, nutritional support, and respiratory support; antibiotic choice is usually **erythromycin**; isolation until 5 days of antibiotic treatment

What antibiotic prophylaxis is given and for how long for people exposed to pertussis?

14 days of erythromycin

Does treatment of infected persons prevent the cough?

Probably not, but those treated early may have a shorter course

How is pertussis prevented?

Vaccination

What are complications of pertussis vaccination?

Some individuals have a febrile reaction, and there are reports of rare CNS complications; the relationship to the vaccine is controversial.

Is protection by pertussis vaccination lifelong?

Not necessarily

Is all whooping cough caused by pertussis?	No. There are viruses and other bacteria (including *Bordetella parapertussis*) that can cause a similar illness.

PARASITIC INFECTIONS AND INFESTATIONS

ROUNDWORM

What is the formal name for roundworm?	*Ascaris lumbricoides*
How big are they?	Adults can be quite large (15–40 cm).
How is roundworm contracted?	Fecal-oral route (i.e., ingest eggs)
Where do the eggs hatch?	Usually in the duodenum
What happens after that?	The larva penetrate the intestinal mucosa and migrate to the lungs and up the trachea, to be swallowed.
Where do the adults live?	Usually in the jejunum
What are symptoms of ascariasis?	May see pulmonary symptoms, including Loffler's pneumonia Common GI findings include abdominal pain, loss of appetite, nausea, and vomiting
What are possible serious complications?	Intestinal obstruction, aberrant migration (to liver, eyes, brain) with inflammatory responses
How is it diagnosed?	Usually by finding the eggs (in feces) or the worm
What is the life span of *Ascaris*?	Usually 2 years
What is the treatment?	Mebendazole Pyrantel pamoate Albendazole
How can it be prevented?	Good hand washing and sanitation

VISCERAL LARVA MIGRANS

What causes visceral larva migrans?
Toxocara canis and *catis*

What are they?
Dog and cat roundworms (intestinal parasites)

How do humans become infected?
Ingestion of eggs (from animal feces, perhaps in dirt)

What happens when humans ingest these eggs?
The eggs hatch in the intestines and migrate to organs (usually the liver)

What are the symptoms?
Symptoms may vary with the tissues involved. Fever, hepatomegaly, or other organ-specific findings may be present.

What are the lab findings?
Eosinophilia, due to the tissue invasiveness of the parasite, is common. Other findings include elevation of isohemagglutinin antibodies, elevated ESR, and positive ELISA.

What is ocular larva migrans?
Eye involvement of visceral larva migrans

What is the treatment of visceral and ocular larva migrans?
Diethylcarbamazine (oral), **mebendazole**, or **albendazole** have been used. Dying organisms may cause an allergic or inflammatory response. Ocular larva migrans may also need **steroid** treatment.

PINWORMS

What is the formal name for pinworms?
Enterobius vermicularis

How is it transmitted?
Hand-to-mouth

What are the symptoms?
Perianal itching, sometimes leading to insomnia

How is it diagnosed?
Demonstration of either pinworms or eggs in the perianal region

What is the tape test?	Use of a clear adhesive tape to pick up eggs or worms from the perianal region; this can be applied by the parents and examined by the physician.
What is the treatment for pinworm infection?	Mebendazole
How is it prevented?	Good hygiene. Cut nails, wash sheets, underwear, and bedclothes daily for several days to prevent reinfection.

WHIPWORM

What is the formal name for whipworm?	*Trichuris trichiura*
How is it spread?	Fecal-oral route
What are the symptoms?	May range from asymptomatic to abdominal pain and flatulence to rectal bleeding and prolapse, depending on the severity of the infestation
How is it diagnosed?	Demonstration of worms or larva in stools
What is the treatment?	Mebendazole
How can it be prevented?	Good hygiene and sanitary disposal of human waste

HOOKWORM

What causes hookworm?	*Necator americanus* (in the United States) and *Ancylostoma duodenale*
What is the epidemiology?	The larva usually burrow through the skin of the feet, enter the bloodstream, and migrate to the lungs, where they ascend and are swallowed; they then reside in the intestines.
What are the complications?	Irritation at the site of skin entry ("**ground itch**"), anemia, hypoproteinemia, nutritional deficiency

How is it diagnosed?	Find ova in stools
What is the treatment?	Pyrantel pamoate or mebendazole
How is it prevented?	Wear shoes; improve sanitation

ATYPICAL MYCOBACTERIA

What are atypical mycobacteria?	Mycobacteria that are nontuberculous
How are they generally acquired?	From the environment, as opposed to person-to-person spread
How are they categorized?	They are categorized into four groups, based on their growth and morphology: 1. Photochromogens 2. Scotochromogens 3. Nonchromogens 4. Rapid growers
What are the most typical infectious manifestations in children?	**Cervical lymphadenitis;** however, children with AIDS are commonly infected systemically with *M. avium*
Can nontuberculous mycobacteria infect other regions of the body?	Yes. Particularly the skin, the lungs, the bones and the joints.
Which *Mycobacterium* accounts for most cases of cervical lymphadenitis?	*M. avium* is responsible in 80% of cases. Most other cases are caused by either *Mycobacterium scrofulaceum* or *kansasii*.
What are typical symptoms of cervical lymphadenitis?	Enlargement of an isolated lymph node or group of nodes; with progressive disease, caseation may occur resulting in drainage to the skin
How is the definitive diagnosis made?	By isolation of the organism from a tissue sample
What is the treatment?	Surgical excision of the involved nodes
Can HIV-positive children who are infected with disseminated *M. avium* be cured of this bacteria?	No, but multiple drug therapy may diminish the effects of the disease.

28

Allergic Diseases

ATOPY

What is it?

It is a category of allergic reaction that implies a hereditary characteristic. These allergic reactions include hay fever, asthma, and eczematoid dermatitis as well as allergic reactions to food, drugs, and insect bites.

What is the pathophysiologic process in an atopic individual?

Selected synthesis of IgE antibodies to common environmental antigens

How is this shown in atopic individuals?

Atopic individuals display a "wheal-and-flare" reaction when their skin is tested with allergenic extracts.

Can nonatopic individuals form IgE antibodies?

Yes—but they do not form them to common environmental substances in the same manner that atopic individuals do

What is the definition of allergy?

It is a specific, acquired host reaction mediated by an immunologic mechanism, causing an undesired physiologic response. A true allergy should be differentiated from adverse reactions to foods or drugs, which do not have a true immunologic basis.

Are antigens and allergens the same?

Not necessarily: Allergens are antigens that provoke a specific immunologic allergic response. All allergens are antigens, although not all are good antigens. Conversely, all antigens are not necessarily allergens.

What laboratory values help confirm allergic diseases?

1. Peripheral blood eosinophilia (> 500 cells/mm^3)
2. Elevated serum IgE
3. Respiratory or gastrointestinal secretions containing > 10% eosinophils
4. Positive allergy skin testing (evidenced by wheals) with prick or intradermal techniques
5. Radioallergosorbent test (RAST) [allergen-specific IgE]
6. Positive food and drug challenges
7. Positive bronchial provocation tests to histamine or methacholine challenge

What are three treatment strategies?

1. Avoidance of irritant
2. Pharmacotherapy, including:
   α-Agonists to reduce edema of mucous membranes
   β-Agonists to dilate airways
   Theophylline to treat asthma
   Cromolyn (smooth muscle relaxant)
   Topical and systemic steroids
   Antihistamines
   Anticholinergics
3. Immunotherapy

FOOD ALLERGIES

What are food allergies?

They are IgE-mediated reactions that usually occur 1–4 hours after ingestion. Symptoms may include nausea, vomiting, diarrhea, anaphylaxis, asthma, eczema, urticaria, and/or angioedema.

What are the causes of nonallergic adverse food reactions?

These types of adverse food reactions, which are more common than allergic ones, can be secondary to toxic substances in food, chemical or bacterial contaminants, endogenous pharmacologic agents, or metabolic diseases in the individual.

What is the most common target organ in IgE-mediated food hypersensitivity?

The **skin**, with onset of urticaria, angioedema, or pruritic rash or eczema

What are the most common foods to which children are allergic?

Milk, eggs, peanuts, soybean, wheat, and fish cause over 90% of the reactions.

How is food sensitivity evaluated?

History and physical exam; skin tests and serum RAST, which are used for measuring IgE antibodies to specific foods, are only helpful in assessing food sensitization.

How is a chemical food allergy confirmed?

Food challenges and, occasionally, **elimination diets**

ALLERGIC RHINITIS

What are the common causes of seasonal allergies?

Outdoor inhalant allergens: tree, grass, cat and dog dander, weed pollens (e.g., ragweed), outdoor mold spores

What are common causes of perennial allergies?

Indoor inhalant allergens: cat and dog dander, dust mites, molds (e.g., *Aspergillus, Penicillium*)

What are the symptoms of allergic rhinitis?

Profuse, watery nasal discharge
Itchy nose
Postnasal drip
Sneezing
Cough
If the eyes are involved, redness, tearing, and itching are observed (**rhinoconjunctivitis**).

What are "allergic shiners"?

Dark discoloration of the infraorbital area caused by **venous stasis** secondary to nasal congestion

What is the pathophysiology of allergic rhinitis?

There is an immediate hypersensitivity response that occurs in the nasal mucosa of a sensitized individual. Specific IgE, which is stimulated by allergens, binds to mast cells. When the patient is reexposed to the allergen, an allergen IgE-antibody reaction occurs, with binding of two or more IgE molecules on the mast cell membrane. This causes mast cell degranulation within minutes and results in the release of mediators (e.g., **histamine, metabolites of the arachidonic acid pathway, and inflammatory cytokines**), which increase vascular permeability, smooth muscle contraction, mucus secretion, and pruritus. Following mast cell degranulation, late-phase reaction occurs because of the infiltration of **eosinophils, neutrophils, and lymphocytes.**

What is the differential diagnosis?

Upper respiratory tract infection, sinusitis, nonallergic rhinitis with eosinophilia, vasomotor rhinitis, rhinitis medicamentosa

What is a Hansel stain?

It is an eosin methylene blue stain that shows eosinophils well. Stained cell preparations that are comprised of > 10% eosinophils are highly suggestive of allergic rhinitis.

How is allergic rhinitis managed?

1. Avoidance of allergens
2. Treatment options include antihistamines, systemic and topical decongestants, intranasal cromolyn or corticosteroids, and immunotherapy

INSECT STINGS AND BITES

What are the common stinging insects?

The hymenoptera order, which includes:
1. **Apidea** family
   Bumble bee
   Honey bee
2. **Vespidea** family
   Yellow jackets
   White-faced hornet
   Yellow hornet
   Wasp
3. **Formicidae** family
   Fire ant

How are reactions classified?

Local: Swelling < **2 cm** and lasts < **24 hours**, often with local erythema and pruritus

Large local: Swelling > **2 cm** and lasts up to **48–72 hours**

Systemic: generalized reactions that may involve diffuse urticaria and pruritus, laryngeal edema, bronchospasm, hypotension, abdominal cramping, nausea, and vomiting

What are toxic reactions?   Nonimmunologic reactions that usually occur with multiple stings and may resemble systemic reactions

What is the typical allergic reaction?   Usually local or large local—most children do not have systemic reactions, and those that do occur are rarely life threatening. Of children who have life-threatening reactions, less than 50% will have a second life-threatening event after another sting.

What is the long-term management of insect allergy?   Education, avoidance, epinephrine-containing kits for acute treatment after a sting, and immunotherapy in children who have experienced a significant systemic reaction

How effective is immunotherapy?   Immunotherapy is at least 95% effective if a maintenance dose of 100 μg venom is achieved, the amount in an average sting.

How long should injection be continued?   Injection shots should be continued for at least 3–5 years in childhood and possibly longer in adults.

29

Genetics

DEFINITIONS

What is the difference between the terms *congenital* and *genetic*?

Congenital means appearing at birth, without regard to the cause, whereas *genetic* implies that the basis of a disease or defect, at least in part, is determined by the genetic makeup of that individual. By definition, all birth defects are congenital, but many are not genetic.

What is a malformation?

A primary defect in the formation or development of a body part or organ

What is a deformation?

A change in the shape, form, or position of a normally formed body part or organ by extrinsic or mechanical forces

What is a disruption?

A defect caused by breakdown in a previously normal body part or organ

What is a syndrome?

A pattern of multiple primary malformations in an individual from a single underlying cause

What is a sequence?

A primary malformation and one or more secondary malformations or deformations

What is an association?

The simultaneous occurrence of two or more traits or abnormalities that cannot be explained by chance

What is the VATER association?

The acronym **VATER** (sometimes called **VACTERL**) is used to describe an association of:
Vertebral defects
Imperforate **A**nus
Tracheo-**E**sophageal fistula
Radial and renal dysplasia
Cardiac and **L**imb anomalies
This is probably the best known pediatric association.

What is an autosome?

A non-sex chromosome (i.e., a chromosome other than X or Y)

What is an autosomal condition?

A condition caused by an abnormality involving a gene on an autosome

What is a mendelian trait or condition?

A genetic condition that is inherited as a *single gene* trait, the occurrence and recurrence of which conforms to Mendel's laws

What is an autosomal recessive trait?

A trait or condition found when the affected person has a pair of mutant genes (i.e., is **homozygous**) for that condition; true autosomal recessive traits have heterozygotes that are free of clinical disease

What is an autosomal dominant trait?

A condition caused by the presence of a single mutant gene, rather than a pair of mutant genes

What is a multifactorial trait?

A trait or condition caused by the interaction of multiple genes as well as additional nongenetic factors; accounts for many common birth defects

What is anticipation?

A phenomenon in which a genetic condition becomes more severe or has an earlier age of onset in succeeding generations; some are associated with expansions of trinucleotide repeats

What is mosaicism?

The presence of two or more genetically different cell lines in the same individual; one is usually normal

COMMON GENETIC SYNDROMES

What is Down syndrome?

A recognizable pattern of malformations caused by the presence of extra chromosome 21 material

What are the features of Down syndrome?

Infants: hypotonia, flattened occiput (brachycephaly), redundant skin (especially on the posterior neck), flattened midface, epicanthal folds, upslanted palpebral fissures, small ears, prominent and/or protruding

tongue, single transverse palmar
creases; congenital heart disease
(particularly AV canal)

Older children: same as those for
infants with associated developmental
delay and/or mental retardation

**What are some of the
other complications?**

Congenital duodenal obstruction
Hirschsprung disease
Hypothyroidism (congenital or acquired)
Congenital heart disease
Increased incidence of respiratory
infections
Increased risk of leukemia

**What causes Down
syndrome?**

Extra material from chromosome 21,
either through trisomy or a translocation;
95% of cases are caused by trisomy 21,
and 5% are caused by unbalanced
translocations occurring in the presence
of extra chromosome 21 material or by
mosaicism

**Is all of chromosome 21
responsible for Down
syndrome?**

Accumulating evidence indicates that a
relatively small portion of the long arm
of chromosome 21 is responsible for
most features of Down syndrome.

**What is the most common
risk factor for Down
syndrome?**

Advanced maternal age (older than 35
years of age at delivery)

**Is there another name for
Down syndrome?**

Trisomy 21 for the nondisjunction types

**What are the features of
trisomy 13?**

Oral/facial clefts
Microphthalmia
Postaxial polydactyly
Apical scalp defects
Intrauterine growth retardation
Congenital heart disease

**What is the prognosis for
trisomy 13?**

Most children die in the first year of
life. Survivors are usually profoundly
retarded.

What are the features of trisomy 18?

Intrauterine growth retardation
Small ears with flattened helices
Small mouth
Congenital heart disease
Omphalocele
Unusual hand positioning (second and fifth fingers overlapping the third and fourth)

What is the prognosis of trisomy 18?

Most children die in the first year of life. Survivors are retarded, although some learn communication skills.

What is Turner syndrome?

Classic Turner syndrome is caused by the **absence of one X chromosome in a female**. About 50% of patients with the Turner syndrome phenotype have a **45, X karyotype**, and about 20%–30% are mosaic. About 10%–20% have a structural rearrangement involving a deletion of part or all of the short arm of one of the two X chromosomes.

What are the features of Turner syndrome?

Girls with Turner syndrome may have:
Short stature
Delayed puberty with primary amenorrhea (caused by gonadal dysgenesis)
Lymphedema of the hands and feet
Coarctation of the aorta (29%)
Kidney malformations (50%)
Webbed neck
Shield (broad) chest
Prominent, posteriorly rotated ears

Are girls with Turner syndrome retarded?

They usually are not retarded, although there may be problems in spatial perceptual ability.

What is Klinefelter syndrome?

A syndrome seen in males who have an extra X chromosome (47, XXY)

What are the features of Klinefelter syndrome?

Young boys with Klinefelter syndrome may have few physical abnormalities. Older patients tend to be taller than average, with testes that are unusually small for their age. Body fat distribution tends to be on the hips and chest, with gynecomastia. Average IQ is reduced, but severe mental retardation is uncommon.

What is fragile X syndrome?

An X-linked condition caused by expansion of a trinucleotide repeat in the FMR1 gene

What are the features of the fragile X syndrome?

Young boys with the full mutation may have developmental delay, large ears, and a long face. Postpubertal boys usually have **enlarged testes**. Boys with the full mutation are usually retarded. Girls with the full mutation may also be retarded, but usually are less severely affected.

What is a premutation?

A premutation for the fragile X syndrome is an increase in the size of the trinucleotide repeat from the normal size (usually < 50 repeats) to about 100–200 repeats. These individuals are usually asymptomatic, but females with the premutation are at risk for having children with a full mutation.

COMMON MUSCULAR DYSTROPHIES

What is Duchenne muscular dystrophy?

An X-linked recessive disorder characterized by progressive muscle weakness, pseudohypertrophy of the calf muscles, and elevation of muscle enzymes (particularly CPK)

What is the molecular defect?

An abnormality (usually a partial deletion) of the **dystrophin gene** on the short arm of the X chromosome.

When does it present?

Usually between 2 and 6 years of age

What is Becker muscular dystrophy?

Another disorder involving the dystrophin gene; it usually has a milder onset and rate of progression

What are three other types of muscular dystrophy?

1. Myotonic
2. Limb-girdle
3. Fascioscapulohumeral

What is spinal muscular atrophy?

A frequently progressive disease of anterior horn cells; usually inherited as autosomal recessive trait

What is Werdnig-Hoffman disease?	Also known as spinal muscular atrophy type I, this is a progressive disorder. Onset is usually before 6 months of age, and survival after 3 years is uncommon.
What is Kugelberg-Welander disease?	A form of spinal muscular atrophy that has a "juvenile" onset; age of onset is usually in first decade, but may be later

OTHER COMMON DISEASES WITH GENETIC CAUSES

What is Wilson disease?	A copper metabolism (transport) disease; also known as hepatolenticular degeneration
When does Wilson disease present?	Clinical disease is uncommon before puberty; most patients present in their early 20s. Presenting signs/symptoms include dystonia, dysarthria, psychiatric symptoms, and parkinsonian movements.
How does Wilson disease present in pediatric patients?	Children are more likely to present with only liver disease.
How is the diagnosis made?	1. Findings of reduced serum copper and ceruloplasmin 2. Increased renal copper excretion (particularly with penicillamine treatment) 3. Liver biopsy, which will show increased copper content, for definitive diagnosis
What is Huntington disease?	It is a progressive autosomal dominant disorder. Onset is usually in adulthood, and it is characterized by progressive chorea, psychiatric problems, and dementia.
How does it present in pediatric patients?	Although pediatric presentations are not common, they do occur. Children with symptomatic disease usually present with psychiatric/behavioral problems and/or rigidity.

What is the cause of Huntington disease?

An expansion of a CAG nucleotide repeat in the "huntington" gene on chromosome 4

What is neurofibromatosis?

An autosomal dominant disorder characterized by hyperpigmented macules (**café au lait spots**) and fibromatous skin tumors

What are common findings?

Multiple (usually more than six) café au lait spots, Lisch nodules of the iris, axillary freckling, cutaneous neurofibromata

What are some complications?

Pseudoarthrosis, scoliosis, meningioma, optic neuroma, seizures, learning disabilities, mental retardation, pheochromocytoma, hypertension, malignant degeneration of a neurofibroma, leukemia

What is tuberous sclerosis?

An autosomal dominant disorder characterized by hamartomas, hypopigmented skin lesions, and an increased risk of seizures and mental retardation

What are the physical findings?

"Ash leaf" hypopigmented macules, shagreen patches, adenoma sebaceum, periungual fibromas, and intracranial lesions, which are sometimes calcified

How does it present in childhood?

Seizures
Developmental delay and/or mental retardation
Skin lesions may not be present or obvious in early infancy; hypopigmented skin lesions may be easier to see if viewed with a Wood's (UV) lamp

What is Rett syndrome?

A progressive degenerative disorder affecting females, marked by loss of purposeful hand movement

What is Reye syndrome?

Metabolic encephalopathy, frequently associated with dysfunction and fatty changes in the liver

What causes Reye syndrome?

The cause is unknown. It is seen following certain viral infections (e.g., varicella, influenza) and it is epidemiologically associated with the use of **aspirin** in some patients.

How is it diagnosed?

Elevated hepatocellular enzymes in serum
Hyperammonemia
Exclusion of other diagnoses (e.g., medium-chain acyl CoA dehydrogenase deficiency)

What is retinoblastoma?

The most common childhood eye tumor

What is the incidence?

About 1/20,000 children

How does it present?

It may present with strabismus and abnormal red reflex

Is it hereditary?

About 40% of cases are familial; the remainder are sporadic.

What causes retinoblastoma?

Loss of function of both copies of the retinoblastoma gene, which is a tumor-suppressor gene on chromosome 13

What other tumors may be seen in these patients?

Osteosarcomas, particularly in patients with hereditary retinoblastoma

Index

Italic numbers indicate figures; *italic t* indicates a table.

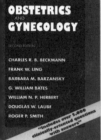
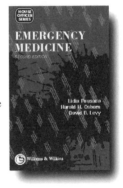
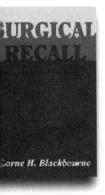